Essentials in Total Knee Arthroplasty

Essentials in Total Knee Arthroplasty

Editor: Zain Ritchie

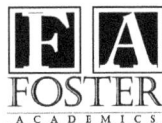

FA FOSTER
ACADEMICS

www.fosteracademics.com

www.fosteracademics.com

FA
FOSTER
ACADEMICS

Cataloging-in-Publication Data

Essentials in total knee arthroplasty / edited by Zain Ritchie.
   p. cm.
Includes bibliographical references and index.
ISBN 978-1-64646-146-2
1. Knee--Surgery. 2. Arthroplasty. 3. Total knee replacement. 4. Knee--Reoperation. I. Ritchie, Zain.
RD561 .E87 2022
617.582--dc23

Foster Academics,
118-35 Queens Blvd., Suite 400,
Forest Hills, NY 11375, USA

ISBN 978-1-64646-146-2 (Hardback)

Contents

Permissions

List of Contributors

Index

Preface

This book has been an outcome of determined endeavour from a group of educationists in the field. The primary objective was to involve a broad spectrum of professionals from diverse cultural background involved in the field for developing new researches. The book not only targets students but also scholars pursuing higher research for further enhancement of the theoretical and practical applications of the subject.

Total knee arthroplasty or total knee replacement surgery is a procedure that is performed in a severely damaged knee joint to restore function and relieve pain. It involves replacing the damaged bone and cartilage from the kneecap, shinbone and thighbone with an artificial joint. The assessment of whether knee arthroplasty is required for a particular condition is determined by assessing the range of motion, strength and stability of the knee. X-ray imaging can offer visual insights to determine the extent of damage. The most common condition that causes knee pain and disability is osteoarthritis. The rate of complication post-surgery is generally low. Most people who have undergone total knee arthroplasty experience a good quality of life, substantial reduction in pain and better mobility. Different approaches, evaluations, methodologies and advanced studies on total knee arthroplasty have been included in this book. Some of the diverse topics covered in this book address the varied techniques and procedures of total knee arthroplasty. This book is a vital tool for all researching or studying orthopedic surgery as it gives incredible insights into emerging trends and concepts.

It was an honour to edit such a profound book and also a challenging task to compile and examine all the relevant data for accuracy and originality. I wish to acknowledge the efforts of the contributors for submitting such brilliant and diverse chapters in the field and for endlessly working for the completion of the book. Last, but not the least; I thank my family for being a constant source of support in all my research endeavours.

Editor

Computer-assisted total knee arthroplasty using mini midvastus or medial parapatellar approach technique

Peter Feczko[1*], Lutz Engelmann[2], Jacobus J. Arts[1] and David Campbell[3]

Abstract

Background: Despite the growing evidence in the literature there is still a lack of consensus regarding the use of minimally invasive surgical technique (MIS) in total knee arthroplasty (TKA).

Methods: A prospective, randomized, international multicentre trial including 69 patients was performed to compare computer-assisted TKA (CAS-TKA) using either mini-midvastus (MIS group) or standard medial parapatellar approach (conventional group).
Patients from 3 centers (Maastricht, Zwickau, Adelaide) with end-stage osteoarthritis of the knee were randomized to either an MIS group with dedicated instrumentation or a conventional group to receive cruciate retaining CAS-TKA without patella resurfacing. The primary outcome was to compare post operative pain and range of motion (ROM). The secondary outcome was to measure the duration of surgery, blood loss, chair rise test, quadriceps strength, anterior knee pain, Knee Society Score (KSS),WOMAC scores, mechanical leg axis and component alignment.

Results: Patients in the MIS group (3.97 ± 2.16) had significant more pain at 2 weeks than patients in the conventional group (2.77 ± 1.43) $p = 0.003$. There was no significant difference in any of the other primary outcome parameters. Surgery time was significantly longer ($p < 0.001$) and there were significantly higher blood loss ($p = 0.002$) in the MIS group as compared to the conventional group. The difference of the mean mechanical leg alignment between the groups was not statistically significant ($-0.43°$ (95 % CI $-1.50 - 0.64$); $p = 0.43$).
There was no significant difference of component alignment between the two surgical groups with respect to flexion/extension ($p = 0.269$), varus/valgus ($p = 0.653$) or rotational alignment ($p = 0.485$) of the femur component and varus valgus alignment ($p = 0.778$) or posterior slope ($p = 0.164$) of the tibial component.

Conclusion: There was no advantage of the MIS approach compared to a conventional approach CAS-TKA in any of the primary outcome measurements assessed, however the MIS approach was associated with longer surgical time and greater blood loss. MIS-TKA in combination with computer navigation is safe in terms of implant positioning.

Keywords: Total knee arthroplasty, Navigation, Minimally invasive surgery, Blood loss, Accuracy

* Correspondence: p.feczko@mumc.nl
[1]Department Orthopaedic Surgery, Research School Capri, Maastricht University Medical Centre, P. Debyelaan 25, 6229 HX Maastricht, The Netherlands
Full list of author information is available at the end of the article

Background

Total knee arthroplasty is a successful surgical treatment for debilitating osteoarthritis of the knee [1–3]. This intervention results excellent long-term survivorship [4–7] and marked improvement in functional capacity and quality of life of the patients [8] . However the conventional medial parapatellar approach is associated with local tissue disruption, interruption of neurovascular tissues, dislocation of the patella and the joint itself [9] resulting in a long hospital stay and long rehabilitation [10, 11]. To ameliorate these issues smaller incisions and muscle preserving approaches have been a prominent trend in total knee arthroplasty in more than 2 decades [12]. Five basic principles of the minimally invasive (MIS) techniques are described [13]: 1. Minimal interruption of nervous tissue and vascular supply. 2. Minimal dissection of muscles, tendons and ligaments. 3. Minimal resection of bone. 4. Minimal blood loss. 5. Minimal pain to the patient. The length of the incision is the least important aspect and should be long enough for the mobile-window technique. Based on the MIS principles, four techniques have become popular in clinical practice and research activities [14, 15]: the mini-subvastus approach [16], the mini-midvastus approach [17], the quadriceps-sparing approach [18, 19] and the mini medial parapatellar approach [20]. Comparative studies have not found a particular MIS approach to be superior or significantly better than anothers [21–23].

The short term results of MIS reported shorter length of hospital stay, better postoperative pain control, less blood loss, better quadriceps function and improved knee flexion compared to a conventional medial parapatellar approach [24–31]. However increased short term adverse event rates and less accuracy of implant position were also reported using MIS approaches [11, 32–36].

Other studies did not find statistical significant differences in pain, range of movement (ROM), Quadriceps strength, Knee Society Score (KSS) [37–40]. The results of meta-analyses are conflicting [28, 36, 41–45].

Computer navigation for total knee arthroplasty was first introduced in Europe in the 1990s, and there has been a widespread increase in its use throughout the world in the last decade. The proposed benefits of computer navigation for total knee arthroplasty include improved accuracy of both tibial and femoral component positioning and overall mechanical alignment [46]. Most studies comparing computer navigation with standard total knee arthroplasty have demonstrated a greater number of patients with coronal mechanical axis alignment within 3 of neutral in the navigation group. The outcome of a previous study showed that CAS-TKA reduced the overall rate of revision and the rate revision for loosening, but it has no effect on the short- and mid-term clinical outcomes [46].

We examined the synergy of combining computer-assisted surgery with a MIS approach with the hypothesis that computer assisted TKA improves component orientation and postoperative limb alignment that has been problematic in some non-computer assisted MIS-TKR studies [47–49]. We examined the hypothesis that minimally invasive, computer-assisted surgery would improve the short-term outcome without compromising the long term survivorship of TKA [50, 51].

The aim of our study was to perform a prospective, randomized multicentre trial to compare computer-assisted TKA using either a mini-midvastus (MIS group) or a medial parapatellar approach (conventional group).

The primary outcome was to compare postoperative pain and range of motion (ROM). The secondary outcome was to compare clinical data including duration of surgery, blood loss, chair rise, quadriceps strength,

Table 1 Demographics & baseline characteristics

	MIS (n = 36)	Conventional (n = 33)	p-value
Sex (F/M)[e]	23/13	22/11	0.81[b]
Age (years)[f]	65.14 ± 8.35	64.88 ± 6.78	0.89[a]
BMI (kg/m²)[f]	28.26 ± 2.81	28.56 ± 2.93	0.67[a]
Side of operation (R/L)[e]	22/14	18/15	0.95[b]
Diagnosis (Primary/Posttraumatic OA)[e]	35/1	33/0	0.52[d]
Chair rise (yes/no)[e]	26/10	25/8	0.74[b]
Anterior knee pain (yes/no)[e]	27/9	26/7	0.71[b]
Quadriceps strength (fair/good – can break/good – can't break)[e]	1/16/19	0/21/12	0.21[c]
KSS[f]	108.91 ± 26.42	99.36 ± 25.02	0.13[a]
WOMAC[f]	78.08 ± 12.92	76.39 ± 10.56	0.56[a]

[a]Student's t-test, [b]Pearson χ^2-test, [c]likelihood ratio χ^2-test and [d]Fisher's Exact test
[e]Value are numbers. [f]Values are mean ± sd

Table 2 Pain. (Likert scale)

	MIS (n = 36)	Conventional (n = 32)	Difference (95 % CI) & p-value[a]
Surgery time (min)	134.53 ± 21.85	103.56 ± 14.93	30.97 (21.79 − 40.14); $p < 0.001$
Intraoperative blood loss (ml)	73.06 ± 99.82	58.06 ± 79.22	14.99 (-29.49 − 59.47); $p = 0.50$
Postoperative blood loss first 24 h (ml)	726.11 ± 471.63	411.09 ± 324.76	315.02 (116.50 − 513.54); $p = 0.002$

[a]Student's t-test

anterior knee pain, Knee Society Score (KSS) and WOMAC scores. Mechanical leg axis and component positioning was also evaluated on radiology and CT investigations respectively.

Methods

Trial design

A prospective, randomized, international multicentre trial including 69 patients was performed according to a standard protocol to compare computer-assisted TKA using either a mini-midvastus (MIS group) or a medial parapatellar approach (conventional group). Patients in 3 centers (Maastricht, Zwickau, Adelaide) with end-stage osteoarthritis of knee were randomized to either an MIS group with dedicated instrumentation or a conventional group.

Ethics

Ethical approval of all centres had been obtained from the local ethical committee of Maastricht (MEC 04-105), Adelaide (RGH 10/04) and Zwickau (EK-MPG-0603) as part of the research program "A prospective comparative, randomized study comparing the MIS computer navigated total knee arthroplasty vs. conventional computer navigated total knee using the Scorpio CR fixed bearing knee and the Stryker navigation system".

Trial Registration Number: ClinicalTrials.gov NCT026 25311 8 December 2015.

Participant selection and consent

Patients were randomized (random permuted blocks of 4) in either the MIS group or the conventional group. A written informed consent was obtained from all participants.

Seventy six participants were included for the study. There were 4 intra-operative exclusions: 3 patients due to problems with the navigation trackers and one patient due to fracture of the tibial plateau.

Three patients were lost to follow up due to unwillingness of the participants. Sixty nine patients completed the 6 months study period.

All cases were performed by a single surgeon in each of the three centres. Before the study, the surgeons participated in training involving multiple cases of cadaver prosthetic implants using the navigation system with the MIS approach and a minimum of ten clinical cases.

Inclusion and exclusion criteria

Patients between 45 and 75 years of age who had an established diagnosis of knee osteoarthritis requiring primary total knee replacement. Exclusion criteria included previous cruciate ligament reconstruction, correction osteotomy of the tibia, patellectomy, BMI greater than 30, flexion contracture greater than 15°, varus or valgus deformity greater than 15°, medio-lateral instability greater than 10° and active inflammation or infection of the knee. In addition, patients were excluded if they were pre-operatively considered to require patellar surface implantation.

Interventions (operative procedure)

The Stryker (Stryker Howmedica Osteonics, Allendale, NJ USA) Navigation System II, version 3.1 was used in all cases. This is an image free, active, cordless system. All knee surgeries were performed using a tourniquet. In the MIS group a 10 cm incision with a flexed knee, mini-midvastus approach was applied per standard protocol and with dedicated instrumentation. In cases where conventional surgical technique was used, a medial parapatellar approach was applied. The navigation system trackers were then attached to the surface of the femur and the tibia. The hip joint rotation center and the center of the ankle joint were established as reference points for leg axis. The rotational position of the femoral component was determined by using the *Whiteside's line*

Table 3 Range of motion

	Time					
	Week 2	Week 3	Week 4	Week 5	Week 6	Week 7
MIS	3.97 ± 2.16	2.97 ± 1.68	3.19 ± 1.43	2.72 ± 1.47	2.20 ± 1.23	1.97 ± 1.10
Conventional	2.77 ± 1.43	2.55 ± 1.71	2.62 ± 1.66	2.10 ± 1.11	1.86 ± 1.09	1.81 ± 1.13
p-value						0.003[a]

[a]Two-way ANOVA. Represents between group p-value for factor 'treatment' (F(1) = 13.32). Post-hoc comparison of between group differences showed a 1.20 (95 % CI 0.27 − 2.12; $p = 0.01$) points difference in favor of the conventional group at week 2

Table 4 Surgery time, intraoperative blood loss & postoperative blood loss (first 24 h)

	Time							
	Week 2	Week 3	Week 4	Week 5	Week 6	Week 7	3 months	6 months
MIS	81.97 ± 16.20	90.97 ± 13.57	92.50 ± 15.49	96.04 ± 14.47	97.69 ± 13.51	97.00 ± 12.40	103.57 ± 13.15	106.67 ± 12.91
Conventional	79.35 ± 14.19	90.65 ± 10.78	93.85 ± 10.49	96.75 ± 8.60	98.40 ± 8.86	101.12 ± 9.16	103.77 ± 10.74	105.97 ± 11.58
p-value								0.12[a]

[a]Two-way ANOVA. Represents between group p-value for factor 'treatment' ($F(1) = 0.73$). No difference between groups

and the transepicondylar line (*TEA*). Tibial rotation was assessed based on the relative positions of the centre of the ankle joint and the medial one third of tibial tubercle. The navigation was accorded with the neutral mechanical axis of the extremity with tibial slope fixed at four degrees. Each resurfacing plane angle was instrumented with dedicated navigation cutting guides and checked with the navigation system following the osteotomy. With both techniques, after determining proper prosthetic size, the collateral ligaments were balanced as required based on ligament tension assessed during functional testing of the prosthetic implant. Patellar surface implantation was not performed. The femoral component was implanted without cementing, whereas the tibial component was cemented with Simplex P (Stryker Howmedica Osteonics, Allendale, NJ USA) containing antibiotics. In each case, a Scorpio (Stryker Howmedica Osteonics, Allendale, NJ USA) CR fixed bearing implant was used without patellar surface implantation.

Outcome measurements

Clinical outcomes were assessed by a blinded independent examiner. All outcome parameters were assessed preoperative and postoperative at 7 weeks, 3 and 6 months. Pain and ROM were also measured weekly between postoperative weeks two to seven.

The primary outcome was to compare postoperative pain and range-of-motion (ROM) of both groups. Pain was assessed using a Likert score [52]. Range of motion (ROM) was measured using a goniometer according to the technique described Norkin [53]. Intra-tester and inter-tester reliability was described by Brosseau [54], the reproducibility by Lenssen [55].

The secondary outcome was to compare duration of surgery, blood loss, chair rise test, quadriceps strength test, anterior knee pain, KSS and WOMAC score. Duration of surgery was measured in minutes from skin incision to closure of the wound. Blood loss was measured intra-operative and during the first 24 h postoperative. All data was recorded in ml. Chair rise test was assessed according to the description of Jones [56]. The patients were sitting on a stool with the hip and knee in 90° of flexion. The patients had to stand up from the stool without using their arms. The test was repeated five times. Quadriceps strength test (fair/good – can break/

good – can't break) [57, 58] and anterior knee pain arising from a chair (yes or no) was assessed by the method described by Insall et al. [58] Knee Society Scores [58] and WOMAC scores [59] were also measured.

The primary hypothesis was that those patients who underwent MIS would benefit from less postoperative pain and higher ROM. The secondary hypothesis was that the use of computer navigation allows MIS-TKA to be performed without increased risk of limb malalignment more than 2° and outliers in component positioning.

Radiological evaluations

The lower limb mechanical axis was measured on long standing radiographs preoperatively and at 3 months postoperatively [60]. Outliers were defined as a coronal mechanical leg alignment of more than 2° from neutral. CT scan was performed three months postoperatively with analysis of component alignment determined by the Perth protocol [61]. The position of femoral component was determined in sagittal, coronal and transverse planes, the tibial component was determined in sagittal and coronal planes. Outliners were defined as the component were positioned more than 2° different than the planned position. Mean values were used for further analyses.

Statistics

Descriptive statistics were used to summarize the data. Categorical data were analyzed using Pearson Chi square test, likelihood Chi square tests or Fisher's Exact tests. For continuous data Student's *t*-test, or two-way ANOVA was used. Analyses were performed using SPSS v19.0. *P*-values < 0.05 were considered statistically significant.

Table 5 Chair rise test (yes/no)

	Time		
	7 weeks	3 months	6 months
MIS	24/12	26/9	26/7
Conventional	22/8	25/5	28/2
p-value	0.56[a]	0.38[a]	0.10[b]

[a]Pearson χ^2-test. [b]Fisher's exact test

Table 6 Anterior knee pain (yes/no)

| | Time | | |
	7 weeks	3 months	6 months
MIS	9/26	2/32	6/27
Conventional	6/24	3/27	1/29
p-value	0.59[a]	0.66[b]	0.11[b]

[a]Pearson χ^2-test. [b]Fisher's Exact test

Boxplots represent 10, 25, 50, 75, and 90 % of data. Outliers are shown as dots. Means are not presented in the boxplots.

Results
Demographics
There was no significant difference between the two surgical groups with respect to sex, age, BMI, side of operation or primary diagnosis at $p > 0.05$ (Table 1).

Primary outcomes
Pain
There was a statistically significant difference in pain scores between groups (two-way ANOVA, $F(1) = 13.32$; $p = 0.003$). Post-hoc comparison of between group differences showed a 1.20 (95 % CI 0.27 – 2.12; $p = 0.01$) points difference in favor of the conventional group at week 2 (MIS 3.97 points $\pm$ 2.16 vs. conventional 2.77 points $\pm$ 1.43). At the other time points, no differences in pain scores between both groups were found (Table 2).

Range of motion
No differences in range of motion between groups were found at the different time points (two-way ANOVA, $F(1) = 0.73$; $p = 0.12$) (Table 3).

Secondary outcomes
Duration of surgery and blood loss
Surgery time was significantly longer (30.97 min (95 % CI 21.79 – 40.14); $p < 0.001$) in the MIS group (134.53 $\pm$ 21.85) as compared to the conventional group (103.56 $\pm$ 14.93) (Table 4). There was no significant difference 14.99 ml (95 % CI 29.49 – 59.47); $p = 0.50$) between MIS group (73.06 $\pm$ 99.82) and conventional group (58.06 $\pm$

Table 7 Quadriceps strength (fair/good – can break/good – can't break)

| | Time | | |
	7 weeks	3 months	6 months
MIS	1/17/18	1/14/20	0/8/25
Conventional	2/16/12	0/17/13	0/6/24
p-value	0.60[a]	0.30[a]	0.69[a]

[a]Likelihood ratio χ^2-test

Table 8 KSS score

| | Time | | |
	7 weeks	3 months	6 months
MIS	141.68 $\pm$ 29.61	156.11 $\pm$ 31.12	168.15 $\pm$ 29.61
Conventional	144.03 $\pm$ 22.89	157.75 $\pm$ 27.98	171.87 $\pm$ 19.05
p-value			0.51[a]

[a]Two-way ANOVA. Represents between group p-value for factor 'treatment' (F(1) = 0.43). No difference between groups

79.22) in intra-operative blood loss. However, the first 24 h blood loss was significantly higher 315.02 ml (95 % CI 116.50 – 513.54); $p = 0.002$) in the MIS group (726.11 ml $\pm$ 471.63) as compared to the conventional group (411.09 ml $\pm$ 324.76) (Table 4).

Chair rise, quadriceps strength and anterior knee pain
At 7 weeks, 3 months and 6 months follow-up, no differences between types of surgery in the ability to rise from a chair (yes/no) ($p = 0.56$, $p = 0.38$, and $p = 0.10$ for 7 weeks, 3 months, and 6 months, respectively; Table 5), between types of surgery in quadriceps strength (fair/good – can break/good – can't break) ($p = 0.60$, $p = 0.30$, and $p = 0.69$ for 7 weeks, 3 months, and 6 months, respectively; Table 6), and between types of surgery in the presence of anterior knee pain (yes/no) were found ($p = 0.59$, $p = 0.66$, and $p = 0.11$ for 7 weeks, 3 months, and 6 months, respectively; Table 7).

Functional scores: KSS and WOMAC
At 7 weeks, 3 months and 6 months follow-up, there were no differences between groups in functional scores (KSS score (two-way ANOVA, $F(1) = 0.43$; $p = 0.51$, Table 8) and WOMAC (Two-way ANOVA; $F(1) = 0.005$; $p = 0.94$, Table 9).

Mechanical leg axis
Limb alignment coronal axis was achieved within a target of 2° equally in both groups (75 % of patients in the MIS group and 78.7 % of patients in the conventional approach group). The mean mechanical leg axis in the conventional group was 0.97° $\pm$ SD 1.87°, in the MIS group 0.54° $\pm$ SD 2.53° (Fig. 1). The difference of the mean mechanical leg alignment between the groups was not statistically significant (-0.43° (95 % CI -1.50 - 0.64); $p = 0.43$).

Table 9 WOMAC score

| | Time | | |
	7 weeks	3 months	6 months
MIS	47.39 $\pm$ 15.41	15.67 $\pm$ 2.52	18.15 $\pm$ 16.51
Conventional	48.48 $\pm$ 13.63	18.00 $\pm$ 2.83	15.57 $\pm$ 12.58
p-value			0.94[a]

[a]Two-way ANOVA. Represents between group p-value for factor 'treatment' (F(1) = 0.005). No difference between groups

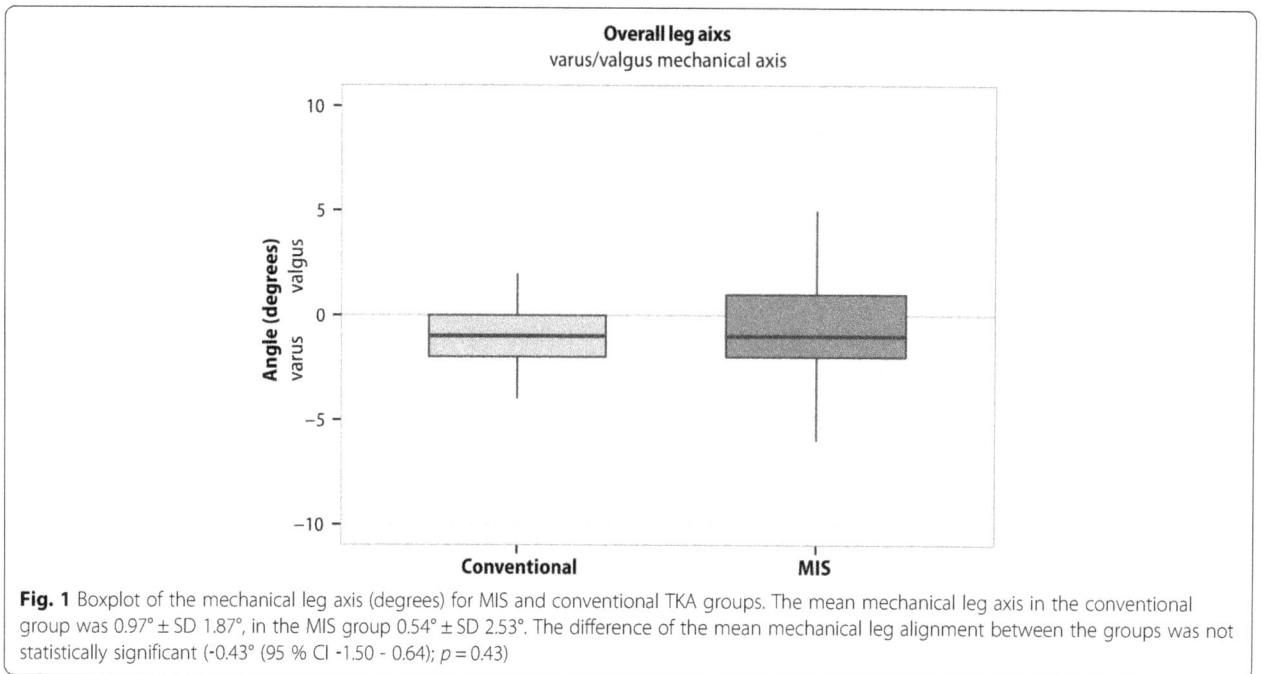

Fig. 1 Boxplot of the mechanical leg axis (degrees) for MIS and conventional TKA groups. The mean mechanical leg axis in the conventional group was 0.97° ± SD 1.87°, in the MIS group 0.54° ± SD 2.53°. The difference of the mean mechanical leg alignment between the groups was not statistically significant (-0.43° (95 % CI -1.50 - 0.64); $p = 0.43$)

Component positioning

There was no significant difference between the two surgical groups with respect to flexion/extension (-0.83° (95 % CI -2.32 - 0.67); $p = 0.27$), rotational alignment of the femur component (-0.45° (95 % CI -1.74 - 0.83); $p = 0.49$) or varus/valgus (-0.18° (95 % CI -0.99 - 0.62); $p - 0.65$) and varus/valgus alignment (-0.16° (95 % CI -1.26 - 0.95); $p = 0.78$) or posterior slope (1.00° (95 % CI -0.43 - 2.42); $p = 0.16$) of the tibial component (Figs. 2, 3, 4, 5 and 6).

Discussion

The primary hypothesis that patients of the MIS group would have less pain and better early ROM was not confirmed by the results of this study.

Most studies comparing MIS-TKA with conventional TKA report lower visual analog pain score [24, 25, 36, 39, 43, 44] and better range of motion [24, 36, 39, 43, 44] in the MIS group in the early postoperative period (2-6 weeks). However, the same studies following this

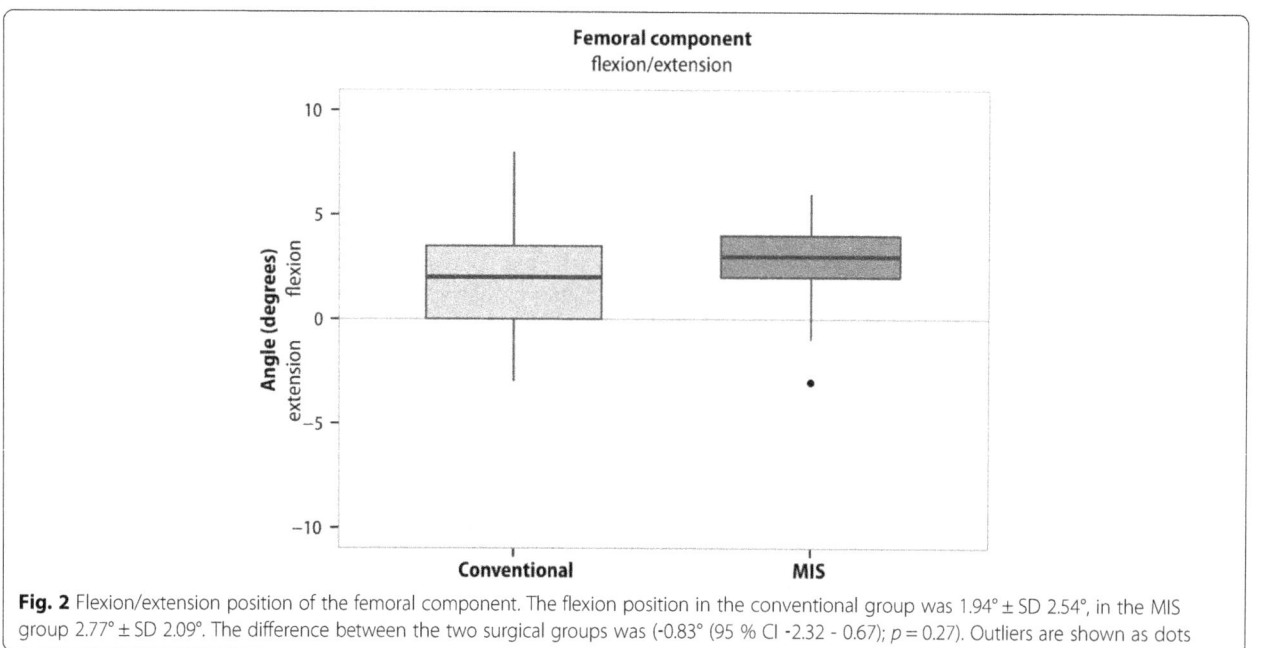

Fig. 2 Flexion/extension position of the femoral component. The flexion position in the conventional group was 1.94° ± SD 2.54°, in the MIS group 2.77° ± SD 2.09°. The difference between the two surgical groups was (-0.83° (95 % CI -2.32 - 0.67); $p = 0.27$). Outliers are shown as dots

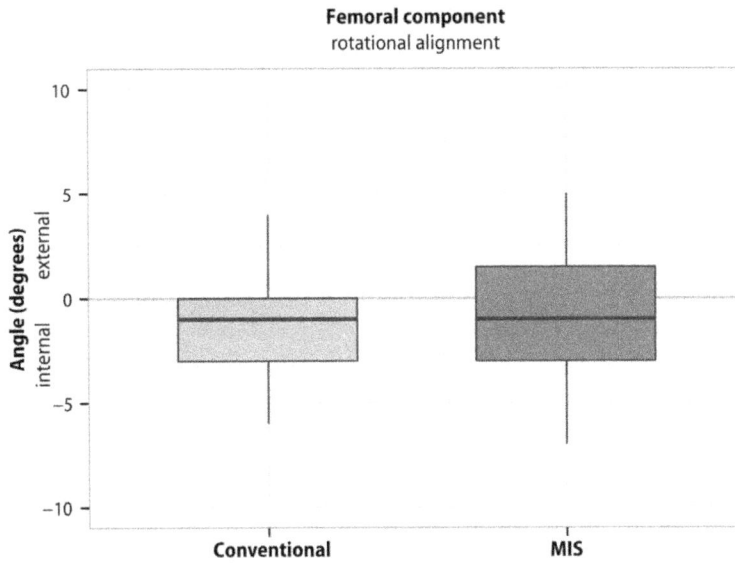

Fig. 3 Rotational position of the femoral component. The rotational position in the conventional group was -1.00° ± SD 2.22°, in the MIS group -0.55° ± SD 2.74°. The difference between the two surgical groups was (-0.45° (95 % CI -1.74 - 0.83); $p = 0.49$). Outliers are shown as dots

variable closely over time report little or no difference between the two groups in subsequent follow-ups (3-6 months). Heekin [40] reported inconsistent pattern in pain and ROM, while other study [41] and meta-analysis [44] found no difference in any of the time points.

The mini-midvastus CAS-TKA resulted in significantly more blood loss as well as an elongated surgery time. Nearly all studies and meta analyses report significant longer duration of surgery in the MIS approach in comparison with medial parapatellar approach. There is no

agreement in previous studies in term of blood loss. Some authors reported significant less blood loss [10, 11, 32, 41, 43, 44] in favor of the minimally invasive approach, while others did not find any differences between techniques [28, 34, 37–39, 42].

One of the most important potential benefits of applying the MIS technique is the ability to avoid manipulation of the extensor apparatus and theoretically a shorter recovery time for quadriceps muscle strength was expected [4, 5, 11]. However, we found no significant

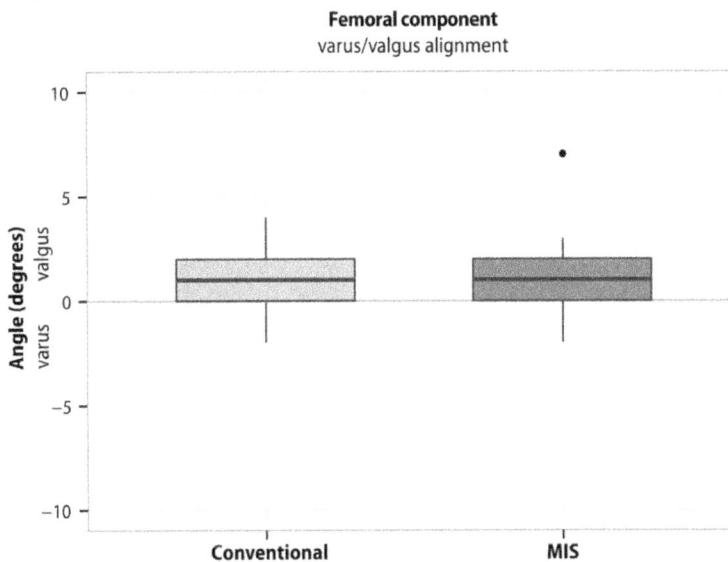

Fig. 4 Varus/valgus position of the femoral component. The varus position in the conventional group was 0.71° ± SD 1.64°, in the MIS group 0.89° ± SD 1.68°. The difference between the two surgical groups was (-0.18° (95 % CI -0.99 - 0.62); $p = 0.65$). Outliers are shown as dots

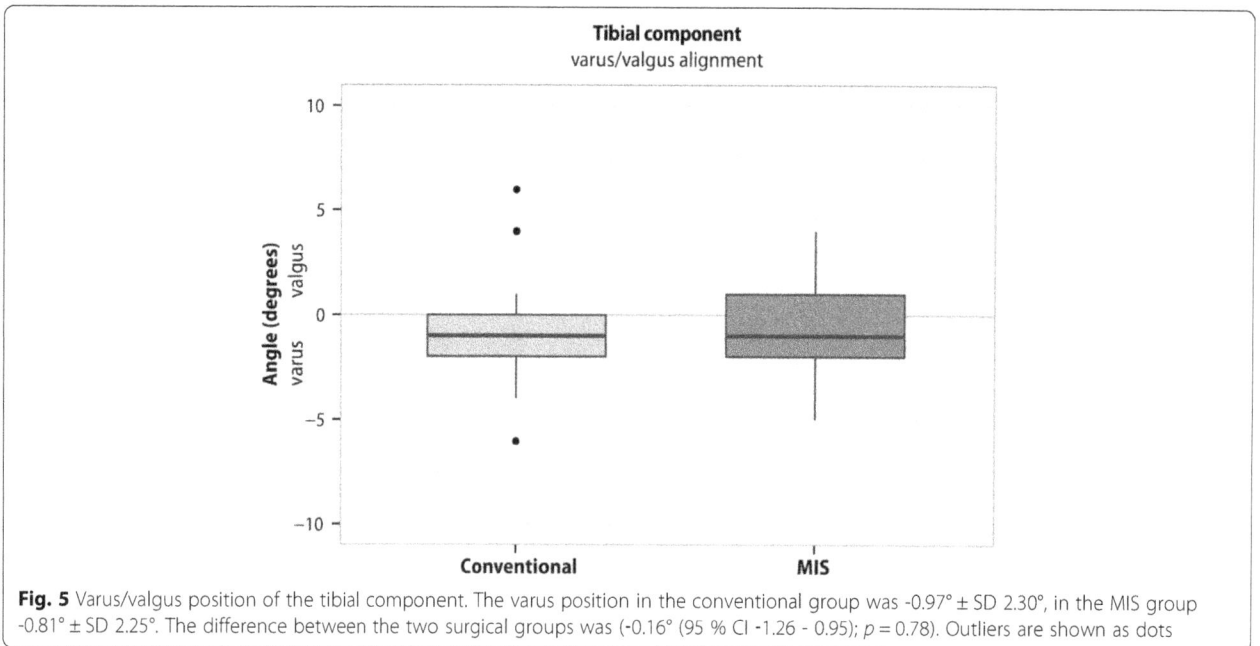

Fig. 5 Varus/valgus position of the tibial component. The varus position in the conventional group was -0.97° ± SD 2.30°, in the MIS group -0.81° ± SD 2.25°. The difference between the two surgical groups was (-0.16° (95 % CI -1.26 - 0.95); $p = 0.78$). Outliers are shown as dots

difference between the groups quadriceps muscle strength assessments, chair rise tests or anterior knee pain. The results measuring quadriceps strength in other studies are also contradictive [25, 31, 34, 44]. There is very few data available in anterior knee pain comparing minimally invasive approach with medial parapatellar approach [23].

The MIS surgery also failed in our study to generate clear advantages in KSS and WOMAC scores. In both groups, there was a marked postoperative improvement of

both KSS and WOMAC scores compared to preoperative values. However, no difference was found between the two groups postoperative values. Similar results are shown in the most publications included meta-analyses [24, 28, 32, 34, 37–40, 42].

The secondary hypothesis was that the use of computer navigation allows MIS-TKA to be performed without increased risk of limb mal-alignment more than 2° and outliners in component positioning [20] was confirmed. The MIS technique did not result in implant

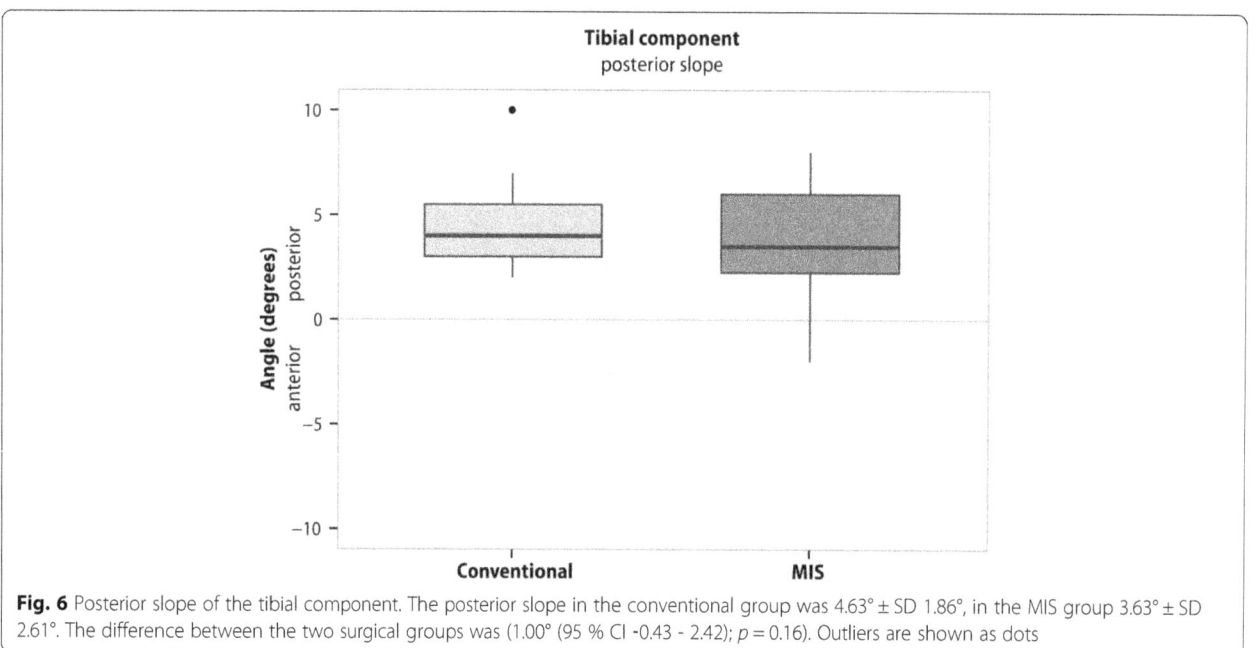

Fig. 6 Posterior slope of the tibial component. The posterior slope in the conventional group was 4.63° ± SD 1.86°, in the MIS group 3.63° ± SD 2.61°. The difference between the two surgical groups was (1.00° (95 % CI -0.43 - 2.42); $p = 0.16$). Outliers are shown as dots

mal-positioning. Component and limb alignment was also comparable between the two surgical approaches and we did not observe an increased incidence of malalignment that has been associated with the restricted access and visualization of the MIS approach [19]. The use of computer assisted navigation can be a useful adjunct to the MIS technique and our results can be confirmed by other authors [46–51].

Conclusion

When comparing the relative merits of the minimally invasive and the conventional approaches we could not confirm any of the short term benefits expected from the minimally invasive technique. There was no advantage of the MIS approach compared to a conventional approach CAS-TKA in any of the primary outcome measurements assessed, however the MIS approach was associated with longer surgical time and greater blood loss. MIS-TKA in combination with computer navigation is safe in terms of implant positioning.

Limitation of the study

The number of patients in our study is rather low and the sample size calculation is missing, however the findings of this study is in line with the findings of previous researches.

Although all of the three surgeons were experienced, high-volume knee surgeons, they had much more experience in medial parapatellar approach than mini-midvastus approach, since the conventional approach was used routinely in all clinics.

The authors did not determine the rotational position of the tibial component since it was not a primary objective of the study and there was no statistical significant difference between groups in terms of component positions in other planes. The rotational alignment of the tibial tray might be theoretically different between groups, however is not in line with the findings of previous studies.

Competing interests
The authors declare that they have no competing interests.

Authors' contributions
FP, EL, CD collected the data, AJ conceived the study, recruited the company, and obtained the funding. FP wrote and submitted the paper. All authors read and approved the final manuscript.

Acknowledgements
The CT investigation and statistical analysis of this study was financially supported by Stryker Corporation. CT investigation cost 20700 euro, de statistical analysis cost 2500 euro. Funding of the CT analysis was necessary because it does take part of the standard health care.

Author details
[1]Department Orthopaedic Surgery, Research School Capri, Maastricht University Medical Centre, P. Debyelaan 25, 6229 HX Maastricht, The Netherlands. Heinrich-Braun-Krankenhaus Zwickau, Städtisches Klinikum, Zwickau, Germany. [3]Repatriation General Hospital, Adelaide, Australia.

References
1. Font-Rodriguez DE, Scuderi GR, Insall JN. Survivorship of cemented total knee arthroplasty. Clin Orthop Relat Res. 1997;345:79–86.
2. Callaghan JJ, O'Rourke MR, Iossi MF, Liu SS, Goetz DD, Vittetoe DA, et al. Cemented rotating-platform total knee replacement. A concise follow up, at a minimum of fifteen years, of a previous report. J Bone Joint Surg Am. 2005;87(9):1995–8.
3. Keating EM, Meding JB, Faris PM, Ritter MA. Long-term followup of nonmodular total knee replacements. Clin Orthop Relat Res. 2002;404:34–9.
4. Gill GS, Joshi AB. Long-term results of cemented, posterior cruciate ligament-retaining total knee arthroplasty in osteoarthritis. Am J Knee Surg. 2001;14(4):209–14.
5. Pavone V, Boettner F, Fickert S, Sculco TP. Total condylar knee arthroplasty: a long-term follow-up. Clin Orthop Relat Res. 2001;388:18–25.
6. Ritter MA, Faris PM, Keating EM, Meding JB. Postoperative alignment of total knee replacement. Its effect on survival. Clin Orthop Relat Res. 1994;299:153–6.
7. Rodriguez JA, Bhende H, Ranawat CS. Total condylar knee replacement: a 20-year followup study. Clin Orthop Relat Res. 2001;388:10–7.
8. Shan L, Shan B, Suzuki A, Nouh F, Saxena A. Intermediate and long-term quality of life after total knee replacement: a systematic review and meta-analysis. J Bone Joint Surg Am. 2015;97(2):156–68.
9. Lotke PA, Lonner JH, editors. Master techniques in orthopaedic surgery: knee arthroplasty. Anterior medial exposure. 3rd ed. Lippincott: Williams & Wilkins; 2009. p. 1–18.
10. Pan WM, Li XG, Tang TS, Qian ZL, Zhang Q, Zhang CM. Mini-subvastus versus a standard approach in total knee arthroplasty: a prospective, randomized controlled study. J Int Med Res. 2010;38(3):890–900.
11. Lai Z, Shi S, Fei J, Wei W. Total knee arthroplasty performed with either a mini-subvastus or a standard approach: a prospective randomized controlled study with a minimum follow-up of 2 years. Arch Orthop Trauma Surg. 2014;134(8):1155–62.
12. Deirmengian CA, Lonner JH. What's new in adult reconstructive knee surgery. J Bone Joint Surg Am. 2010;92(16):2753–64.
13. Goble EM, Justin DF. Minimally invasive total knee replacement: principles and technique. Orthop Clin North Am. 2004;35(2):235–45.
14. Scuderi GR. Minimally invasive total knee arthroplasty: surgical technique. Am J Orthop (Belle Mead NJ). 2006;35(7 Suppl):7–11.
15. Lonner JH. Minimally invasive approaches to total knee arthroplasty: results. Am J Orthop (Belle Mead NJ). 2006;35(7 Suppl):27–9.
16. Hofmann AA, Plaster RL, Murdock LE. Subvastus (Southern) approach for primary total knee arthroplasty. Clin Orthop Relat Res. 1991;269:70–7.
17. Engh GA, Holt BT, Parks NL. A midvastus muscle-splitting approach for total knee arthroplasty. J Arthroplasty. 1997;12(3):322–31.
18. Tria Jr AJ, Coon TM. Minimal incision total knee arthroplasty: early experience. Clin Orthop Relat Res. 2003;416:185–90.
19. Alan RK, Tria Jr AJ. Quadricpes-sparing total knee arthroplasty using the posterior stabilized TKA design. J Knee Surg. 2006;19(1):71–6.
20. Tenholder M, Clarke HD, Scuderi GR. Minimal-incision total knee arthroplasty: the early clinical experience. Clin Orthop Relat Res. 2005;440:67–76.
21. Satterly T, Neeley R, Johnson-Wo AK, Bhowmik-Stoker M, Shrader MW, Jacofsky MC, et al. Role of total knee arthroplasty approaches in gait recovery through 6 months. J Knee Surg. 2013;26(4):257–62.
22. Lin SY, Chen CH, Fu YC, Huang PJ, Lu CC, Su JY, et al. Comparison of the clinical and radiological outcomes of three minimally invasive techniques for total knee replacement at two years. Bone Joint J. 2013;95-B(7):906–10.
23. Pongcharoen B, Yakampor T, Charoencholvanish K. Patellar tracking and anterior knee pain are similar after medial parapatellar and midvastus approaches in minimally invasive TKA. Clin Orthop Relat Res. 2013;471(5):1654–60.
24. Laskin RS, Beksac B, Phongjunakorn A, Pittors K, Davis J, Shim JC, et al. Petersen Minimally invasive total knee replacement through a mini-midvastus incision: an outcome study. Clin Orthop Relat Res. 2004;428:74–81.
25. Tashiro Y, Miura H, Matsuda S, Okazaki K, Iwamoto Y. Minimally invasive versus standard approach in total knee arthroplasty. Clin Orthop Relat Res. 2007;463:144–50.
26. Schroer WC, Dieffeld PJ, Reedy ME, LeMarr AR. Mini-subvastus approach for total knee arthroplasty. J Arthroplasty. 2008;23(1):19–25.

27. Bonutti PM, Mont MA, McMahon M, Ragland PS, Kester M. Minimally invasive total knee arthroplasty. J Bone Joint Surg Am. 2004;86-A Suppl 2:26–32.

28. Cheng T, Liu T, Zhang G. Does minimally invasive surgery improve short-term recovery in total knee arthroplasty? Clin Orthop Relat Res. 2010;468:1635–48.

29. Schroer WC, Diesfeld PJ, Reedy ME, LeMarr AR. Isokinetic strength testing of MinimallyInvasive total knee arthroplasty recovery. J Arthroplasty. 2010;25(2):274–9.

30. Tasker A, Hassaballa M, Murray J, Lancaster S, Artz N, Harries W, et al. Minimally invasive total knee arthroplasty; a pragmatic randomised controlled trial reporting outcomes up to 2 year follow up. Knee. 2014;21(1):189–93.

31. Kim JG, Lee SW, Ha JK, Choi HJ, Yang SJ, Lee MY. The effectiveness of minimally invasive total knee arthroplasty to preserve quadriceps strength: a randomized controlled trial. Knee. 2011;18:443–7.

32. Hernandez-Vaquero D, Noriega-Fernandez A, Suarez-Vazquez A. Total knee arthroplasties performed with a mini-incision or a standard incision. Similar results at six months follow-up. BMC Musculoskelet Disord. 2010;6:11–27.

33. Schroer WC, Diesfeld PJ, Reedy ME, LeMarr AR. Surgical accuracy with the mini-subvastus total knee arthroplasty - a computer tomography scan analysis of postoperative implant alignment. J Arthroplasty. 2008;23(4):543–9.

34. Kolisek FR, Bonutti PM, Hozack WJ, Purtill J, Sharkey PF, Zelicof SB, et al. Clinical experience using a minimally invasive surgical approach for total knee arthroplasty: early results of a prospective randomized study compared to a standard approach. J Arthroplasty. 2007;22(1):8–13.

35. Dalury DF, Dennis DA. Mini-incision total knee arthroplasty can increase risk of componentmalalignment. Clin Orthop Relat Res. 2005;440:77–81.

36. Gandhi R, Smith H, Lefaivre KA, Davey RD, Mahomed NN. Complications after minimally invasive total knee arthroplasty as compared with traditional incision techniques - a meta-analysis. J Arthroplasty. 2011;26(1):29–35.

37. Xu SZ, Lin XJ, Tong X, Wang XW. Minimally invasive midvastus versus standard parapatellar approach in total knee arthroplasty: a meta-analysis of randomized controlled trials. PLoS One. 2014;9(5), e95311.

38. Heekin RD, Fokin AA. Mini-midvastus versus mini-medial parapatellar approach for minimally invasive total knee arthroplasty: outcomes pendulum is at equilibrium. J Arthroplasty. 2014;29(2):339–42.

39. Dayton MR, Bade MJ, Muratore T, Shulman BC, Kohrt WM, Stevens-Lapsley JE. Minimally invasive total knee arthroplasty: surgical implications for recovery. J Knee Surg. 2013;26(3):195–201.

40. Guy SP, Farndon MA, Conroy JL, Bennett C, Grainger AJ, London NJ. A prospective randomized study of minimally invasive midvastus total knee arthroplasty compared with standard total knee arthroplasty. Knee. 2012;19(6):866–71.

41. Li C, Zeng Y, Shen B, Kang P, Yang J, Zhou Z, et al. A meta-analysis of minimally invasive and convetional medial parapatellar approaches fpr primary total knee arthroplasty. Knee Surg Sports Traumatol Arthrosc. 2015;23(7):1971–85.

42. Alcelik I, Sukeik M, Pollock R, Misra A, Naguib A, Haddad FS. Comparing the mid-vastus and medial parapatellar approaches in total knee arthroplasty: a meta-analysis of short-term outcomes. Knee. 2012;19(4):229–36.

43. Khanna A, Gougoulias N, Longo UG, Maffulli N. Minimally invasive total knee arthroplasty: a systematic review. Orthop Clin North Am. 2009;40(4):479–89.

44. Liu Z, Yang H. Comparison of the minimally invasive and standard approaches for total knee arthroplasty: systematic review and meta-analysis. J Int Med Res. 2011;39(5):1607–17.

45. Smith TO, King JJ, Hing CB. A meta-analysis of randomized controlled trials comparing the clinical and radiological outcomes following minimally invasive to conventional exposure for total knee arthroplasty. Knee. 2012;19(1):1–7.

46. de Steiger RN, Liu YL, Graves SE. Computer navigation for total knee arthroplasty reduces revision rate for patients less than sixty-five years of age. J Bone Joint Surg Am. 2015;97:635–42.

47. Bauwens K, Matthes G, Wich M, Gebhard F, Hanson B, Ekkernkamp A, et al. Navigated total knee replacement. A meta-analysis. J Bone Joint Surg Am. 2007;89(2):261–9.

48. Mason JB, Fehring TK, Estok R, Banel D, Fahrbach K. Meta-analysis of alignment outcomes in computer-assisted total kne arthroplasty surgery. J Arthroplasty. 2007;22(8):1097–106.

49. Hernandez-Vaquero D, Noriega-Fernandez A, Fernandez-Carreira JM, Fernandez-Simon JM, Llorens de Los Rios J. Computer-assisted surgery improves rotational positioning of the femoral component but not the tibial component in total knee arthroplasty. Knee Surg Sports Traumatol Arthrosc. 2014;22(12):3127–34.

50. Dutton AQ, Yeo SJ. Computer-assisted minimally invasive total knee arthroplasty compared with standard total knee arthroplasty. Surgical technique. J Bone Joint Surg Am. 2009;91 Suppl 2 Pt 1:116–30.

51. Khakha RS, Chowdhry M, Norris M, Kheiran A, Patel N, Chauhan SK. Five-year follow-up of minimally invasive computer assisted total knee arthroplasty (MICATKA) versus conventional computer assisted total knee arthroplasty (CATKA) - a population matched study. Knee. 2014;21(5):944–8.

52. Guyatt GH, Townsend M, Berman LB, Keller JL. A comparison of Likert and visual analogue scales for measuring change in function. J Chronic Dis. 1987;40(12):1129–33.

53. Norkin CC, White DJ. Measurement of joint motion; a guide to goniometry. F.A. Davis Company; 4th ed. 2009.

54. Brosseau L, Tousignant M, Budd J, Chartier N, Duciaume L, Plamondon S, et al. Intratester and intertester reliability and criterion validity of the parallelogram and universal goniometers for active knee flexion in healthy subjects. Physiother Res Int. 1997;2(3):150–66.

55. Lenssen AF, van Dam EM, Crijns YH, Verhey M, Geesink RJ, van den Brandt PA, et al. Reproducibility of goniometric measurement of the knee in the in-hospital phase following total knee arthroplasty. BMC Musculoskelet Disord. 2007;8:83.

56. Jones SE, Kon SS, Canavan JL, Patel MS, Clark AL, Nolan CM, et al. The five-repetition sit-to-stand test as a functional outcome measure in COPD. Thorax. 2013;68(11):1015–20.

57. Evanich CJ, Tkach TK, von Glinski S, Camargo MP, Hofmann AA. 6- to 10-year experience using countersunk metal-backed patellas. J Arthroplasty. 1997;12(2):149–54.

58. Insall JN, Dorr LD, Scott RD, Scott WN. Rationale of the knee society clinical rating system. Clin Orthop Relat Res. 1989;248:13–4.

59. Bellamy N, Buchanan WW, Goldsmith CH, Campbell J, Sitt L. Validation study of WOMAC: a health status instrument for measuring clinically-important patient-relevant outcomes following total hip or knee arthroplasty in osteoarthritis. J Orthop Reuth. 1988;1:95–108.

60. Ewald FC. The knee society total knee arthroplasty roentgenographic evaluation and scoring system. Clin Orthop Relat Res. 1989;248:9–12.

61. Chauhan SK, Clark GW, Lloyd S, Scott RG, Breidahl W, Sikorski JM. Computer-assisted total knee replacement. A controlled cadaver study using a multi-parameter quantitative CT assessment of alignment (the Perth CT Protocol). J Bone Joint Surg Br. 2004;86(6):818–23.

2

Comparison of continuous infusion versus bolus injection of factor concentrates for blood management after total knee arthroplasty in patients with hemophilia

Young Shil Park[1], Won-Ju Shin[2] and Kang-Il Kim[3*]

Abstract

Background: Total knee arthroplasty (TKA) has become the treatment of choice for end-stage hemophilic arthropathy of the knee. Theoretically in hemophilia A, perioperative continuous infusion (CI) of factor VIII (FVIII) would provide a more consistent FVIII level than general bolus injections (BI) in TKA. Current study was designed to evaluate the effectiveness of CI of coagulation factor concentrates during the perioperative period compared to BI.

Methods: A total of 42 TKAs were performed in 31 patients with severe hemophilia A. Under the supervision of a multidisciplinary hemophilia team, CI and BI were monitored during application of a standardized regimen. Perioperative clinical parameters including postoperative hemoglobin drop, drained blood volume, transfusion rate, total consumption of FVIII, and perioperative complications were assessed.

Results: The difference in the postoperative hemoglobin drop was significant between two groups with a lower decrease in the CI group ($p = 0.002$). The drained blood volume for postoperative 24 h was significantly lower in the CI than the BI groups ($p = 0.037$). Total consumption of factor concentrates for postoperative 5 days was greater in the CI group than in the BI group ($p = 0.000$). One postoperative hematoma and wound dehiscence occurred in BI group and no other complication developed.

Conclusions: Although good control of hemostasis could be achieved using either method during the perioperative period of TKA, CI seems more tolerable and effective than BI to provide perioperative blood management undergoing TKA in patients with hemophilia.

Keywords: Hemophilia a, Total knee arthropathy, Continuous infusion, Bolus injection, Blood

Background

Blood management has been an issue in perioperative care in general TKA and especially in hemophilia, inappropriate perioperative blood management in the hip and knee arthroplasty is the most important cause of affecting the clinical outcome [1–4]. Control of bleeding episodes, and the management of perioperative bleeding in patients with hemophilia, is attained via the administration of plasma-derived or recombinant coagulation factors. Most often, these factors are given at regular intervals as a bolus injection (BI) to attain hemostasis [5]; however, there has been growing interest in the use of continuous infusions (CI) of clotting factors during major surgery to maintain constant factor concentrations, thus reducing the risk of bleeding caused by overly low factor trough levels [5–8]. Compared with BI, the CI method is believed to reduce the total FVIII dose required and also the incidence of severe bleeding events. However, there has been paucity in the literature regarding comparison between these two

* Correspondence: khuknee@daum.net
[3]Department of Orthopedic Surgery, Kyung Hee University Hospital at Gangdong, School of Medicine, Kyung Hee University, 892, Dongnam-ro, Gangdong-Gu, Seoul 05278, Korea
Full list of author information is available at the end of the article

different methods of coagulation factor replacement for major surgery in patients with hemophilia. Therefore, we questioned whether CI has superiority in terms of perioperative bleeding control and consumption of FVIII following TKA. This study was performed to explore the effectiveness and safety of CI in hemophilia A patients that underwent TKA, by comparing CI with BI.

Methods

This prospective study involved 42 TKAs performed in 31 patients with severe hemophilia A, admitted to undergo TKA by a single institute. The inclusion criteria were severe hemophilia A (FVIII: C < 1%), more than 150 exposure days (EDs) to any FVIII product before enrolment, no previous history of inhibitors, and good compliance. Each group consisted of 21 cases. Since this disease entity is rare compared to primary osteoarthritis, we assumed that the same infusion protocol in consecutive patients would be better to manage in hemophilia teams. The BI protocol was applied to the former half of the cases in the period between July 2010 and December 2013 and the CI protocol was applied to the latter half of cases during the period between January 2014 and July 2016.

Hemostatic treatment

Under the supervision of a multidisciplinary hemophilia team of our institute, CI followed a standardized protocol. On the day of surgery, 30 min before the incision, a bolus of FVIII concentrates was administered. The first bolus CI dose was 50 IU/kg, affording FVIII plasma levels of 100%. The infusion rate commenced at 4 IU/kg/h and was adjusted to the clinical situation by measuring FVIII levels daily. Factor concentrates were administered without additional dilution, changing the syringes every 8 h (using peripheral venous access). CI was performed for 5 days. During the first 3 days after the operation, FVIII infusion rates were controlled to achieve an FVIII level of 100%. After the first 3 days of operation, the infusion rate was decreased to achieve target FVIII levels of 80% and tailored based on the patient status. In some cases with lower FVIII levels relative to target factor levels, a BI was prescribed in parallel. BI was also administered using the standard protocol of our center; the first bolus of 50 IU/kg was given 30 min before surgery to achieve a preoperative FVIII level of 100%; BI continued for 3 days after operation [9]. Approximately 50% of the initial dose was administered every 8 h. The doses were changed depending on the patient's postoperative status, and the dosing intervals were increased to 12 h after postoperative 7 days. From postoperative 6 days, all patients were applied to BI protocol for easier rehabilitation.

The total consumption of coagulation factor concentrates during hospitalization was recorded for each

procedure. An elastic compression stocking was applied to prevent deep vein thrombosis. No other chemical antithrombotic prophylaxis was prescribed.

Procedures

All operations were performed by a single surgeon (corresponding author) under the general anesthesia with use of a tourniquet. Conventional cemented TKA prostheses were used in all cases. Postoperative drainage was constant and maintained for 2 days. Postoperative rehabilitation began as soon as patients returned to their rooms, using a passive mobilization device. Identical peri- and post-operative care was delivered to both groups. All patients had same postoperative rehabilitation and recommended to discharge at postoperative 10 days.

Evaluation of outcomes and complications

The level of hemoglobin was evaluated the day before TKA, on the operation day, and on postoperative days 1, 2, and 5. To evaluate postoperative blood loss, the volume of drained blood was assessed from patient records. Data collected on short-term complications included hemarthrosis, acute infection, and CI-related complications (such as inhibitor development and thrombotic event) till the postoperative 6 months.

Statistical analysis

All eligible patients were enrolled and their data used to evaluate efficacy and safety. Student's t-test and Fisher's exact test (the chi-squared test) were employed for between-group comparisons. A P value <0.05 was considered statistically significant.

Results

Patient characteristics

In total, 42 cases in 31 patients with severe hemophilia A were evaluated. The mean age of patients at the time of operation was 39.4 ± 9.332 years (range: 26.0–64.0 years). Eleven patients had bilateral TKAs, while one of these patients underwent TKA under BI once and under CI at another time. The first consecutive 21 patients underwent TKA under BI and the latter 21 patients under CI. Recombinant FVIII concentrates were infused to three patients in the CI group, and plasma-derived FVIII concentrates were administered in other cases.

Comparison between BI and CI groups

The mean age of patients at the time of operation in each group was 43.33 ± 9.593 years (range: 27.0–64.0 years) in the CI group and 35.47 ± 7.646 years (range: 26.0–62.0 years) in the BI group. Comparison of the patient characteristics of the two groups revealed no difference in underlying viral status or operation direction. The clinical characteristics of both groups are listed in Table 1.

Table 1 Patient characteristics of the continuous infusion group and bolus injection group

	Continuous infusion (n = 21)	Bolus injection (n = 21)	p
Age (years)			
Mean ± SD	43.33 ± 9.593	35.47 ± 7.646	0.006
BMI			
Mean ± SD	21.67 ± 3.028	23.67 ± 3.201	0.044
Hemoglobin (g/dL)			
Mean ± SD	14.71 ± 0.864	15.05 ± 1.963	0.468
Patient's viral status			
HBV+	1	1	1.000
HCV+	13	13	1.000
TKA (n)			
Right	13	11	
Left	8	10	0.111

SD Standard deviation, BMI Body mass index, HBV+ Hepatitis virus B, HCV Hepatitis virus B, TKA Total knee arthroplasty
*p < 0.05

Table 2 Comparison between the continuous infusion group and bolus injection group

	Continuous infusion (n = 21)	Bolus injection (n = 21)	p
Total amount of coagulation factor concentrates (IU/kg)			
Mean ± SD			
Operation day 0–3	460.23 ± 72.721	359.19 ± 86.686	0.000*
Operation day 0–5	604.03 ± 112.836	467.85 ± 101.157	0.000*
Hemoglobin (g/dL)			
Mean ± SD			
Pre-operation	14.71 ± 0.864	15.05 ± 1.963	0.468
Operation day (post)	13.66 ± 1.188	12.79 ± 1.891	0.081
Hemoglobin drop	1.14 ± 0.961	2.26 ± 1.238	0.002*
Drained blood volume at postoperation day 1 (mL)	574.76 ± 286.855	788.33 ± 351.494	0.037*
Mean ± SD			
Packed RBC transfusion			
No. (n)	1 / 21	5 / 21	0.184
Volume (mL/kg)	0.81 ± 3.740	3.56 ± 7.015	0.120

SD Standard deviation, RBC Red blood cell
*p < 0.05

A surgery-related decrease in hemoglobin was observed in both groups. The average preoperative hemoglobin and hemoglobin on the operation day did not differ between the groups, but comparison of the difference between the two values (hemoglobin drop) in both groups revealed a significant difference (1.14 ± 0.961 g/dL in the CI group vs. 2.26 ± 1.238 g/dL in the BI group; $p = 0.002$). The volume of drained blood during the first 24 h postoperatively differ significantly between the two groups ($p = 0.037$) (Table 2). One patient in the CI group, and five patients in the BI group, required transfusion after TKA during the perioperative period. Total consumption of factor concentrates from operation day to postoperative day 5 was 604.03 ± 112.86 IU/kg in the CI group and 467.85 ± 105.157 IU/kg in the BI group ($p = 0.000$).

Complications and safety
During hospitalization, one patient in the BI group had a postoperative hematoma that required aspiration. Another patient, in the BI group, presented with wound dehiscence which healed after re-closure. No acute periprosthetic joint infection or other thrombotic events were observed in either group. There was no thrombotic event despite the absence of antithrombotic prophylaxis. In addition, no new inhibitor development occurred in either the BI or CI group during the postoperative 6 months.

Discussion
Postoperative hemorrhagic complications in hemophilia patients are quite common and may lead to serious consequences after TKA [10–13]. In patients with hemophilia, coagulation factor concentrates can be administered by way of CI or BI as the perioperative blood management

[14]. While several studies have shown that the CI method is safe and effective due to maintaining constant level of the coagulation factor in the blood during the perioperative periods [15–17], most studies practically have utilized a simple BI method [2, 12, 18]. Furthermore, no comparative study regarding CI and BI methods following total joint replacement for of hemophilia could be found. Therefore the authors attempted to evaluate whether the CI could show efficacy and advantages compared to the BI especially undergoing a relatively common major surgery, such as TKA by way of prospective comparative study. We confirmed that CI could lead to a significant decrease in both postoperative hemoglobin drop and drained blood volume following TKA.

CI has been established that coagulation factor concentrates are stable and microbiologically safe at room temperature [19, 20]. Moreover, it has been known that Cl is a cost-effective drug delivery approach, compared with BI [6, 21]. In this study, the average consumption of coagulation factor concentrates with CI for 5 days was 604.03 ± 112.84 IU/kg, in comparison with 467.85 ± 1.16 IU/kg of BI for the same period after undergoing TKA. There was a discrepancy in our results vis-à-vis the theoretically-advantageous aspect of CI. The discrepancy seems to be coming from the dissimilar BI protocols implemented by different institutions. In this study, the target peak level of factor concentrates administered via BI was 100% at Day 0–3 and 80% at Day 4–6. This regimen required a less amount of factor concentrates than other regimens as reported from various centers [22–26]. Unlike CI that maintains the peak level for 24 h a day, BI achieves the peak level only for a certain duration of just injected time. Afterward, the FVIII levels, given by BI, continue to decline for the half-life of FVIII, 8–12 h, until FVIII level rises after administration of a dose to reach the peak level again. The fact of the matter is that the peak level using a BI method is maintained not 100%, but just 75% for 3 days, in comparison with the conception applicable to CI method. Therefore, the total factor dose administered by BI might be lesser than that of CI, which would maintain the peak level 100% throughout the 24 h-duration. However, the presumption is that the inability to maintain the peak level for 100% of the time would lead to the inferior results of BI, as shown by the decline in hemoglobin level or blood drainage volume, as well as by the increased frequency of blood infusion. Furthermore, a less dose of factor concentrates was administered via BI in this same regimen, in comparison with hemophilia patients who had undergone total hip arthroplasty [9]. This would be the rationale behind CI showing greater consumption of FVIII than BI in this investigation. Further study on various protocols, including cost-effectiveness, is necessary.

The initial concern for prolonged CI was focused on factor stability and safety when the products were kept at room temperature for some period of time [27]. However, such a concern has been addressed in several articles [19, 20, 23]. The potential for inhibitor development has been a recent issue in the context of CI; as such development renders FVIII replacement therapy ineffective and makes it difficult to control bleeding [14, 28, 29]. At the end of our study, we found that no patient had developed inhibitors of FVIII. However, at the time of enrollment, all subjects had over 150 EDs FVIII with no history of prior development of inhibitors were taken. Other studies also reported that inhibitors were absent in previously treated patients who underwent CI during surgery [22].

Another issue with CI is a thromboembolism. Recent reviews on CI found that venous thrombosis developed in 1.39%–3.8% of patients who had received FVIII via CI during various surgeries [16, 30]. In this study, no symptomatic thrombotic event was noted, although we did not use chemoprophylaxis. Also, neither saline dilution nor heparin addition was not carried out during the CI. The suggestion is that CI would not increase the risk of postoperative thrombosis. No saline dilution was prepared for CI in this study, while the syringe was changed at 8 h intervals. CI was carried out at the infusion rate of 4 IU/kg/h of clotting factor concentrates.

In current study, the patients in the BI group showed a significant drop in hemoglobin levels after TKA. Moreover, there was a significant difference between the CI and BI groups in drained blood volume for postoperative 24 h. The frequency number of postoperative transfusions given by BI was larger than that provided by CI. Meanwhile, the patient age and body mass index before surgery were not similar between these two groups. During the investigational period, the study was conducted in sequence of patient's hospital admission. The difference of the mean ages of these two groups might inadvertently contribute to bias. It appears to be an issue, attributing to the scarcity of the disease and that of patients. How this may affect the bleeding management of patients with hemophilia remains unclear, but the difference between the two groups was the limitation in this study. Another limitation of this study was the fact that it had not been a randomized study. However, it was prospectively designed and followed up. Finally, this study was carried out among patients in Asian population and there could be ethnic differences. Further study regarding Western population would be interesting.

Conclusions

Good control of hemostasis could be achieved using either infusion method during the perioperative period of TKA in patients with hemophilia. However, CI seems more tolerable and effective than BI to reduce perioperative blood loss in these cohorts undergoing TKA.

Abbreviations
BI: bolus injections; CI: continuous infusion; EDs: exposure days; FVIII: factor VIII; TKA: Total knee arthroplasty

Acknowledgements
Not applicable

Funding
This research was supported by the Korea Hemophilia Foundation.

Authors' contributions
KIK and YSP contributed significantly to the study design and analysis and interpretation of data. WJS helped to perform the study and collect data. All authors contributed to the critical review and revision processes, and approved the final version for submission.

Consent for publication
Not applicable

Competing interests
The authors' declare that they have no competing interests.

Author details
[1]Department of Pediatrics, Kyung Hee University Hospital at Gangdong, School of Medicine, Kyung Hee University, 892, Dongnam-ro, Gangdong-Gu, Seoul 05278, Korea. [2]Department of Orthopedic Surgery, Kyung Hee

University Medical Center, 23, Kyungheedae-ro, Dongdaemun-gu, Seoul 0244, Korea. [3]Department of Orthopedic Surgery, Kyung Hee University Hospital at Gangdong, School of Medicine, Kyung Hee University, 892, Dongnam-ro, Gangdong-Gu, Seoul 05278, Korea.

References

1. Goddard NJ, Mann HA, Lee CA. Total knee replacement in patients with endstage haemophilic arthropathy: 25-year results. J Bone Joint Surg Br. 2010;92:1085–9.
2. Panotopoulos J, Ay C, Trieb K, Schuh R, Windhager R, Wanivenhaus HA. Outcome of total knee arthroplasty in hemophilic arthropathy. J Arthroplast. 2014;29:749–52.
3. Silva M, Luck JV Jr. Long-term results of primary total knee replacement in patients with hemophilia. J Bone Joint Surg Am. 2005;87:85–91.
4. Westberg M, Paus AC, Holme PA, Tjønnfjord GE. Haemophilic arthropathy: long-term outcomes in 107 primary total knee arthroplasties. Knee. 2014;21:147–50.
5. Batorova A, Martinowitz U. Intermittent injections vs. continuous infusion of factor VIII in haemophilia patients undergoing major surgery. Br J Haematol. 2000;110:715–20.
6. Martinowitz U, Schulman S, Gitel S, Horozowski H, Heim M, Varon D. Adjusted dose continuous infusion of factor VIII in patients with haemophilia a. Br J Haematol. 1992;82:729–34.
7. Martinowitz UP, Schulman S. Continuous infusion of factor concentrates: review of use in hemophilia a and demonstration of safety and efficacy in hemophilia B. Acta Haematol. 1995;94(Suppl. 1):35–42.
8. Meijer K, Rauchensteiner S, Santagostino E, Platokouki H, Schutgens RE, Brunn M, Tueckmantel C, Valeri F, Schinco PC. Continuous infusion of recombinant factor VIII formulated with sucrose in surgery: non-interventional, observational study in patients with severe haemophilia a. Haemophilia. 2015;21:e19–25.
9. Yoo MC, Cho YJ, Kim KI, Ramteke A, Chun YS. The outcome of cementless total hip arthroplasty in haemophilic hip arthropathy. Haemophilia. 2009;15:766–73.
10. Rana NA, Shapiro GR, Green D. Long-term follow-up of prosthetic joint replacement in hemophilia. Am J Hematol. 1986;23:329–37.
11. Karthaus RP, Novakova IR. Total knee replacement in haemophilic arthropathy. J Bone Joint Surg Br. 1988;70:382–5.
12. Figgie MP, Goldberg VM, Figgie HE 3rd, Heiple KG, Sobel M. Total knee arthroplasty for the treatment of chronic hemophilic arthropathy. Clin Orthop Relat Res. 1989;248:98–107.
13. Dingli D, Gastineau DA, Gilchrist GS, Nichols WL, Wilke JL. Continuous factor VIII infusion therapy in patients with haemophilia a undergoing surgical procedures with plasma-derived or recombinant factor VIII concentrates. Haemophilia. 2002;8:629–34.
14. Wong JM, Mann HA, Goddard NJ. Perioperative clotting factor replacement and infection in total knee arthroplasty. Haemophilia. 2012 Jul;18:607–12.
15. McMillan CW, Webster WP, Roberts HR, Blythe WB. Continuous intravenous infusion of factor VIII in classic haemophilia. Br J Haematol. 1970;18:659–67.
16. Batorova A, Martinowitz U. Continuous infusion of coagulation factors: current opinion. Curr Opin Hematol. 2006;13:308–15.
17. Takedani H. Continuous infusion during total joint arthroplasty in Japanese haemophilia a patients: comparison study among two recombinants and one plasma-derived factor VIII. Haemophilia. 2010;16:740–6.
18. Wallny TA, Strauss AC, Goldmann G, Oldenburg J, Wirtz DC, Pennekamp PH. Elective total knee arthroplasty in haemophilic patients. Proposal for a clinical pathway. Hamostaseologie. 2014;34(Suppl. 1):S23–9.
19. Schulman S, Gitel S, Martinowitz U. Stability of factor VIII concentrates after reconstitution. Am J Hematol. 1994;45:217–23.
20. Schulman S, Varon D, Keller N, Gitel S, Martinowitz U. Monoclonal purified F VIII for continuous infusion: stability, microbiological safety and clinical experience. Thromb Haemost. 1994;72:403–7.
21. Lee M, Morfini M, Negrier C, Chamouard V. The pharmacokinetics of coagulation factors. Haemophilia. 2006;12(Suppl. 3):1–7.
22. Peersman G, Laskin R, Davis J, Peterson M. Infection in total knee replacement: a retrospective review of 6489 total knee replacements. Clin Orthop Relat Res. 2001;392:15–23.
23. Martinowitz U, Luboshitz J, Bashari D, Ravid B, Gorina E, Regan L, Stass H, Lubetsky A. Stability, efficacy, and safety of continuously infused sucrose-formulated recombinant factor VIII (rFVIII-FS) during surgery in patients with severe haemophilia. Haemophilia. 2009;15:676–85.
24. Rahmé M, Ehlinger M, Faradji A, Gengenwin N, Lecocq J, Sibilia J, Bonnomet F. Total knee arthroplasty in severe haemophilic patients under continuous infusion of clotting factors. Knee Surg Sports Traumatol Arthrosc. 2012;20:1781–6.
25. Auerswald G, Bade A, Haubold K, Overberg D, Masurat S, Moorthi C. No inhibitor development after continuous infusion of factor concentrates in subjects with bleeding disorders undergoing surgery: a prospective study. Haemophilia. 2013;19:438–44.
26. Rodriguez-Merchan EC. Special features of total knee replacement in hemophilia. Expert Rev Hematol. 2013;6:637–42.
27. Belgaumi AF, Patrick CC, Deitcher SR. Stability and sterility of a recombinant factor VIII concentrate prepared for continuous infusion administration. Am J Hematol. 1999;62:13–8.
28. von Auer C, Oldenburg J, von Depka M, Escuriola-Ettinghausen C, Kurnik K, Lenk H, Scharrer I. Inhibitor development in patients with hemophilia a after continuous infusion of FVIII concentrates. Ann N Y Acad Sci. 2005;1051:498–505.
29. Eckhardt CL, Mauser-Bunschoten EP, Peters M, Leebeek FW, van der Meer FJ, Fijnvandraat K. Inhibitor incidence after intensive FVIII replacement for surgery in mild and moderate haemophilia a: a prospective national study in the Netherlands. Br J Haematol. 2012;157:747–52.
30. Chevalier Y, Dargaud Y, Lienhart A, Chamouard V, Negrier C. Seventy-two total knee arthroplasties performed in patients with haemophilia using continuous infusion. Vox Sang. 2013;104:135–43.

3

The relationship between pain with walking and self-rated health 12 months following total knee arthroplasty

Maren Falch Lindberg[1,2], Tone Rustøen[2,3], Christine Miaskowski[4], Leiv Arne Rosseland[3,5] and Anners Lerdal[1,2]*

Abstract

Background: A subgroup of patients continue to report pain with walking 12 months after total knee arthroplasty (TKA). The association between walking pain and self-rated health (SRH) after TKA is not known. This prospective longitudinal study aimed to investigate the association between a comprehensive list of preoperative factors, postoperative pain with walking, and SRH 12 months after TKA.

Methods: Patients ($N = 156$) scheduled for TKA completed questionnaires that evaluated demographic and clinical characteristics, symptoms, psychological factors, and SRH. SRH was re-assessed 12 months after TKA. Clinical variables were retrieved from medical records. Pain with walking was assessed before surgery, at 6 weeks, 3, and 12 months after TKA. Subgroups with distinct trajectories of pain with walking over time were identified using growth mixture modeling. Multiple linear regression was used to investigate the relationships between pain with walking and other factors on SRH.

Results: Higher body mass index, a higher number of painful sites at 12 months, recurrent pain with walking group membership, ketamine use, higher depression scores, and poorer preoperative self-rated health were associated with poorer SRH 12 months after TKA. The final model was statistically significant ($p = 0.005$) and explained 56.1% of the variance in SRH 12 months after surgery. SRH improved significantly over time. Higher C-reactive protein levels, higher number of painful sites before surgery, higher fatigue severity, and more illness concern was associated with poorer preoperative SRH.

Conclusions: In patients whose walking ability decreases over time, clinicians need to assess for unreleaved pain and decreases in SRH. Additional research is needed on interventions to improve walking ability and SRH.

Keywords: Self-rated health, Walking, Postoperative pain, Total knee arthroplasty, Fatigue

Background

Osteoarthritis (OA) of the knee is a common disorder that leads to pain and restricted mobility. Total knee arthroplasty (TKA) for OA aims to relieve pain and improve function when conservative treatment is no longer effective. Although the procedure is highly effective in terms of prosthesis-related outcomes [1] and quality of life [2], some patients continue to report a higher degree of functional limitations 1 year after TKA compared to healthy age matched controls [3]. Of note, in a recent systematic review [4], approximately 20% of patients reported little or no improvement in terms of pain relief.

The mechanisms that underlie this variability in TKA outcomes are likely to be multifactorial and complex [5]. For example, poorer self-efficacy with walking skills [6], more preoperative walking limitations, higher body mass index (BMI), slower 1 month gait speed, contralateral knee pain, and use of quadstick before surgery [7] were associated with poorer walking outcomes 6 months after TKA. Recently, our research group demonstrated that one in five patients reported no improvements in pain

* Correspondence: anners.lerdal@medisin.uio.no
[1]Department of Surgery, Lovisenberg Diakonale Hospital, Pb 4970 Nydalen, 0440 Oslo, Norway
[2]Department of Nursing Science, Institute of Health and Society, Faculty of Medicine, University of Oslo, Pb 1072 Blindern, 0316 Oslo, Norway
Full list of author information is available at the end of the article

interference with walking 1 year after TKA [8]. In that study, pain interference with walking was measured at repeated intervals during the first year. In a growth mixture modeling, two subgroups of patients with different trajectories of pain with walking were identified. While one group of patients (i.e., Continuous Improvement group, 78%) improved steadily during the first year, a second group of patients (i.e., Recurrent Interference group, 22%) was characterized by initial improvements followed by recurrent pain interference with walking after the first 3 months, resulting in no improvements in terms of pain interference with walking 12 months after surgery. Patients in the Recurrent Interference group were characterized by higher preoperative pain, fatigue, and depression scores and poorer illness perceptions compared to Continuous Improvers. The current study builds on these results to further investigate how walking outcomes and a comprehensive set of predictors are related to a general health outcome (i.e., self-rated health (SRH) at 12 months after TKA.

Walking difficulties seem to influence patients' future health. For example, walking difficulties were associated with higher mortality rates 10 years after TKA [9]. In addition, walking difficulty and shorter walking distance predicted higher health care costs, disability, and mortality [10] as well as poorer self-rated health [11] in the general population.

SRH is a global measure of general health status [12] and is considered a reliable predictor of a variety of outcomes including mortality and morbidity, recovery after disease, and use of health care resources in various patient populations [13–15]. In addition, SRH is used as an outcome measure in population-based studies [16] and was associated with walking speed and walking difficulties [11]. Because SRH was responsive to changes in health and mental well-being during recovery after TKA [17], Peruccio and colleagues suggested that the use of this simple measure could identify patients who might benefit from targeted interventions to improve general health. However, to our knowledge, no studies have investigated the association between pain with walking, other pre- and perioperative factors, and SRH 1 year after TKA. Therefore, the aims of this study were to (1) describe changes in SRH from before until 12 months after TKA, (2) identify preoperative factors associated with poorer preoperative SRH, and (3) investigate the key predictors of poorer SRH 12 months after TKA.

Methods

Data collection for this longitudinal study was performed between October 2012 and September 2014 at a high volume surgical clinic in Norway. The clinic serves patients from all regions of Norway. Patients ≥18 years of age were eligible for inclusion if they were scheduled for TKA for

OA, agreed to participate, and did not have a diagnosis of dementia. Patients undergoing unicompartmental or revision surgery were excluded. The study was approved by the Regional Medical Research Ethics Committee of Health South East of Norway (# 2011/1755).

Patients and procedures

Written information was distributed to all patients considered for eligibility prior to or on the day of admission. A nurse approached patients who met the inclusion criteria and invited them to participate. Written consent regarding questionnaires and extraction of data from the medical records was obtained from all patients before completing the baseline questionnaire that assessed demographic, clinical, symptom and psychological characteristics, as well as health-related quality of life and pain interference with walking. Follow-up assessments of pain interference with walking were performed at postoperative day (POD) 4, 6 weeks, 3 months, and 12 months after surgery. Health-related quality of life follow-up questionnaires were completed 12 months after surgery. All questionnaires were returned in sealed envelopes. Non-responders received a reminder by mail or phone.

Perioperative procedures

The surgical department had a standardized regimen for anesthesia, surgery and postoperative pain management. All patients received the same posterior cruciate-retaining fixed modular-bearing implant for the TKA using an intraoperative tourniquet and with drains that were removed on POD 1. The full regimen for pain management was described in detail elsewhere [8]. Patients were allowed full weight bearing starting on POD 1 and were followed up with weekly physical therapy for 4 to 6 months after surgery. Most patients were prescribed a combination of acetaminophen and tramadol at discharge.

Measurements

Self-rated health: Patients rated their own perceived overall health status today (i.e., SRH) on a numeric rating scale from the well validated EuroQol-5D-3 L [18]. The scale ranges from 0 (worst imaginable health status) to 100 (best imaginable health status).

Clinical variables

Data on comorbidities, BMI, American Society of Anesthesiologists (ASA) classification score, blood pressure, type of anesthesia, type of implant, length of surgery, length of stay, C-reactive protein (CRP), and creatinine values were extracted from the medical records. Data on opioid consumption and use of ketamine were obtained through chart review.

Pain and interference with function measures

The Brief Pain Inventory (BPI) was used to measure pain and interference with walking [11]. The BPI consists of four items that evaluate pain intensity rated on a numeric rating scale (NRS) from 0 (no pain) to 10 (pain as bad as you can imagine); seven items that evaluate pain interference with seven domains of life (i.e., general activity, mood, walking ability, normal work, relations to other people, sleep, enjoyment of life) rated from 0 (no interference) to 10 (interferes completely); and a body map that evaluates pain locations. The validity and reliability of the Norwegian version of the BPI is well established [12].

For this study, pain interference with walking was a factor of particular interest and was assessed on the day before surgery, on POD 4, at 6 weeks, 3 months, and 12 months after surgery. This final endpoint was chosen because the largest gains in functional improvement typically occur within 1–3 years after TKA [19, 20]. In our previous study [21], two subgroups of patients with distinct trajectories of pain interference with walking following TKA were identified. The first group (i.e., Continuous Improvement group) reported significant improvements in pain with walking from before to 12 months after surgery. The second group (i.e., Recurrent Interference group) reported significant improvements in pain interference with walking from before until 3 months after surgery, followed by a distinct worsening returning to preoperative scores 12 months after surgery. This subgroup classification was included in this study as a potential predictor of SRH. Details about this subgroup analysis are published elswhere [21].

Symptom measures
Fatigue severity
Fatigue severity was evaluated using the 5-item Lee Fatigue Scale (LFS). Each item was rated on a 0 to 10 NRS. A mean score using all items was calculated with higher scores indicating higher fatigue severity. The LFS has satisfactory validity and reliability [13]. In this study, its Cronbach's alpha was .92.

Fatigue interference
Fatigue interference during the past week was measured using the 7-item Fatigue Severity Scale (FSS-7). Patients used a 7 point Likert scale to rate their agreement with 7 statements. A total mean score using all seven items was calculated. Scores can range from 1 to 7 with higher scores indicating higher levels of interference. Psychometric properties of the Norwegian version of the FSS-7 were good [14]. In this study, its Cronbach's alpha was .92.

Mood states
The Hospital Anxiety and Depression Scale (HADS) [15] was used to evaluate symptoms of depression and anxiety. HADS consists of two subscales with 7 items for

depression and 7 items for anxiety. Separate mean scores for anxiety and depression were calculated, using all the specific items for each subscale [22]. Each subscale can range from 0 to 21 with higher scores indicating higher levels of anxiety and depression. The Norwegian version of the HADS has excellent psychometric properties [16]. In this study, the Cronbach's alphas for the depression and the anxiety subscales were .78 and .86, respectively.

Psychological measure
The Brief Illness Perception Questionnaire (BIPQ) [17] was used to measure self-reported perceptions of illness. The scale consists of eight items that each measure one dimension of illness perceptions (i.e., consequences, timeline, personal control, treatment control, identity, illness concern, coherence, and emotional response). Each item was rated on a 0 to 10 NRS. For this study, the patients rated their illness perceptions in relation to their OA knee. Five items from the BIPQ (i.e., consequences, personal control, identity, concern, emotional response) were used in the statistical analyses because these specific items were sensitive to changes over time in patients with traumatic injuries [18].

Data analysis
Data analysis was performed using Statistical Package for Social Science version 22 (IBM, Armonk, NY). Growth mixture modeling (GMM) with full maximum likelihood estimation using Mplus Version 7.3 [23] was performed to identify subgroups of patients with distinct trajectories based on their experience with pain interference with walking before through 12 months after TKA. The statistical procedure for this analysis is described in detail elsewhere [21].

For the current analysis, descriptive statistics were generated on sample characteristics, pain, and health related quality of life. A paired t-test was done to evaluate for changes in SRH from prior to until 12 months after TKA. Exploratory analyses using Pearson's bivariate correlation coefficients were performed to select potential variables for inclusion in the multivariate analyses. Non-significant variables were excluded from further testing. Separate regression analyses were performed for preoperative SRH and SRH at 12 months. For both analyses, age, sex and number of comorbidities were included as covariates since these variables were associated with SRH in various populations [24–26].

Preoperative SRH
Variables with a statistically significant association with preoperative SRH in the exploratory analysis (Table 1) were entered into a blockwise multiple linear regression using backwards entry in the following blocks: demographic characteristics, clinical characteristics, pain

Table 1 Potential predictors to self-rated health prior to surgery and 12 months following total knee arthroplasty – Pearsons bivariate correlation coefficient

	Pearsons correlation coefficient			
	Prior to surgery	P-value	12 months	P-value
Demographic characteristics				
Age	0.21+	**	0.19+	*
Sex (male as reference)	−0.20+	*	0.02+	
Cohabitation status (living with partner as reference)	0.08		−0.03	
Employment status (paid work as reference)	0.11		0.01	
Education level (less than 14 years as reference)	0.01		0.04	
Clinical characteristics				
Body mass index	−0.18+	*	−0.30+	**
Number of comorbidities (0–5)	−0.20+	*	−0.26+	**
American Society of Anesthesiologists' physical status classification (1–3)	0.01		−0.05	
Systolic blood pressure	0.17+	*	0.09	
C-reactive protein	−0.30+	**	−0.15	
Creatinine	0.17+	*	0.08	
Pain characteristics				
Average pain prior to surgery	−0.31+	**	−0.16+	*
Worst pain prior to surgery	−0.35+	**	−0.31+	**
Pain interference with function prior to surgery	−0.43+	**	−0.36+	**
Number of painful sites prior to surgery	−0.33+	**	−0.27+	**
Number of painful sites 12 months	n/a		−0.35+	**
Contralateral knee pain 12 months	n/a		−0.06	
Pain interference with walking group (Continuous improvement group as reference)	n/a		−0.55+	**
Perioperative characteristics:				
Type of anesthesia (regional anesthesia as reference)	0.01		−0.17+	*
Length of surgery (minutes)	n/a		−0.06	
Length of stay (days)	n/a		−0.06	
Ketamine (no as reference)	n/a		−0.24+	**
Average dose of opioids over 4 days	n/a		−0.10	
Preoperative symptoms				
Fatigue severity (Lee fatigue scale total score)	−0.44+	**	−0.33+	**
Fatigue interference (Fatigue Severity Scale)	−0.38+	**	−0.36+	**
Depression	−0.32+	**	−0.43+	**
Anxiety	−0.32+	**	−0.31+	**
Psychological characteristics***				
Consequences	−0.35+	**	−0.21+	**
Personal control	−0.20+	*	−0.31+	**
Identity	−0.29+	**	−0.21+	**
Illness concern	−0.43+	**	−0.31+	**
Emotional response	−0.37+	**	−0.23+	**
Health characteristics				
Self-rated health prior to surgery	n/a		0.46+	**

*Correlation is significant at the 0.05 level (2 tailed)
** Correlation is significant at the 0.01 level (2 tailed)
*** Single item scores from the Brief Illness Perception Questionnaire
n/a = not applicable
+Selected for inclusion in linear regressions

characteristics, preoperative symptoms, and psychological characteristics. Then, variables with the least association (i.e. highest *p*-value) with the dependent variable were excluded one by one and nested models were repeated until the final model was determined.

SRH 12 months
Variables with a statistically significant association with SRH at 12 months in the exploratory analysis (Table 1) were entered into a blockwise multiple linear regression using backwards entry using the following blocks: demographic characteristics, clinical characteristics, pain characteristics, perioperative characteristics, preoperative symptoms, psychological characteristics, and health characteristics. Then, variables with the least association (i.e. highest *p*-value) with the dependent variable were excluded one by one and nested models were repeated until the final model was determined. For both analyses, the blocks were created based on the framework used in our previous studies [21, 27, 28] that investigated the impact of demographic, clinical, symptom, and psychological characteristics on acute pain and pain interference with walking after TKA.

Results
Demographic and clinical characteristics
A total of 245 patients were invited to participate in the study, of which 33 declined to participate and six had their surgery cancelled. A total of 206 consenting patients were enrolled in the study. Two patients were later excluded due to postoperative disorientation, one patient died, and 47 had incomplete data on several of

the variables of interest, leaving a total of 156 patients in this analysis. No significant differences were found between responders and non-responders based on any of the preoperative characteristic used in this study.

As displayed in Table 2, the majority of the sample was female (67.9%), lived with a partner (61%), and were not employed (64%). The mean age was 69 (SD 9.1) years and 49% had completed higher education. SRH improved significantly over time ($p < .001$, $t = 9.15$) from before surgery (mean 60.9, SD 19.7) until 12 months after surgery (mean 74.7, SD 16.0).

Predictors of SRH prior to surgery
The final model for preoperative SRH is shown in Table 3. The final model was statistically significant ($p = .002$) and explained 37.0% of the variance in SRH prior to surgery. Higher levels of CRP, a higher number of painful sites before surgery, higher fatigue severity, and higher illness concern were significantly associated with poorer SRH, after controlling for age, sex, and number of comorbidities.

Predictors of SRH at 12 months after TKA
The final model for SRH 12 months after surgery is shown in Table 3. The final model was significant ($p = 0.005$) and explained 56.1% of the variance in SRH 12 months after surgery. Higher BMI, higher number of painful sites 12 months after surgery, Recurrent Interference group membership, perioperative use of ketamine, higher preoperative depression score, higher perceived personal control, and poorer preoperative SRH were associated with poorer SRH 12 months after TKA, after controlling for age, sex and number of comorbidities. Among all associated factors, pain interference walking group membership had the strongest association with SRH at 12 months ($Beta = -0.33$). Patients who had no improvement in pain with walking scored 12.45 points (CI: −17.67 to −7.24) lower on SRH 12 months after TKA, compared to patients whose pain with walking decreased.

Discussion
This study aimed to investigate key predictors associated with poorer SRH 12 months after TKA. Findings from this study suggest that lack of improvement in walking during the first year following TKA was the strongest predictor of poorer SRH scores 12 months after surgery. After controlling for demographic, clinical, and personal factors, membership in the Recurrent Interference group was associated with a 12 point lower SRH score, well above the minimally clinically important difference of 8 points for this scale [29]. In addition, a number of pre- and perioperative factors (i.e., higher number of painful sites, higher BMI, perioperative use of ketamine as supplemental pain medication, higher preoperative

depression scores and poorer preoperative SRH) were associated with poorer SRH scores after TKA. In contrast, poorer preoperative SRH was associated with higher levels of CRP, a higher number of painful sites, higher fatigue severity, and more illness concern related to the osteoarthritic knee.

The preoperative SRH scores in our sample were comparable to OA patients awaiting joint replacement and TKA patients [30, 31]. As expected, overall the sample's SRH score improved significantly during the first year, with a large effect size (Cohen's d = 0.77). An improvement of almost 14 points is well above the clinically important difference of 8 points for this scale [29], which suggests that this improvement is clinically meaningful. This result is in line with previous studies that suggested that TKA has a high success rate for the majority of patients [2]. The improvement in SRH found at 1 year after surgery is similar to a previous report [31].

Consistent with other studies [9, 32], the association between poorer trajectories of pain interference with walking and poorer SRH 1 year after TKA suggests that walking ability is an important predictor of future health. For example, postoperative walking disability was linked to higher mortality rates 10 years after TKA [9]. In the general population, poorer walking performance among older adults was associated with a higher risk for future incidence of cardiovascular disease, mortality, and mobility disabilities [32]. Patients in our study received physical therapy for up to 6 months after surgery. While rehabilitation programs for TKA patients tend to focus on muscle strengthening and range of motion of the joint, assuming that this approach will in turn improve patients' ability to walk, these programs seem to have limited effect on walking ability [33]. Although physical activity levels tend to increase after TKA, patients do not reach the same functional levels as the healthy population, and postsurgical activity levels seem to be influenced mainly by patients' physical activity levels prior to surgery [34]. However, a recent study of a rehabilitation program that used walking and weight bearing exercises had better results for walking speed six months after TKA compared to usual physical therapy [35]. In addition, a 3 month hiking program resulted in improved walking speed and quality of life [36]. Improvements in walking and pain are among the most important outcomes for patients [37], but a substantial number of patients experience reduced walking distance and difficulty climbing stairs [38]. These persistent problems may potentially lead to a less active life and reduced quality of life. Additional studies are needed to determine the effect of improved walking skills on SRH after TKA.

Interestingly, higher preoperative BMI was associated with poor SRH at 12 months after surgery, but not with

Table 2 Demographic, clinical, symptom, and psychological characteristics of patients (N =156) prior to surgery

Demographic characteristics		Mean	SD
Age	Years	68.9	9.1
		n	%
Sex	Female	106	67.9
Cohabitation status	Married/partnered	95	60.9
Employment status	Unemployed/retired	100	64.1
Education level	College/university	76	48.7
Clinical characteristics		Mean	SD
	Body mass index (BMI)	29.2	4.6
		n	%
	Obese (BMI ≥30 kg/m^2)	61	39.1
	Morbidly obese (BMI ≥40 kg/m^2)	4	2.6
		Mean	SD
	Number of comorbidities (0–5)	1.2	1.0
	American Society of Anesthesiologists' physical status classification score	2.0	0.5
	Systolic blood pressure	138.6	16.1
	C-reactive protein	3.3	3.0
	Creatinine	77.6	23.0
Pain characteristics			
	Average pain prior to surgery (0–10)	5.3	1.8
	Worst pain prior to surgery (0–10)	5.5	2.1
	Pain interference with function (0–10)	4.4	2.0
Number of painful sites	Prior to surgery	2.1	1.6
	12 months after surgery	2.0	1.2
		n	%
	Contralateral knee pain 12 months – yes (n = 130)	40	30.8
Pain interference walking group			
	Recurrent interference group	36	23.1
	Continuous improvement group	120	76.9
Perioperative characteristics:			
Anesthesia	Regional anesthesia	132	84.6
	Total intravenous anesthesia	24	15.4
		Mean	SD
	Length of surgery (minutes)	65	13.0
	Length of stay (days)	4.6	1.1
Pain management	Average dose of opioids (mg)[a]	12.6	6.2
		n	%
	Ketamine - yes	22	14.1

Table 2 Demographic, clinical, symptom, and psychological characteristics of patients (N =156) prior to surgery (Continued)

Preoperative symptoms		Mean	SD
	Fatigue severity (1–10)	2.6	2.2
	Fatigue interference (1–7)	3.9	1.5
	Depression (0–21)	3.4	3.1
	Anxiety (0–21)	4.6	3.7
Psychological characteristics[b]			
	Consequences (0–10)	6.2	1.8
	Personal control (0–10)	5.4	2.3
	Identity (0–10)	6.6	1.7
	Concern (0–10)	5.1	2.6
	Emotional response (0–10)	4.5	2.6
Health status			
	Preoperative self-rated health	60.9	19.7
	Self-rated health, 12 months	74.7	16.0

[a]All opioids were converted to intravenous morphine equivalents. Value is the average dose of opioids over 4 days
[b]Single item scores from the Brief Illness Perception Questionnaire

SRH preoperatively. Obesity is considered a modifiable risk factor for OA [39] and weight gain is a risk factor for undergoing TKA [40]. With the global increase of obesity [41], the number of overweight patients undergoing TKA is likely to increase. Obesity is associated with a variety of short and long term complications after TKA [42]. Consistent with our finding, in a systematic review [2], obesity was associated with a poorer quality of life after TKA. A recent study found that patients with a BMI ≥30 kg/m^2 are at increased risk for poorer knee function, revision surgery within 5 years, superficial infection and deep venous thrombosis [43]. In addition, compared to non-obese patients, a systematic review found that patients with a BMI ≥40 kg/m^2 had significantly lower implant survivorship and lower function scores. However, this association was not seen in patients with a BMI ≥30 kg/m^2 [44]. Based on these findings, a cutoff BMI ≥40 kg/m^2 may guide patient selection for TKA. However, Kulkarni and colleagues argued that because all patients are unique, the decision to perform surgery should not rely solely on a patient's BMI but consider each patient's potential risks and benefits [42]. Patients in this category may need counselling about weight reduction and other treatment alternatives for painful OA of the knee. Obese patients with BMI ≥30 kg/m^2 needs to be informed about the risk of a poorer outcomes including SRH, prior to deciding to undergo TKA.

Patients with a higher number of painful sites before and 12 months after surgery were more likely to report poorer SRH, both prior to surgery and 12 months after

Table 3 Multiple linear regression analyses of demographic, clinical, symptom, and psychological factors on pre- and postoperative self-rated health in patients undergoing total knee arthroplasty (TKA)

Independent variables	Beta	B	95% CI	Explained variance (R^2)	Change of variance (R^2 –change)	P-value
Self-rated health prior to surgery						
Step 1. Demographic characteristics				8.5%	8.5%	.001
Age	.06	.12	−.18 to .42			
Sex (male as reference)	−.08	−3.39	−9.16 to 2.39			
Step 2. Clinical characteristics				18.2%	9.7%	<.001
Number of comorbidities	−.05	−1.02	−3.69 to 1.66			
C-reactive protein	**−.25**	**−1.63**	−2.51 to−.74			
Step 3. Pain characteristics				25%	6.8%	<.001
Number of painful sites before surgery	**−.18**	**−2.17**	−3.88 to−.46			
Step 4 Preoperative symptoms				32.7%	7.7%	<.001
Fatigue severity (higher = more fatigue)	**−.22**	**−1.99**	−3.45 to−.54			
Step5 Psychological characteristics				37.0%	4.3%	.002
Illness concern (higher = more concern)	**−.24**	**−1.82**	−2.97 to−.66			
Self-rated health 12 months after TKA						
Step 1. Demographic characteristics				3.5%	3.5%	.12
Age	−.02	−.04	−.27 to .20			
Sex (male as reference)	.06	1.99	−2.53 to 6.52			
Step 2. Clinical characteristics				15.8%	12.3%	<.001
Body mass index	**−.15**	**−.53**	−.98 to−.07			
Number of comorbidities	.07	−1.11	−3.19 to .96			
Step 3. Pain characteristics				42.9%	27.1%	<.001
Number of painful sites 12 months after surgery	**−.17**	**−2.18**	−3.93 to−.42			
Pain interference walking group (Continuous improvement group as reference)	**−.33**	**−12.45**	-.17.67 to -7.24			
Step 4 Perioperative characteristics				45.3%	2.4%	.025
Ketamine Yes/No – No as reference	**−0.15**	**−6.95**	−12.80 to −1.10			
Step 5 Preoperative symptoms				51.0%	5.7%	<.001
Depression	**−.21**	**−1.08**	−1.80 to −.37			
Step 6 Psychological characteristics				52.9%	1.8%	.04
Personal control	−.12	−.84	−1.74 to .07			
Step 7 Health characteristics				56.1%	3.2%	.005
Preoperative self-rated health	**.21**	**.17**	.05 to .29			

Statistically significant defined as $p \leq 0.05$. Bold coefficient = statistically significant
Abbreviations: Beta standardized beta coefficient, *B* unstandardized coefficient, *CI* confidence interval, *SE* standard error

TKA. This characteristic was the only factor common to both time points. Interestingly, number of comorbidities correlated with number of painful sites prior to surgery (.22, *p* = .008) but not with number of painful sites after 12 months (.10, *p* = .23). It is well known that patients with OA have a large number of painful sites often accompanied by pain sensitization [45] which can be linked to increased symptom severity. A higher number of painful sites as well as higher total symptom load was associated with persistent pain after TKA [46], lower functional scores [47], poor improvements in walking

after TKA [21], poor overall health and sleep quality, female gender [48], and poorer health-related quality of life [49]. While preoperative widespread pain was associated with higher pain severity prior to and 12 months after joint replacement surgery [50], patients seem to gain the same amount of pain relief [50] and functional improvements [51] from their TKA compared to patients without widespread pain. Thus, multiple painful sites prior to surgery should be regarded as a risk factor for decreases in walking ability and poorer SRH 12 months after TKA.

Our study revealed that patients with higher preoperative depression scores were more likely to report poorer SRH at 12 months after TKA. This finding complements a systematic review of the literature stating that poorer mental health is associated with worse pain and functional outcomes 1 year after TKA [52]. However, in a recent study, depressed patients improved at the same or better rate as non-depressed patients and had similar satisfaction rates 1 year after TKA [53]. However, depressive symptoms are risk factors for poorer adherence with physical therapy [54]. Thus, identification of depressed patients may be important to individualize care plans and optimize their treatment outcomes.

Poorer SRH prior to surgery was significantly associated with poorer SRH 12 months after TKA. Similarly, poorer preoperative SRH was found to be predictive of poorer health outcomes and SRH 6 months following total hip and knee replacement surgery [55]. While in other samples, SRH was used as a predictor that captured a variety of future health outcomes [13–15], its use as a predictor in joint replacement surgery is limited. Because this simple tool is easy and non-demanding for clinical use, it could be considered for inclusion as part of a screening tool to assess patients at risk for poor outcomes after TKA surgery. However, more research is needed to establish its usefulness in conjunction with other risk factors.

Except for number of painful sites, the factors associated with SRH prior to surgery were not the same as the factors associated with SRH 12 months after TKA. Prior to surgery, SRH scores were associated with higher fatigue scores and higher levels of the inflammatory marker CRP. A systematic review found that higher CRP levels in OA patients were significantly associated with pain, decreased physical function, but not with radiographic OA, suggesting that low-grade systemic inflammation may increase patients' symptomatology [56]. Patients with hip and knee OA are characterized by multiple co-occuring symptoms including pain, fatigue, and depression [57], which may impact their activity levels [58]. Hawker et al [59] found that fatigue contributed to lower physical activity and increased pain in OA patients, which in turn may lead to poorer SRH. However, as these findings were not factors in the model for SRH 12 months after TKA, they may be linked mainly to the OA condition and do not significantly impact the trajectory of recovery after surgery.

This study has several limitations. While our sample was recruited from one single hospital, the surgical department is a high volume surgical clinic which admits patients from all regions of Norway, which we believe increases the generalizability of our findings. No data were available on previous injuries that may have caused the OA condition. Other factors not accounted for in

our study may contribute to long-term outcomes after TKA (e.g., inflammation, reactions to metal and polyethylene). More specific details on other chronic diseases 12 months after surgery may have provided us with more detailed information about other factors that impact patients' SRH. Finally, the use of objective measures of walking ability may have provided additional insight.

The prospective design and relatively large sample are advantages with our study. In addition, all patients received the same type of implant and a standardized regimen for pain management and mobilization. Finally all of the patients received physical therapy for 4–6 months after TKA.

Conclusions

In conclusion, patients with no improvements in terms of pain interference with walking report poorer SRH 12 months after TKA. In addition, poorer SRH after TKA was associated with higher BMI, a higher number of painful sites, higher depression scores and poorer preoperative SRH. Patients whose pain with walking over time does not improve need to be followed closely and may need additional physical therapy to improve their general health status. While a screening tool may enable clinicians to detect patients who need additional follow-up, more research is needed to develop and test such a screening tool. Finally, more research is needed to determine what type and dose of physical therapy is needed to improve TKA patients' walking ability.

Abbreviations
BIPQ: Brief Illness perception questionnaire; BMI: Body mass index; BPI: Brief pain inventory; CRP: C-reactive protein; FSS-7: Fatigue severity scale; GMM: Growth mixture modeling; HADS: Hospital anxiety and depression scale; LFS: Lee fatigue scale; NRS: Numeric rating scale; OA: Osteoarthritis; POD: Postoperative day; SRH: Self-rated health; TKA: Total knee arthroplasty

Acknowledgements
We would like to thank the Orthopedic Research Group at Lovisenberg Diakonale Hospital for their cooperation. We would like to thank Bruce A. Cooper for his assistance with the statistical analysis.

Funding
The study was funded by Lovisenberg Diakonale Hospital. The PhD fellowship for M.F.Lindberg was provided by Lovisenberg Diakonale Hospital, the Norwegian Nursing Organization, and Fulbright Foundation. None of the funders were involved in the study at any time.

Author's contributions
TR, CM, LAR, AL and MFL collaborated on the development and the design of the study. MFL and AL performed the literature search and performed the statistical analyses. All authors were responsible for the data interpretation and preparation of the manuscript and have read and approved the final manuscript.

Competing interests
The authors declare that they have no competing interests.

Consent for publication
Not applicable.

Author details
[1]Department of Surgery, Lovisenberg Diakonale Hospital, Pb 4970 Nydalen, 0440 Oslo, Norway. [2]Department of Nursing Science, Institute of Health and Society, Faculty of Medicine, University of Oslo, Pb 1072 Blindern, 0316 Oslo, Norway. [3]Department of Research and Development, Division of Emergencies and Critical Care, Oslo University Hospital, Pb 4956 Nydalen, 0424 Oslo, Norway. [4]School of Nursing, University of California, San Francisco, UCSF, Box 0610, San Francisco, CA 94143, USA. [5]Institute of Clinical Medicine, University of Oslo, Pb 1072 Blindern, 0316 Oslo, Norway.

References
1. Callahan CM, Drake BG, Heck DA, Dittus RS. Patient outcomes following tricompartmental total knee replacement. A meta-analysis. JAMA. 1994;271(17):1349–57.
2. da Silva RR, Santos AA, de Sampaio Carvalho Junior J, Matos MA. Quality of life after total knee arthroplasty: systematic review. Rev Bras Ortop. 2014;49(5):520–7.
3. Noble PC, Gordon MJ, Weiss JM, Reddix RN, Conditt MA, Mathis KB. Does total knee replacement restore normal knee function? Clin Orthop Relat Res. 2005;431:157–65.
4. Beswick AD, Wylde V, Gooberman-Hill R, Blom A, Dieppe P. What proportion of patients report long-term pain after total hip or knee replacement for osteoarthritis? A systematic review of prospective studies in unselected patients. BMJ Open. 2012;2(1):e000435.
5. Wylde V, Dieppe P, Hewlett S, Learmonth ID. Total knee replacement: is it really an effective procedure for all? Knee. 2007;14(6):417–23.
6. Hiyama Y, Wada O, Nakakita S, Mizuno K. Factors Affecting Mobility after Knee Arthroplasty. J Knee Surg. 2016. doi:10.1055/s-0036-1584562. (Epub ahead of print).
7. Pua YH, Seah FJ, Clark RA, Poon CL, Tan JW, Chong HC. Development of a prediction model to estimate the risk of walking limitations in patients with total knee arthroplasty. J Rheumatol. 2016;43(2):419–26.
8. Lindberg MF, Miaskowski C, RustoEn T, Rosseland LA, Cooper BA, Lerdal A. Factors that can predict pain with walking, 12 months after total knee arthroplasty. Acta Orthop. 2016;87(6):600–6.
9. Lizaur-Utrilla A, Gonzalez-Parreno S, Miralles-Munoz FA, Lopez-Prats FA. Ten-year mortality risk predictors after primary total knee arthroplasty for osteoarthritis. Knee Surg Sports Traumatol Arthrosc. 2015;23(6):1848–55.
10. Hardy SE, Kang Y, Studenski SA, Degenholtz HB. Ability to walk 1/4 mile predicts subsequent disability, mortality, and health care costs. J Gen Intern Med. 2011;26(2):130–5.
11. Jylha M, Guralnik JM, Balfour J, Fried LP. Walking difficulty, walking speed, and age as predictors of self-rated health: the women's health and aging study. J Gerontol A Biol Sci Med Sci. 2001;56(10):M609–617.
12. Wu S, Wang R, Zhao Y, Ma X, Wu M, Yan X, He J. The relationship between self-rated health and objective health status: a population-based study. BMC Public Health. 2013;13(1):320.
13. Idler EL, Benyamini Y. Self-rated health and mortality: a review of twenty-seven community studies. J Health Soc Behav. 1997;38(1):21–37.
14. Latham K, Peek CW. Self-rated health and morbidity onset among late midlife U.S. adults. J Gerontol B Psychol Sci Soc Sci. 2013;68(1):107–16.
15. Smith PM, Glazier RH, Sibley LM. The predictors of self-rated health and the relationship between self-rated health and health service needs are similar across socioeconomic groups in Canada. J Clin Epidemiol. 2010;63(4):412–21.
16. Ree E, Odeen M, Eriksen HR, Indahl A, Ihlebaek C, Hetland J, Harris A. Subjective health complaints and self-rated health: are expectancies more important than socioeconomic status and workload? Int J Behav Med. 2014;21(3):411–20.
17. Perruccio AV, Badley EM, Hogg-Johnson S, Davis AM. Characterizing self-rated health during a period of changing health status. Soc Sci Med. 2010;71(9):1636–43.
18. EuroQol Group. EuroQol–a new facility for the measurement of health-related quality of life. Health Policy. 1990;16(3):199–208.
19. Nilsdotter AK, Toksvig-Larsen S, Roos EM. A 5 year prospective study of patient-relevant outcomes after total knee replacement. Osteoarthr Cartil. 2009;17(5):601–6.
20. Jones CA, Beaupre LA, Johnston DW, Suarez-Almazor ME. Total joint arthroplasties: current concepts of patient outcomes after surgery. Rheum Dis Clin North Am. 2007;33(1):71–86.
21. Lindberg MKF, Miaskowski C, Rustøen T, Rosseland LA, Cooper BA, Lerdal A. Factors predicting pain with walking 12 months after total knee arthroplasty - a trajectory analysis of 202 patients. Acta Orthop. 2016;87:600–6.
22. Mykletun A, Stordal E, Dahl AA. Hospital anxiety and depression (HAD) scale: factor structure, item analyses and internal consistency in a large population. Br J Psychiatry. 2001;179:540–4.
23. Muthén LKM BO. (1998-2015) mplus User's guide. 7th ed. Los Angeles: Muthen & Muthen; 2015.
24. Unden AL, Elofsson S. Do different factors explain self-rated health in men and women? Gend Med. 2006;3(4):295–308.
25. Mavaddat N, Valderas JM, van der Linde R, Khaw KT, Kinmonth AL. Association of self-rated health with multimorbidity, chronic disease and psychosocial factors in a large middle-aged and older cohort from general practice: a cross-sectional study. BMC Fam Pract. 2014;15:185.
26. Lindberg MF, Grov EK, Gay CL, Rustoen T, Granheim TI, Amlie E, Lerdal A. Pain characteristics and self-rated health after elective orthopaedic surgery - a cross-sectional survey. J Clin Nurs. 2013;22(9-10):1242–53.
27. Lindberg MF, Miaskowski C, Rustøen T, Rosseland LA, Paul SM, Cooper BA, Lerdal A. The Impact of Demographic, Clinical, Symptom and Psychological Characteristics on the Trajectories of Acute Postoperative Pain After Total Knee Arthroplasty. Pain Med. 2016;1-16. doi:10.1093/pm/pnw080.
28. Lindberg MKF, Miaskowski C, Rustøen T, Rosseland LA, Paul SM, Lerdal A. Preoperative pain, symptoms, and psychological factors related to higher acute pain trajectories during hospitalization for total knee arthroplasty. PLoS One. 2016;11(9):1-20. doi:10.1371/journal.pone.0161681.
29. Zanini A, Aiello M, Adamo D, Casale S, Cherubino F, Della Patrona S, Raimondi E, Zampogna E, Chetta A, Spanevello A. Estimation of minimal clinically important difference in EQ-5D visual analog scale score after pulmonary rehabilitation in subjects with COPD. Respir Care. 2015;60(1):88–95.
30. Conner-Spady BL, Marshall DA, Bohm E, Dunbar MJ, Loucks L, Al Khudairy A, Noseworthy TW. Reliability and validity of the EQ-5D-5L compared to the EQ-5D-3L in patients with osteoarthritis referred for hip and knee replacement. Qual Life Res. 2015;24(7):1775–84.
31. W. Dahl A, Robertsson O. Similar outcome for total knee arthroplasty after previous high tibial osteotomy and for total knee arthroplasty as the first measure. Acta Orthop. 2016;87(4):1-6.
32. Newman AB, Simonsick EM, Naydeck BL, Boudreau RM, Kritchevsky SB, Nevitt MC, Pahor M, Satterfield S, Brach JS, Studenski SA, et al. Association of long-distance corridor walk performance with mortality, cardiovascular disease, mobility limitation, and disability. JAMA. 2006;295(17):2018–26.
33. Minns Lowe CJ, Barker KL, Dewey M, Sackley CM. Effectiveness of physiotherapy exercise after knee arthroplasty for osteoarthritis: systematic review and meta-analysis of randomised controlled trials. BMJ. 2007;335(7624):812.
34. Brandes M, Ringling M, Winter C, Hillmann A, Rosenbaum D. Changes in physical activity and health-related quality of life during the first year after total knee arthroplasty. Arthritis Care Res. 2011;63(3):328–34.
35. Bruun-Olsen V, Heiberg KE, Wahl AK, Mengshoel AM. The immediate and long-term effects of a walking-skill program compared to usual physiotherapy care in patients who have undergone total knee arthroplasty (TKA): a randomized controlled trial. Disabil Rehabil. 2013;35(23):2008–15.
36. Hepperger C, Gfoller P, Hoser C, Ulmer H, Fischer F, Schobersberger W, Fink C. The effects of a 3-month controlled hiking programme on the functional abilities of patients following total knee arthroplasty: a prospective, randomized trial. Knee Surg Sports Traumatol Arthrosc. 2016. DOI: 10.1007/s00167-016-4299-3. (Epub ahead of print).
37. Yoo JH, Chang CB, Kang YG, Kim SJ, Seong SC, Kim TK. Patient expectations of total knee replacement and their association with sociodemographic factors and functional status. J Bone Joint Surg (Br). 2011;93(3):337–44.
38. Heiberg K, Bruun-Olsen V, Mengshoel AM. Pain and recovery of physical functioning nine months after total knee arthroplasty. J Rehabil Med. 2010;42(7):614–9.
39. Zheng H, Chen C. Body mass index and risk of knee osteoarthritis: systematic review and meta-analysis of prospective studies. BMJ Open. 2015;5(12):e007568.

40. Apold H, Meyer HE, Nordsletten L, Furnes O, Baste V, Flugsrud GB. Weight gain and the risk of knee replacement due to primary osteoarthritis: a population based, prospective cohort study of 225,908 individuals. Osteoarthritis Cartilage. 2014;22(5):652–8.

41. NCD Risk Factor Collaboration (NCD-RisC). Trends in adult body-mass index in 200 countries from 1975 to 2014: a pooled analysis of 1698 population-based measurement studies with 19.2 million participants. Lancet. 2016; 387(10026):1377–96.

42. Kulkarni K, Karssiens T, Kumar V, Pandit H. Obesity and osteoarthritis. Maturitas. 2016;89:22–8.

43. Si HB, Zeng Y, Shen B, Yang J, Zhou ZK, Kang PD, Pei FX. The influence of body mass index on the outcomes of primary total knee arthroplasty. Knee Surg Sports Traumatol Arthrosc. 2015;23(6):1824–32.

44. McElroy MJ, Pivec R, Issa K, Harwin SF, Mont MA. The effects of obesity and morbid obesity on outcomes in TKA. J Knee Surg. 2013;26(2):83–8.

45. Fingleton C, Smart K, Moloney N, Fullen BM, Doody C. Pain sensitization in people with knee osteoarthritis: a systematic review and meta-analysis. Osteoarthritis Cartilage. 2015;23(7):1043–56.

46. Lewis GN, Rice DA, McNair PJ, Kluger M. Predictors of persistent pain after total knee arthroplasty: a systematic review and meta-analysis. Br J Anaesth. 2015;114(4):551–61.

47. Bruusgaard D, Tschudi-Madsen H, Ihlebaek C, Kamaleri Y, Natvig B. Symptom load and functional status: results from the Ullensaker population study. BMC Public Health. 2012;12:1085.

48. Kamaleri Y, Natvig B, Ihlebaek CM, Benth JS, Bruusgaard D. Number of pain sites is associated with demographic, lifestyle, and health-related factors in the general population. Eur J Pain. 2008;12(6):742–8.

49. Lacey RJ, Belcher J, Rathod T, Wilkie R, Thomas E, McBeth J. Pain at multiple body sites and health-related quality of life in older adults: results from the North Staffordshire Osteoarthritis Project. Rheumatology (Oxford). 2014;53(11):2071–9.

50. Wylde V, Sayers A, Lenguerrand E, Gooberman-Hill R, Pyke M, Beswick AD, Dieppe P, Blom AW. Preoperative widespread pain sensitization and chronic pain after hip and knee replacement: a cohort analysis. Pain. 2015;156(1):47–54.

51. Bican O, Jacovides C, Pulido L, Saunders C, Parvizi J. Total knee arthroplasty in patients with fibromyalgia. J Knee Surg. 2011;24(4):265–71.

52. Vissers MM, Bussmann JB, Verhaar JA, Busschbach JJ, Bierma-Zeinstra SM, Reijman M. Psychological factors affecting the outcome of total hip and knee arthroplasty: a systematic review. Semin Arthritis Rheum. 2012;41(4):576–88.

53. Perez-Prieto D, Gil-Gonzalez S, Pelfort X, Leal-Blanquet J, Puig-Verdie L, Hinarejos P. Influence of depression on total knee arthroplasty outcomes. J Arthroplasty. 2014;29(1):44–7.

54. Jack K, McLean SM, Moffett JK, Gardiner E. Barriers to treatment adherence in physiotherapy outpatient clinics: a systematic review. Man Ther. 2010;15(3-2):220–8.

55. Perruccio AV, Davis AM, Hogg-Johnson S, Badley EM. Importance of self-rated health and mental well-being in predicting health outcomes following total joint replacement surgery for osteoarthritis. Arthritis Care Res (Hoboken). 2011;63(7):973–81.

56. Jin X, Beguerie JR, Zhang W, Blizzard L, Otahal P, Jones G, Ding C. Circulating C reactive protein in osteoarthritis: a systematic review and meta-analysis. Ann Rheum Dis. 2013;1-8. doi:10.1136/annrheumdis-2013-204494.

57. Murphy SL, Lyden AK, Phillips K, Clauw DJ, Williams DA. Subgroups of older adults with osteoarthritis based upon differing comorbid symptom presentations and potential underlying pain mechanisms. Arthritis Res Ther. 2011;13(4):R135.

58. Murphy SL, Alexander NB, Levoska M, Smith DM. Relationship between fatigue and subsequent physical activity among older adults with symptomatic osteoarthritis. Arthritis Care Res (Hoboken). 2013;65(10):1617–24.

59. Hawker GA, Gignac MA, Badley E, Davis AM, French MR, Li Y, Perruccio AV, Power JD, Sale J, Lou W. A longitudinal study to explain the pain-depression link in older adults with osteoarthritis. Arthritis Care Res (Hoboken). 2011;63(10):1382–90.

4

Anterior tibial curved cortex is a reliable landmark for tibial rotational alignment in total knee arthroplasty

Joong Il Kim[1], Jak Jang[2], Ki Woong Lee[2], Hyuk Soo Han[2], Sahnghoon Lee[2] and Myung Chul Lee[2]*

Abstract

Background: Rotational alignment of the tibial component is important for long-term success of total knee arthroplasty (TKA). This study aimed to compare five axes in normal and osteoarthritic (OA) knees to determine a reliable landmark for tibial rotational alignment in TKA.

Methods: One hundred twenty patients with OA knees and 40 with normal knees were included. The angle between a line perpendicular to the surgical transepicondylar axis and each of five axes were measured on preoperative computed tomography. The five axes were as follows: a line from the center of the posterior cruciate ligament (PCL) to the medial border of the patellar tendon (PCL-PT), medial border of the tibial tuberosity (PCL-TT1), medial one-third of the tibial tuberosity (PCL-TT2), and apex of the tibial tuberosity (PCL-TT3), as well as the anteroposterior axis of the tibial prosthesis along the anterior tibial curved cortex (ATCC).

Results: For all five axes tested, the mean angles were smaller in OA knees than in normal knees. In normal knees, the angle of the ATCC axis had the smallest mean value and narrowest range (1.6° ± 2.8°; range, −1.7°–7.7°). In OA knees, the mean angle of the ATCC axis (0.8° ± 2.7°; range, −7.9°–9.2°) was larger than that of the PCL-TT1 axis (0.3° ± 5.5°; range, −19.7°–10.6°) (P = 0.461), while the angle of the ATCC axis had the smallest SD and narrowest range.

Conclusion: The ATCC was found to be the most reliable and useful anatomical landmark for tibial rotational alignment in TKA.

Keywords: Total knee arthroplasty, Rotational alignment, Tibial component rotation, Anatomical landmark, Anterior tibial curved cortex

Background

Total knee arthroplasty (TKA) is considered a definitive treatment option for severe osteoarthritic (OA) knee [1]. Although most patients who receive TKA show successful functional outcomes, some patients have persistent knee pain, limited range of motion, and instability after TKA, eventually requiring revision TKA [2–4]. While multiple factors are relevant for achieving successful functional outcomes after TKA, the rotational alignment of the tibial component is particularly important, since malrotation can cause patellar maltracking [5–7], tibiofemoral joint instability in flexion [8–10], and premature wear of the polyethylene components, which eventually affects implant longevity [11–13].

In contrast to the transepicondylar axis (TEA), which is generally accepted as a reliable landmark for determining the rotational alignment of the femur [14–16], no gold standard has been established for determining the rotational alignment of the tibia, despite its critical relevance in the outcomes of TKA. Therefore, many anatomical landmarks on the proximal tibia have been used to determine tibial rotational alignment in TKA, including the medial one-third of the tibial tuberosity, medial border of the tibial tuberosity, apex of the tibial tuberosity, midsulcus line, and medial border of the patellar tendon [17–27]. However, these landmarks are difficult to identify after cutting the tibia and vary greatly among patients [20, 21, 28]. Indeed, Siston et al. [22]

* Correspondence: leemc@snu.ac.kr
2Department of Orthopaedic Surgery, Seoul National University Hospital, 101 Daehak-ro, Jongno-gu, Seoul 110-744, Korea
Full list of author information is available at the end of the article

reported substantial deviations in tibial rotational alignment after TKA, which ranged from 44° of internal rotation to 46° of external rotation, depending on the surgeon's ability.

Recently, Baldini et al. [17] proposed that the anterior tibial curved cortex (ATCC) represents a reproducible and reliable landmark for tibial rotational alignment. The approach using the ATCC as a landmark proceeds as follows: after cutting the proximal tibia, the anterior surface of the tibial baseplate is matched with the ATCC of the proximal tibia. However, the study by Baldini et al. was based on normal knees, and their measurements were not evaluated at the standard resection level for primary TKA. In addition, there has been no comprehensive comparison between the usefulness of the ATCC landmark and that of other potential landmarks. Therefore, in this study, we aimed to determine the most useful landmark for assessing tibial rotational alignment in TKA. For this reason, we considered five axes on the proximal tibia in normal and OA knees, at the standard resection level for primary TKA using preoperative computed tomography (CT). We hypothesized that, compared with the other four axes assessed, the ATCC is the most reliable landmark for optimal tibial rotational alignment, in both normal and OA knees.

Methods

Between June and September 2010, 120 patients with OA knees and 40 with normal knees were recruited for this study. Patients who were candidates for TKA and had OA knees (grade 3 or 4 on the Kellgren-Lawrence scale) were included. Patients with inflammatory arthritis, previous open knee surgery, or infective arthritis (active or chronic) were excluded. The normal knee group comprised 40 patients without OA knees and with no ligament instability, who had been scheduled for simple meniscectomy. All patients were informed of the risk of exposure to radiation during computed tomography (CT), and written informed consent was obtained. This study was approved by our institutional review board (H-0906-044-283). Table 1 summarizes the demographic characteristics of the study participants.

To determine tibial rotational alignment, transverse CT scans (Siemens Somatom; Siemens Medical Solutions, Malvern, PA, USA) were obtained at 1.0- or 1.3-mm intervals from the hip to the ankle, with the knee in full extension, as described previously [24, 29]. Digital Imaging and Communications in Medicine images were processed using a three-dimensional image-reconstruction/analysis program (OnDemand3D; CyberMed, Irvine, CA, USA), and the best image of the femur showing the lateral and medial epicondylar prominences was selected. In addition, a transverse image of the proximal tibia at the optimal osteotomy level

Table 1 The demographic characteristics of the study population

	Normal knee	OA knee
Number of knees	40	120
Gender (M/F)	4:36	7:113
Mean age (year)[a]	32.1 ± 9.7	70.0 ± 7.2
BMI (kg/m^2)[a]	25.9 ± 3.4	26.7 ± 3.2
Height (mm)[a]	163 ± 7.4	161 ± 5.4
Mechanical Tibiofemoral angle (°)[a]	varus 0.8 ± 0.4	varus 6.4 ± 3.8

[a]The values are presented as mean and standard deviation

(10 mm below the highest point of the lateral plateau) was also selected. The reference axis was defined as a line perpendicular to the surgical TEA (sTEA; a line from the tip of the lateral epicondyle to the sulcus of the medial epicondyle) of the femur (Fig. 1a). Tibial rotational alignment was measured as the angle between the reference axis and each of five anteroposterior (AP) axes, at the level of tibial osteotomy. The five axes were identified and defined as follows: (1) a line from the center of the posterior cruciate ligament (PCL) to the medial border of the patellar tendon (PCL-PT; Fig. 1b) [18]; (2) a line from the center of the PCL to the medial border of the tibial tuberosity (PCL-TT1; Fig. 1c) [19]; a line from the center of the PCL to the medial one-third of the tibial tuberosity (PCL-TT2; Fig. 1d) [20]; (4) a line from the center of the PCL to the apex of the tibial tuberosity (PCL-TT3; Fig. 1e) [27]; and (5) the AP axis of the tibial prosthesis, using a tibial prosthesis template (LPS-Flex; Zimmer, Warsaw, IN, USA), along the ATCC (Fig. 1f) [17]. Internal rotation was shown as a negative value, while external rotation was shown as a positive value.

Statistical Analysis

A priori sample size analysis using G*Power version 3.1.2 showed that 30 cases per group were required to detect a statistically significant between-group difference with 1° precision in terms of tibial component rotation (α = 0.05, β = 0.8). For descriptive analysis, data are presented as mean values with standard deviations (SDs) and ranges. All data were tested for normal distribution using the Kolmogorov-Smirnov test. When a normal distribution was present, the Student's t test was used to evaluate the relationship within each group, and the paired t test was used to examine the significance of the difference for each axis. Radiographic parameters were measured twice by two independent observers (JJ and JIK), with a two-week interval between measurements. Intra- and interobserver reliability were assessed using intraclass correlation coefficients (ICCs). Statistical analyses were performed using

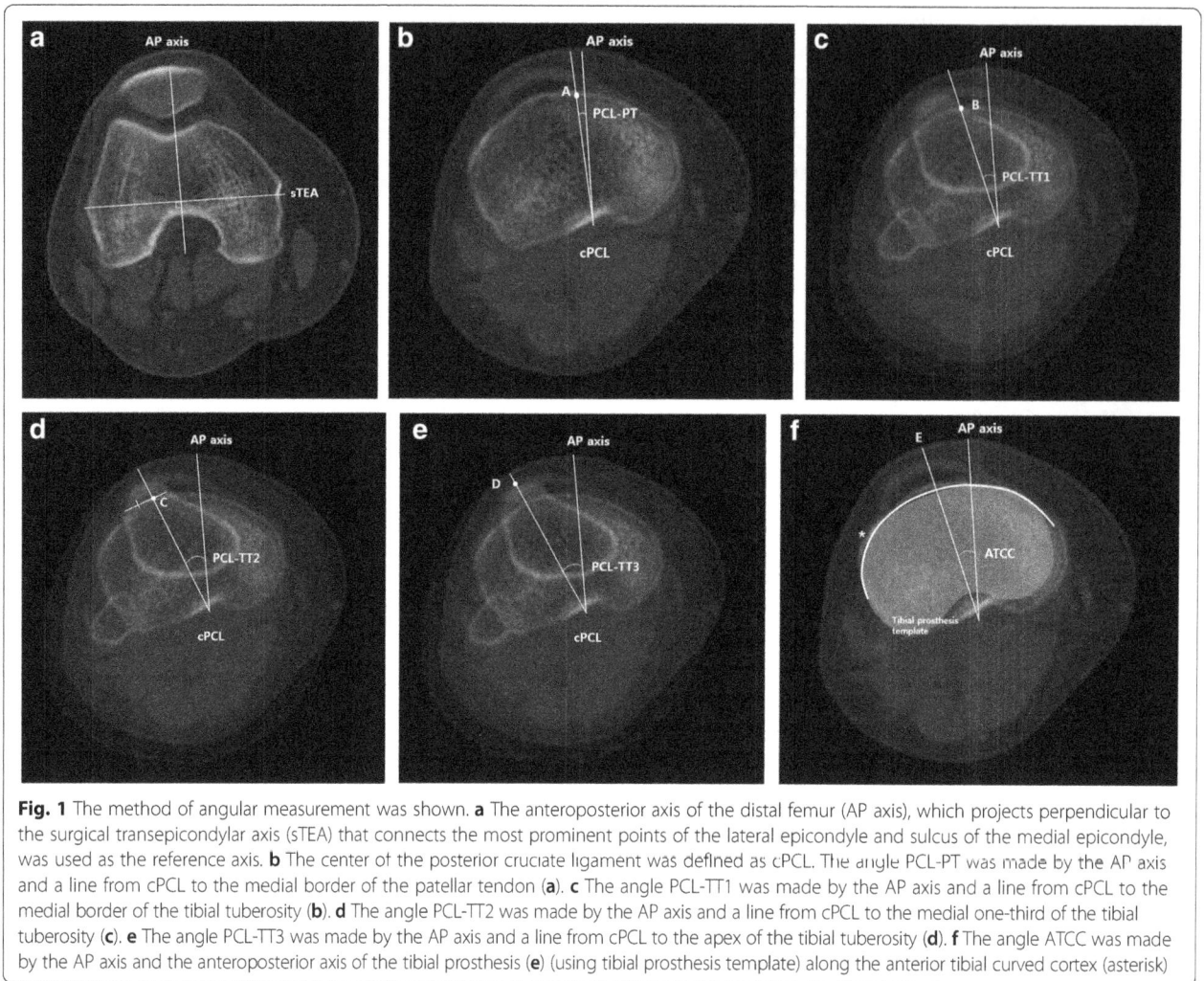

Fig. 1 The method of angular measurement was shown. **a** The anteroposterior axis of the distal femur (AP axis), which projects perpendicular to the surgical transepicondylar axis (sTEA) that connects the most prominent points of the lateral epicondyle and sulcus of the medial epicondyle, was used as the reference axis. **b** The center of the posterior cruciate ligament was defined as cPCL. The angle PCL-PT was made by the AP axis and a line from cPCL to the medial border of the patellar tendon (**a**). **c** The angle PCL-TT1 was made by the AP axis and a line from cPCL to the medial border of the tibial tuberosity (**b**). **d** The angle PCL-TT2 was made by the AP axis and a line from cPCL to the medial one-third of the tibial tuberosity (**c**). **e** The angle PCL-TT3 was made by the AP axis and a line from cPCL to the apex of the tibial tuberosity (**d**). **f** The angle ATCC was made by the AP axis and the anteroposterior axis of the tibial prosthesis (**e**) (using tibial prosthesis template) along the anterior tibial curved cortex (asterisk)

SPSS version 20.0 (IBM Corporation, Armonk, NY, USA), with P values of <0.05 considered significant.

Results

For all five axes tested, the mean angles were smaller in OA knees than in normal knees ($P < 0.05$). The AP axes of the proximal tibia showed greater internal rotation in OA knees than in normal knees. The difference in the mean angle of the ATCC axis between OA and normal knees was smaller than that of the other axes tested ($P = 0.047$). In normal knees, the angle of the ATCC axis had the smallest mean value and narrowest range (1.6° ± 2.8°; range, −1.7°–7.7°). In OA knees, the angle of the PCL-TT1 axis (0.3° ± 5.5°; range, −19.7°–10.6°) had the smallest mean value, but the SD and range exceeded those of the angle of the ATCC axis (0.8° ± 2.7°; range, −7.9°–9.2°). The mean angle of the ATCC axis was larger than that of the PCL-TT1 axis, but the difference was not significant ($P = 0.461$). The angle of the ATCC axis had the smallest SD and narrowest range (Table 2). The ICCs for inter- and intraobserver reliability were >0.8 for

all measurements, ranging from 0.81 to 0.92, which indicated that all measurements had good reliability.

Discussion

The most important findings of this study were as follows: (1) the AP axes of the proximal tibia showed greater internal rotation in OA knees than in normal knees, and (2) although the mean angle of the ATCC axis was larger than that of the PCL-TT1 axis, the angle of the ATCC axis had the smallest SD and narrowest range noted for OA knees.

Based on previous reports, the nature of OA-related rotational deformity of the tibia with respect to the corresponding position in normal knees is debatable. In a CT study, Matsui et al. [30] reported that the tibia tends to be externally rotated in OA knees with varus deformity. Similarly, using magnetic resonance imaging, Sahin et al. [31] showed that, in OA knees with varus deformity, the tibia tends to rotate externally relative to the orientation noted in normal knees. On the contrary, in the present study, although the absolute values of the

Table 2 The tibial component rotational alignment in normal and OA knees

| | Tibial Component Rotational Alignment | | | | |
| | Normal knees (n = 40) | | OA knees (n = 120) | | |
	Mean ± SD (°)[a]	Range (°)[a]	Mean ± SD (°)[a]	Range (°)[a]	P value[b]
PCL-PT	2.8 ± 4.9	−8.2 ~ 13.2	−1.2 ± 4.7	−13.8 ~ 10.0	< 0.001
PCL-TT1	4.0 ± 4.7	−6.2 ~ 12.2	0.3 ± 5.5	−19.7 ~ 10.6	< 0.001
PCL-TT2	14.7 ± 5.0	5.4 ~ 23.5	9.8 ± 5.4	−8.1 ~ 21.9	< 0.001
PCL-TT3	19.9 ± 5.4	8.4 ~ 28.7	14.8 ± 5.4	0.3 ~ 27.8	< 0.001
ATCC	1.6 ± 2.8	−1.7 ~ 7.7	0.8 ± 2.7	−7.9 ~ 9.2	0.047

[a]Internal rotation was denoted as a negative value, and external rotation as a positive value
[b]Student's t-test

angles of the AP axes indicated external rotation compared with the reference axis (except for the PCL-PT axis), OA knees were found to show a tendency to rotate internally relative to the orientation noted in normal knees. This finding is consistent with that of Khan et al. [32], who showed greater external rotation in normal knees than in OA knees. This aspect is important clinically because, if information regarding tibial rotational alignment in normal knees is applied to OA knees, the tibial component might rotate externally and result in malrotation-related adverse outcomes after TKA.

Rotational alignment of the tibia is important for the long-term success and good functional outcome of TKA. However, the tibial component may malrotate intraoperatively due to a lack of distinct landmarks after cutting the tibia or anatomic variability [20, 21, 28]. Several authors reported that excessive internal rotation of the tibial component causes patellar maltracking and persistent anterior knee pain [5–7]. Other reports also mentioned flexion and mid-flexion instability due to poor matching between the tibial and femoral components through the range of motion [8–10]. Some authors expressed particular concern regarding the association between the malrotation of the tibial component and premature wear of the polyethylene components, leading to component loosening [11–13]. Moreover, Su et al. [33] reported that malrotation of the tibial component is one of the causes of knee stiffness, whereas Barrack et al. [2] reported that even small deviations (6.2°) towards internal rotation of the tibial component were associated with increased postoperative pain. Finally, the mechanism underlying the detrimental effect of malrotation of the tibial component was confirmed not only in clinical studies but also in a biomechanical study, which showed that malrotation is implicated in increased biomechanical stress induced by AP translations [34].

To determine the rotational alignment of the tibial component in TKA, several anatomical landmarks on the proximal tibia have been proposed [17–27]. Many studies have shown that the tibial tuberosity is a reliable landmark [24, 35–37]. However, there is some concern

that employing the tibial tuberosity as a landmark results in malrotation of the tibial component. As for the medial one-third of the tibial tuberosity, Dalury et al. [19] reported that the tibial tray should be rotated externally to the medial one-third of the tibial tuberosity to maximize function. In addition, Eckhoff et al. [20] demonstrated that an average of 19° of external rotation of the tibial component relative to the femoral component occurred when the medial one-third of the tibial tuberosity was used as a reference for tibial rotational alignment. As for the medial border of the tibial tuberosity, Huddleston et al. [21] evaluated a neutral point on the rotating tibial insert and reported that this point was approximately 5° external to the medial border of the tibial tuberosity. In this study, the mean angles of these landmarks varied greatly compared with the others, indicating that isolated use of this landmark could result in tibial malrotation.

The PCL-PT axis also has been suggested as a reliable reference line for tibial rotational alignment [19]. This landmark was initially proposed by Akagi et al. [18], who reported that the mean angle between this line and a line perpendicular to the clinical epicondylar axis of the femur in normal knees was 0°, ranging from 6.3° of internal rotation to 5.2° of external rotation. Sahin et al. [31] also reported that Akagi's line was the least affected by interobserver inconsistency, and, therefore, provided the best guidance for determining tibial rotational alignment. Our result using the PCL-PT axis as a landmark in OA knees (−1.2° ± 4.7°) is similar to reported findings [18, 24, 31, 38]; however, the SD was greater, indicating more variability than the angle of the ATCC axis (0.8° ± 2.7°).

In our study, we found that the ATCC axis had a narrow SD with the least variability. The mean angle of the ATCC axis (0.8° ± 2.7°) was larger than that of the PCL-TT1 axis (0.3° ± 5.5°), but the difference was not significant. Additionally, use of the ATCC as a landmark has several advantages over the other axes. First, a single area is more readily identifiable than a single point or line. The ATCC can be palpated after tibial cutting during TKA, and, thus, proper positioning of the tibial component can be achieved intraoperatively. Unfortunately, many sagittal axes are not easily identifiable during surgery. Second, if preoperative CT images are obtained to improve positioning of the tibial component, the ATCC can offer a simple and accurate method to predict tibial rotational alignment after TKA by applying the tibial prosthesis template on the CT image at the desired osteotomy level. Therefore, we believe that the ATCC is a reliable and useful anatomical landmark for tibial rotational alignment.

There are several limitations to our study. First, this study only addressed tibiofemoral conformity with the knee in extension, and not through the arc of flexion, during which the degree of matching may change. However, in their biplanar image-matching study, Asano et al. [14] reported that the flexion-extension axis of the knee corresponded to an sTEA of 0° to 90°. Because the present study compared the usefulness of five axes with reference to the sTEA, we believe that tibiofemoral conformity in flexion would be better with use of the ATCC axis because this axis has less deviation from the sTEA. Second, with the advent of mobile bearings systems and customized devices, the importance of landmarks for rotation alignment of tibia may decreased. However, even with mobile bearing systems, obtaining accurate tibial component rotation remains of key importance because substantial malrotations may not be entirely corrected using mobile bearing systems. Thus, it is more feasible to obtain tibial component rotation as precise as possible, and correct some minor errors by mobile bearing systems. Customization has certain disadvantages such as increased inconvenience and economic cost. Therefore, rather than implementing customization in routine clinical practice, we believe that it is better to use customized devices only when severe deformity exists. The ATCC-based method for determining tibial rotational alignment is simple and accurate, because the ATCC can be palpated after tibial cutting and, thus, proper positioning of the tibial component can be achieved easily even without customized devices.

Finally, the number of normal knees was small compared with the number of OA knees, and the patients' characteristics such as age and mechanical tibiofemoral angle were not matched between the groups. However, OA is more prevalent at older ages, while normal knees are rarer; therefore, it is difficult to match the age. In addition, although the mechanical tibiofemoral angles were not matched between groups, it should be noted that, in each group, the angles of five axes were compared under the same mechanical tibiofemoral angle. Therefore, we believe that ATCC is the most accurate landmark for determining the rotational alignment of the tibia in both normal and mild-to-moderate varus alignment.

Conclusion

In this study, we compared the usefulness of five anatomical landmarks on the proximal tibia for determining tibial rotational alignment in TKA. Compared to the observations in normal knees, these AP axes showed greater internal rotation relative to sTEA in OA knees. The ATCC was found to be the most reliable and useful anatomical landmark for determining tibial rotational alignment in TKA.

Abbreviations
AP: Anteroposterior; ATCC: Anterior tibial curved cortex; CT: Computed tomography; OA: Osteoarthritic; PCL: Posterior cruciate ligament; PT: Patellar tendon; SD: Standard deviation; sTEA: Surgical transepicondylar axis; TKA: Total knee arthroplasty; TT: Tibial tuberosity

Acknowledgement
The authors thank Medical Research Collaborating Center of Seoul National University Hospital for support in the statistical analysis.

Funding
There was no external funding for this study.

Authors' contributions
JLK collected the data, performed the measurement and analysis, participated in the study design and drafted the manuscript. HSH and SL participated in the study design, supervised the analysis and helped to draft the manuscript. JJ collected the data, performed the measurement. KWL helped to draft the manuscript and review the manuscript. MCL designed the study, supervised the whole study process and helped to draft and review the manuscript. All authors read and approved the final manuscript.

Competing interests
The authors declared that they have no competing interests.

Consent for publication
Not applicable.

Author details
[1]Department of Orthopaedic Surgery, Hallym University Kangnam Sacred Heart Hospital, 1, Singil-ro, Yeongdeungpo-gu, Seoul 150-950, Korea. [2]Department of Orthopaedic Surgery, Seoul National University Hospital, 101 Daehak-ro, Jongno-gu, Seoul 110-744, Korea.

References
1. Insall JN, Kelly M. The total condylar prosthesis. Clin Orthop Relat Res. 1986; 205:43–8.
2. Barrack RL, Schrader T, Bertot AJ, Wolfe MW, Myers L. Component rotation and anterior knee pain after total knee arthroplasty. Clin Orthop Relat Res. 2001;392:46–55.

3. Mulhall KJ, Ghomrawi HM, Scully S, Callaghan JJ, Saleh KJ. Current etiologies and modes of failure in total knee arthroplasty revision. Clin Orthop Relat Res. 2006;446:45–50.
4. Ritter MA, Lutgring JD, Davis KE, Berend ME. The effect of postoperative range of motion on functional activities after posterior cruciate-retaining total knee arthroplasty. J Bone Joint Surg Am. 2008;90(4):777–84.
5. Akagi M, Matsusue Y, Mata T, Asada Y, Horiguchi M, Iida H, et al. Effect of rotational alignment on patellar tracking in total knee arthroplasty. Clin Orthop Relat Res. 1999;366:155–63.
6. Nagamine R, Whiteside LA, White SE, McCarthy DS. Patellar tracking after total knee arthroplasty. The effect of tibial tray malrotation and articular surface configuration. Clin Orthop Relat Res. 1994;304:262–71.
7. van Gennip S, Schimmel JJ, van Hellemondt GG, Defoort KC, Wymenga AB. Medial patellofemoral ligament reconstruction for patellar maltracking following total knee arthroplasty is effective. Knee Surg Sports Traumatol Arthrosc. 2014;22(10):2569–73.
8. Anouchi YS, Whiteside LA, Kaiser AD, Milliano MT. The effects of axial rotational alignment of the femoral component on knee stability and patellar tracking in total knee arthroplasty demonstrated on autopsy specimens. Clin Orthop Relat Res. 1993;287:170–7.
9. Romero J, Duronio JF, Sohrabi A, Alexander N, MacWilliams BA, Jones LC, et al. Varus and valgus flexion laxity of total knee alignment methods in loaded cadaveric knees. Clin Orthop Relat Res. 2002;394:243–53.
10. Van Damme G, Defoort K, Ducoulombier Y, Van Glabbeek F, Bellemans J, Victor J. What should the surgeon aim for when performing computer-assisted total knee arthroplasty? J Bone Joint Surg Am. 2005;87(Suppl 2):52–8.
11. Hofmann S, Romero J, Roth-Schiffl E. Albrecht T. [Rotational malalignment of the components may cause chronic pain or early failure in total knee arthroplasty]. Orthopade. 2003;32(6):469–76.
12. Lewis P, Rorabeck CH, Bourne RB, Devane P. Posteromedial tibial polyethylene failure in total knee replacements. Clin Orthop Relat Res. 1994; 299:11–7.
13. Wasielewski RC, Galante JO, Leighty RM, Natarajan RN, Rosenberg AG. Wear patterns on retrieved polyethylene tibial inserts and their relationship to technical considerations during total knee arthroplasty. Clin Orthop Relat Res. 1994;299:31–43.
14. Asano T, Akagi M, Nakamura T. The functional flexion-extension axis of the knee corresponds to the surgical epicondylar axis: in vivo analysis using a biplanar image-matching technique. J Arthroplast. 2005;20(8):1060–7.
15. Churchill DL, Incavo SJ, Johnson CC, Beynnon BD. The transepicondylar axis approximates the optimal flexion axis of the knee. Clin Orthop Relat Res. 1998;356:111–8.
16. Miller MC, Berger RA, Petrella AJ, Karmas A, Rubash HE. Optimizing femoral component rotation in total knee arthroplasty. Clin Orthop Relat Res. 2001; 392:38–45.
17. Baldini A, Indelli PF, DEL L, Mariani PC, Marcucci M. Rotational alignment of the tibial component in total knee arthroplasty: the anterior tibial cortex is a reliable landmark. Joints. 2013;1(4):155–60.
18. Akagi M, Oh M, Nonaka T, Tsujimoto H, Asano T, Hamanishi C. An anteroposterior axis of the tibia for total knee arthroplasty. Clin Orthop Relat Res. 2004;420:213–9.
19. Dalury DF. Observations of the proximal tibia in total knee arthroplasty. Clin Orthop Relat Res. 2001;389:150–5.
20. Eckhoff DG, Metzger RG, Vandewalle MV. Malrotation associated with implant alignment technique in total knee arthroplasty. Clin Orthop Relat Res. 1995;321:28–31.
21. Huddleston JI, Scott RD, Wimberley DW. Determination of neutral tibial rotational alignment in rotating platform TKA. Clin Orthop Relat Res. 2005; 440:101–6.
22. Siston RA, Goodman SB, Patel JJ, Delp SL, Giori NJ. The high variability of tibial rotational alignment in total knee arthroplasty. Clin Orthop Relat Res. 2006;452:65–9.
23. Ikeuchi M, Yamanaka N, Okanoue Y, Ueta E, Tani T. Determining the rotational alignment of the tibial component at total knee replacement: a comparison of two techniques. J Bone Joint Surg Br. 2007;89(1):45–9.
24. Incavo SJ, Coughlin KM, Pappas C, Beynnon BD. Anatomic rotational relationships of the proximal tibia, distal femur, and patella: implications for rotational alignment in total knee arthroplasty. J Arthroplast. 2003;18(5):643–8.
25. Sahin N, Atici T, Kurtoglu U, Turgut A, Ozkaya G, Ozkan Y. Centre of the posterior cruciate ligament and the sulcus between tubercle spines are

reliable landmarks for tibial component placement. Knee Surg Sports Traumatol Arthrosc 2012.
26. Sun T, Lu H, Hong N, Wu J, Feng C. Bony landmarks and rotational alignment in total knee arthroplasty for Chinese osteoarthritic knees with varus or valgus deformities. J Arthroplast. 2009;24(3):427–31.
27. Berger RA, Crossett LS, Jacobs JJ, Rubash HE. Malrotation causing patellofemoral complications after total knee arthroplasty. Clin Orthop Relat Res. 1998;356:144–53.
28. Akagi M, Mori S, Nishimura S, Nishimura A, Asano T, Hamanishi C. Variability of Extraarticular Tibial Rotation References for Total Knee Arthroplasty. Clinical Orthopaedics and Related Research 2005;436:172–176.
29. Kim D, Seong SC, Lee MC, Lee S. Comparison of the tibiofemoral rotational alignment after mobile and fixed bearing total knee arthroplasty. Knee Surg Sports Traumatol Arthrosc. 2012;20(2):337–45.
30. Matsui Y, Kadoya Y, Uehara K, Kobayashi A, Takaoka K. Rotational deformity in varus osteoarthritis of the knee: analysis with computed tomography. Clin Orthop Relat Res. 2005;433:147–51.
31. Sahin N, Atici T, Ozturk A, Ozkaya G, Ozkan Y, Avcu B. Accuracy of anatomical references used for rotational alignment of tibial component in total knee arthroplasty. Knee Surg Sports Traumatol Arthrosc. 2012;20(3):565–70.
32. Khan MS, Seon JK, Song EK. Rotational profile of lower limb and axis for tibial component alignment in varus osteoarthritic knees. J Arthroplast. 2012;27(5):797–802.
33. Su EP, Su SL, Della Valle AG. Stiffness after TKR: how to avoid repeat surgery. Orthopedics. 2010;33(9):658.
34. Thompson JA, Hast MW, Granger JF, Piazza SJ, Siston RA. Biomechanical effects of total knee arthroplasty component malrotation: a computational simulation. J Orthop Res. 2011;29(7):969–75.
35. Coughlin KM, Incavo SJ, Churchill DL, Beynnon BD. Tibial axis and patellar position relative to the femoral epicondylar axis during squatting. J Arthroplast. 2003;18(8):1048–55.
36. Graw BP, Harris AH, Tripuraneni KR, Giori NJ. Rotational references for total knee arthroplasty tibial components change with level of resection. Clin Orthop Relat Res. 2010;468(10):2734–8.
37. Uehara K, Kadoya Y, Kobayashi A, Ohashi H, Yamano Y. Bone anatomy and rotational alignment in total knee arthroplasty. Clin Orthop Relat Res. 2002; 402:196–201.
38. Aglietti P, Sensi L, Cuomo P, Ciardullo A. Rotational position of femoral and tibial components in TKA using the femoral transepicondylar axis. Clin Orthop Relat Res. 2008;466(11):2751–5.

5

Comparison of fixed and mobile-bearing total knee arthroplasty in terms of patellofemoral pain and function

P. Z. Feczko[1]* ⓘ, L. M. Jutten[1], M. J. van Steyn[2], P. Deckers[3], P. J. Emans[1] and J. J. Arts[1]

Abstract

Background: Despite growing evidence in the literature, there is still a lack of consensus regarding the use of the mobile-bearing (MB) design total knee arthroplasty (TKA).

Methods: In a prospective, comparative, randomised, single centre trial, 106 patients with end-stage osteoarthritis of the knee were randomised to either an MB or fixed-bearing (FB) group to receive posterior stabilised (PS)-TKA using a standard medial parapatellar approach and patellar resurfacing with follow-up (FU) for 5 years. The primary outcome was anterior knee pain (AKP) during the chair rise test and the stair climb test 5 years after surgery. The secondary outcome was the ability to rise from a chair and to climb stairs, range of motion (ROM), Knee Society Score (KSS), RAND-36 scores and radiological analysis of the patellar tilt.

Results: No statistically significant difference was found between the two groups at 5 years FU in terms of median AKP during the chair rise test and the stair climb test ($p = 0.5$ and $p = 0.8$, respectively). There was no significant difference in any of the other secondary outcome parameters between the groups at 5 years FU.

Conclusion: A mobile-bearing TKA does not decrease AKP compared to fixed bearings.

Level of evidence: II

Keywords: Total knee arthroplasty, Anterior knee pain, Mobile bearing, Fixed bearing

Background

Total knee arthroplasty (TKA) is a successful surgical treatment for osteoarthritis of the knee [1–3]. This intervention results in excellent long-term survivorship [4–7] and marked improvement in functional capacity and quality of life for the patients [8]. However anterior knee pain (AKP) is present in 4 to 40% of all cases [9–11] independently of patellar resurfacing, restricting the patients in climbing stairs, rising from a chair, cycling, or, in worst case scenarios, walking normally. The causes of AKP are multifactorial and can be divided into non-modifiable and

modifiable factors [12, 13]. Non-modifiable factors are young age, female gender, ethnicity and low pain threshold [14–17]. Modifiable factors can be patient related, like anxiety, depression, pain processing problems [18, 19], muscle imbalance and dynamic valgus during gate [12]. A wide range of non-patient related, modifiable factors are published in the literature to explain and treat AKP after TKA [12–17]. Van Jonbergen [20] found inflammatory changes in the Hoffa and local peripatellar synovitis. Van Jonbergen and coworkers reported a positive effect on AKP by resection of the Hoffa and peripatellar synovectomy. Patellar clunk syndrome [21–23] and the degree of wear of the patellar cartilage [24] were also linked with AKP. There is also growing evidence that prosthetic design features such as the morphology of the anterior flange of the femoral component, gender femoral component, single or

* Correspondence: p.feczko@mumc.nl
[1]Department of Orthopaedic Surgery, CAPHRI Research School, Maastricht University Medical Centre, P. Debyelaan 25, 6229 HX Maastricht, the Netherlands
Full list of author information is available at the end of the article

multi radius design, and post-cam mechanism can have an influence on AKP [14, 15, 25–29]. The literature mostly reports on surgery-related factors after TKA. The application of circumpatellar electrocautery does not lessen the incidence of AKP [30, 31]. Resurfacing the patella also remains controversial [32–34]. According to Heergaard [35] TKA leads in nearly all cases to different patellar tracking and increased patellofemoral contact pressures. In contrast to the healthy knee in which conformity between the articular surfaces is optimal, the patellofemoral contact zones are significantly reduced after TKA [35]. Restoration of the standard patellar thickness and central positioning of the patella may minimise the contact forces [36, 37]. There is good experimental and clinical evidence that poor femoral or tibial rotational alignment can adversely affect patellar tracking and kinematics [35, 38–40]. The question is how to achieve optimal tibio-femoral and patellofemoral kinematics.

The mobile-bearing (MB) design TKA was introduced in the United States in 1980 first with the meniscal bearing concept, followed by the rotating platform design. The MB-TKA was developed to reduce polyethylene contact stresses and wear resulting in a lower rate of aseptic loosening. The other design goal was to create a self-aligning nature for the implants to provide an improved, more natural prosthetic knee joint and alignment with better functional results [41–46]. The MB design TKA was theoretically a revolutionary and attractive concept, however the clinical benefit is still controversial. Most meta-analyses could not show any benefit for the use of the MB-TKA [42, 47–50] in terms of clinical scores, loosening, ROM, pain, complications, quality of life, patient satisfaction and revision rate. There is no data in the meta-analyses for MB- versus fixed-bearing (FB) TKA in terms of AKP. Theoretically the MB design offers the potential advantage of self-correction of a rotational mismatch between the tibia and femur providing an optimization of patellofemoral mechanics and a potential reduction in AKP [51, 52] Most studies examine the kinematics of the patellofemoral joint in MB-TKA. Stiehl et al. [53] suggested that the MB design may reduce the patellofemoral maltracking resulting from the femoral component malposition conditions. Colwell [54] stated that the MB design can compensate for the malrotation of the femoral component on a limited basis. Sawaguchi [55] found in an intraoperative study where the medial shift and lateral tilt of the patella were significantly smaller in MB-TKA compared with FB-TKA. Lower patellofemoral contact stresses were found in MB-TKA compared with FB-TKA, however both designs had increased contact stress compared with native knees [56]. The New-Zealand Joint Registry study found a higher rate of revision for secondary resurfacing of the patella in the FB-TKA group [57].

The aim of the study was to collect more clinical data for AKP in MB- vs. FB-TKA patients. A prospective, comparative, randomised, single centre, trial including 106 patients was performed to compare mobile-bearing (MB) and fixed-bearing (FB) posterior stabilised (PS) TKA with patella resurfacing at 5 years follow-up (FU).

The primary outcome was anterior knee pain during the chair rise test and the stair climb test 5 years after surgery. The secondary outcome was the ability to rise from a chair and to climb stairs, range of motion (ROM), Knee Society Score (KSS), RAND-36 scores and radiological analysis of the patellar tilt 5 years after surgery.

The null hypothesis was that patients in the MB-TKA group do not exhibit less AKP during rising from a chair or climbing stairs.

The alternative hypothesis (H1) was that patients in the MB-TKA group do exhibit less AKP during rising from a chair or climbing stairs.

Method
Trial design
A prospective, comparative, randomised, single centre trial that included 106 patients was performed to compare MB and FB PS-TKA with patella resurfacing at 5 years follow-up (FU). Patients with end-stage osteoarthritis of the knee were randomised to either an MB or FB group to receive PS-TKA using a standard medial parapatellar approach.

Ethics, participant selection and consent
Ethical approval was obtained from the local ethical committee of Maastricht (METC 08–055), as part of the research program, "Should my knee rotate? A randomised controlled trial to compare fixed and mobile-bearing total knee arthroplasty using the Scorpio PS SuperFlex and Scorpio + PS Mobile Bearing knee systems". Patients were randomised (random permuted blocks of changing size) in either the MB or the FB group. The randomization process was computer generated using SPSS software. The randomization scheme ensured that during the enrolment period the ratio of the number of cases in the two groups remained constant. A written informed consent was obtained from all participants. All data was collected at the Department of Orthopaedics of Maastricht University Medical Centre. All patients and the researcher, who collected the data, was blinded. The surgeons were not blinded (see also author's contribution).

Trial Registration Number: ClinicalTrials.gov NCT02892838 Retrospectively registered (2 Sep 2016).

Inclusion and exclusion criteria
Inclusion criteria included patients between 21 and 80 years of age who had an established diagnosis of knee osteoarthritis or post-traumatic arthritis requiring primary

total knee replacement. Exclusion criteria included medio-lateral instability greater than 10 degrees, active inflammation or infection of the knee, and patients with diagnosed systemic disease (such as bone diseases, immunologically suppressed conditions, neuromuscular deficits, Complex Regional Pain Syndrome (CRPS) that would have affected the overall outcome of the study. In addition, patients were excluded if they we unable to receive a patella component (e.g., old patella fracture, too thin patella, etc.).

Interventions (operative procedure)

The aim of the operation was to achieve neutral coronal limb alignment ±2° and a stable knee defined as having a maximum of 0–3 mm laxity of the collateral ligaments [58].

All knee surgeries were performed by two surgeons. A medial parapatellar approach was applied in all cases using a tourniquet. The rotational position of the femoral component was determined by using the *Whiteside's line* and the transepicondylar line (TEA) [59, 60]. The rotational position of the tibial tray was determined by using the medial one third of the tibial tubercle [61, 62]. The tibial slope was corrected to 0 degrees. With both techniques, after determining proper prosthetic size, the collateral ligaments were balanced as required based on ligament tension assessed during functional testing of the prosthetic implant [63]. Patients younger than 70 years of age received cementless femoral and tibial components, while patients older than 70 years of age received cemented implants using Simplex-P (Stryker Howmedica Osteonics, Allendale, NJ USA) containing antibiotics. Cemented patellar surface implantation was performed in every case. In each case, a Scorpio (Stryker Howmedica Osteonics, Allendale, NJ USA) PS implant was used with fixed- or mobile-bearing inserts.

Outcome measurements

Clinical outcomes were assessed by a blinded independent examiner. All clinical outcome parameters were assessed preoperatively and postoperatively at 6 weeks, 3 and 6 months, 1, 2 and 5 years.

The primary outcome was AKP during the chair raise test and the stair climb test measured on a visual analogue scale (VAS) [64, 65] 5 years after surgery. The secondary outcome was the ability to rise from a chair and to climb stairs, range of motion (ROM), Knee Society Score (KSS), RAND-36 scores and radiological analysis of the patellar tilt 5 years after surgery.

The chair rise test was assessed according to the Jones' description [66]. The initial sitting position during the chair rise test was standardised. The patients were sitting on an adjustable chair with the hip and knee in 90° of flexion. The patients had to stand up from the chair without using their arms. The test was repeated five times and patients were asked to report pain and location of the pain. It was noted whether the patients were able to rise (yes or no) and the VAS was used to measure AKP.

In order to standardise the movement during stair climbing, the same stairs were used by each individual patient. The patients had to walk up and down 10 steps with alternating legs without using the handrail. It was noted whether the patients were able to rise (yes or no) and VAS was used to measure AKP. ROM was measured during physical examination using a goniometer according to the technique described by Norkin [67]. Intra-tester and inter-tester reliability was described by Brosseau [68], the reproducibility by Lenssen [69]. Knee Society Scores [70] and RAND-36 scores [71, 72] were also measured.

Radiological evaluations

Standard plain radiographs with Merchant 30/60/90° views were performed preoperatively and postoperatively at 6 weeks, 3 and 6 months, 1, 2 and 5 years. The position of the patella was measured from the Merchant view producing an angle between a line through the most prominent parts of the femur and a line through the backside of the patellar component (cement–component interface) [73]. Mean and median values were used for further analyses.

Statistics and sample size analysis

Descriptive statistics were used to summarise the data. Differences between 'fixed' and 'mobile' at 5 years were tested using Mann–Whitney U tests for continuous variables as normal distribution could not be assumed and chi-squared tests or Fisher's Exact tests for categorical variables. Statistical analyses were performed using R version 3.3.1 (R Foundation, Vienna, Austria). P-values <0.05 were considered statistically significant.

A sample size estimation showed that 37 knees per group would be required to detect a clinically relevant difference of 1 point with a standard deviation of 1.5 points in the anterior knee pain VAS score, with an alpha of 0.05 and a power of 80%.

Results

Flowchart

One hundred six participants were included for the study. Due to administrative protocol deviations, three patients from both groups were immediately excluded. Three additional patients of the MB group received wrong implant. Forty-seven patients in the MB and 50 patients in the FB group were available for the baseline data. Forty-two patients in the MB group and 48 patients in the FB group were available for the 5-year follow-up (Fig. 1).

C O N S O R T
TRANSPARENT REPORTING of TRIALS

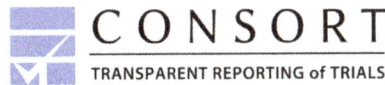

CONSORT 2010 Flow Diagram

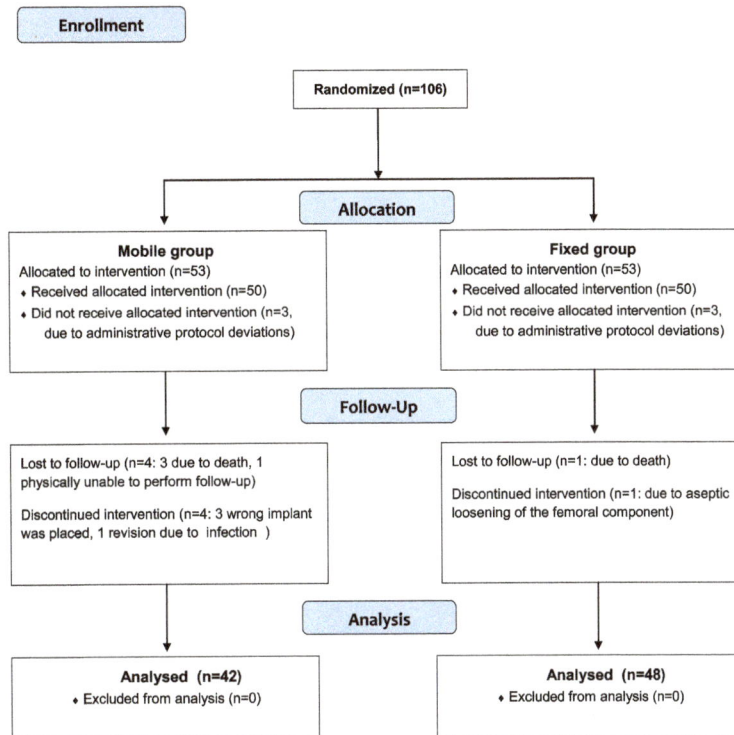

Fig. 1 Flow-chart of participants. One hundred six participants were included for the study. Due to administrative protocol deviations, three patients from both groups were immediately excluded. Three additional patients of the MB group received wrong implant. Forty-seven patients in the MB and 50 patients in the FB group were available for the baseline data. Forty-two patients in the MB group and 48 patients in the FB group were available for the 5-year follow-up

Demographics
There was no significant difference between the two surgical groups with respect to gender, age, BMI, side of operation or primary and secondary outcome measurements (Table 1).

Primary outcomes
At 5 years follow-up, median AKP scores during chair rise and during stair climb in the 'fixed' group were 0 (range 0–7) and 0 (range 0–8), respectively. In the 'mobile' group median pain scores during chair rise and stair climb were both zero (range 0–7). No statistically significant difference in anterior knee pain during chair rise ($p = 0.5$) and anterior knee pain during stair climb ($p = 0.8$) between the two surgical groups was found (Table 2). There was no significant difference between groups in terms of percentage of participants having AKP during chair rise (FB group 22% vs. MB group 14.9%, $p = 0.3$) or during stair climb (16% vs. 17%, respectively, $p = 0.9$).

Secondary outcomes
The ability to climb stairs and to rise from a chair, ROM, KSS scores, RAND-36 scores and patellar tilt were not statistically different between the two surgical groups (Table 2).

There was no statistically significant difference between the FB and MB groups in terms of ability to rise from a chair ($p = 0.6$, 97.9% vs. 95.2%, respectively) or ability to climb stairs ($p = 0.6$ 97.9% vs. 97.9%, respectively).

There was no statistically significant difference between the FB and MB groups in terms of median ROM ($p = 0.9$, 110° (70–130) vs. 110° (85–130), respectively).

There was no statistically significant difference between the FB and MB groups in terms of total KSS and RAND-36 (Table 2).

There was no statistically significant difference between the FB and MB groups in terms of patellar tilt at 30°, 60°, 90° degrees of flexion ($p = 0.4$, 2.56 ± 3.62 vs. 1.98 ± 3.58, $p = 0.6$, 1.96 ± 3.15 vs. 1.80 ± 3.82, $p = 0.4$, 1.81 ± 3.25 vs. 1.40 ± 3.42, respectively).

Table 1 Baseline characteristics and pre-operative values of outcomes

	Fixed (n = 50)	Mobile (n = 47)
BMI (kg/m^2)	30.1 (±4.5)	28.7 (±4.2)
Side (L/R)	22/28	25/22
AKP during chair rise (VAS 0–10 median)	5 (0–10)	4 (0–8)
AKP during chair rise (yes/no %)	80/20	85.1/14.9
AKP during stair climb (VAS 0–10 median)	5.5 (0–10)	5 (0–9)
AKP during stair climb (yes/no %)	90/10	83/17
Ability to rise from a chair (able/unable %)	72/28	82.9/17.1
Ability to climb stairs (able/unable%)	97.9/2.1	95.3/4.7
Range of motion (ROM) (degrees)		
Flexion	110 (85–140)	110 (75–140)
Extension	−5 (−20–5)	−5 (−35–5)
Total	105 (70–140)	110 (65–140)
KSS		
Pain	48 (11–92)	49 (11–83)
Function	55 (0–80)	60 (0–90)
Total	101 (31–157)	106 (25–151)
RAND-36		
Physical functioning	30 (5–75)	35 (5–90)
Social role functioning	62 (0–100)	62 (0–100)
Physical role functioning	0 (0–100)	0 (0–100)
Emotional role functioning	33 (0 100)	50 (0 100)
Mental health	60 (4–100)	70 (8–96)
Vitality	50 (15–95)	55 (0–90)
Bodily pain	40 (0–80)	40 (0–80)
General health perceptions	60 (15–95)	62.5 (20–100)
General health change	50 (0–75)	50 (0–100)
Patellar tilt median (degrees)		
30 degrees flexion	2 (0–25)	2 (−1–13)
60 degrees flexion	2 (0–13)	2 (0–11)
90 degrees flexion	1 (0–11)	2 (0–10)
Patella tilt mean (degrees + SD)		
30 degrees of flexion	2.70 ± 4.06	3.0 ± 3.39
60 degrees of flexion	2.26 ± 2.72	2.72 ± 2.73
90 degrees of flexion	1.58 ± 2.17	2.29 ± 2.51

Table 2 Primary and secondary outcomes

	Fixed (n = 48)	Mobile (n = 42)	p-value
Primary outcomes			
AKP during chair rise median (VAS 0–10)	0 (0–7)	0 (0–7)	0.5
AKP during chair rise (yes/no %)	22/78	14.9/85.1	0.3
AKP during stair climb median (VAS 0–10)	0 (0–8)	0 (0–7)	0.8
AKP during stair climb (yes/no %)	16/84	17/83	0.9
Secondary outcomes			
Ability to rise from chair (able/unable %)	97.9/2.1	95.2/4.8	0.6*
Ability to climb stairs (able/unable%)	97.9/2.1	97.9/4.8	0.6*
Range of motion (ROM) (degrees)			
Flexion	110 (80–130)	110 (85–130)	0.9
Extension	0 (−10–5)	−0 (−10–5)	0.7
Total	110 (70–130)	110 (85–130)	0.9
KSS			
Pain	94.0 (62–100)	95 (61–100)	0.8
Function	80 (30–100)	87.5 (5–100)	0.8
Total	174.5 (102–200)	178.5 (95–200)	0.8
RAND-36			
Physical functioning	55 (5 100)	55 (0 100)	0.6
Social role functioning	75 (25–100)	75 (0–100)	0.7
Physical role functioning	25 (0–100)	25 (0–100)	0.7
Emotional role functioning	100 (0–100)	67 (0–100)	0.3
Mental health	68 (4–100)	72 (20–100)	0.5
Vitality	60 (0–100)	65 (15–90)	0.9
Bodily pain	67 (12–100)	67 (0–100)	0.7
General health perceptions	65 (10–95)	55 (10–95)	0.6
General health change	50 (25–75)	50 (0–100)	0.6
Patellar tilt median (degrees)			
30 degrees flexion	1 (0–15)	0.5 (0–17)	0.4
60 degrees flexion	0 (0–15)	0 (0–20)	0.6
90 degrees flexion	0 (0–16)	0 (0–20)	0.4
Patellar tilt mean (degrees + SD)			
30 degrees flexion	2.56 ± 3.62	1.98 ± 3.58	
60 degrees flexion	1.96 ± 3.15	1.80 ± 3.82	
90 degrees flexion	1.81 ± 3.25	1.40 ± 3.42	

*Fisher's Exact test

Discussion

Compared to the FB-TKA patients, patients in the MB-TKA group did not benefit from less anterior knee pain during rising from a chair or climbing stairs at 5 years follow-up in this study. This outcome is in line with the finding of previous meta-analyses, however AKP was not mentioned specifically. Only two meta-analyses [50, 74] reported lower pain scores in the MB group, but the quality of evidence was moderate to low [50, 74].

Price [75] and Breugem [76] reported lower pain scores in the MB group in the short term, but the same outcome was not confirmed in the long term [76, 77] nor did it differentiate AKP from general knee pain. The study by Biau [78] also showed a lower AKP in the MB group, however the difference was not statistically significant. This study showed 22% and 16% of patients had AKP during chair rise and stair climb in the FB group, meanwhile the AKP was 14.9% and 17% in the MB group during the same activities. Popovic [9] reported a much higher rate of AKP (49.2%) in posterior stabilised MB-TKA. The outcome was explained with the suboptimal trochlear design of the type of prosthesis. Wyatt et al. [57] reported a significantly higher rate of revision for secondary resurfacing of the patella in FB-PS-TKA designs compared with MB-TKA, which is not in line with the result of this study, however Wyatt reported a retrospective study.

AKP is known to cause the most problems in daily activities such as rising from a chair, or climbing stairs. Theoretically a larger percentage of patients who received MB-TKA would be able to rise from a chair and climb stairs compared with patients from the FB-TKA group, and while less patellar compression pain was expected in the MB group, it could not be confirmed. Little evidence can be found in the literature in terms of the ability to rise from a chair or climb stairs. Pais-Brito [79] found no differences between the MB- and FB-TKA groups in the ability to ascend and descend stairs. Woolson [80] stated that more patients in the MB group required aid to climb stairs compared with patients in the FB group, however this finding was statistically not significant. The meta-analysis by Smith [81] found no significant difference between groups based on nine studies.

Theoretically the MB design could lead to better ROM during daily activities [82]. We observed no difference in ROM between patients in either group. Most meta-analyses [42, 47, 48, 50, 81] also reported no significant differences between groups. Carothers [83] found no difference in ROM between groups, but the MB groups were significantly better in increase of ROM compared with the pre-operative function. Aglietti [84] found better ROM in the MB group while Haas [82] reported better ROM in the FB group. Kim [85] found minimally better ROM in the MB group although the difference was not statistically significant. The variation in design of the MB produced differences in ROM between the MB- and FB-TKA [49]. Since several MB designs are available (pure rotation, pure translation, combined rotation-translation and meniscal bearing) the results of meta-analyses can be influenced. A MB insert stops moving at flexion deeper than 90° and after this point the MB prostheses performs essentially as a fixed-bearing implant [49]. The question is how mobile is the bearing in MB prosthesis design during the stance phase of stair climbing and during rising from a chair if the flexion of the knee is less than 90°? The mobile-bearing insert can act as a fixed-bearing, but it is not proven. Studies utilising fluoroscopic techniques have demonstrated that knee joint kinematics are highly unpredictable in MB prostheses [86]. If mobile bearing insert act as a fixed bearing it could be an explanation why no differences were found between the two type of prostheses.

Stryker Scorpio PS MB and FB design was used in this study. The femoral components are the same in both prostheses with slightly different inserts. Both knees have single radius design and according to the manufacturer the Scorpio PS has great internal and external rotational freedom throughout the full range of motion. The design is not conforming between femoral component and tibial insert and as far as the authors know, there is no difference in conformity between the MB and FB design.

Most studies and meta-analyses [42, 47–50, 81, 83, 87, 88] reported no significant differences in clinical scores (KSS, HSS, WOMAC, OKS) between the MB and FB design TKA. Only two studies found significant differences in KSS is favour of the MB design TKA. The meta-analysis by van der Voort [49] reported significantly better physical SF-12 scores. The RAND-36 in our study was not different between groups.

No significant differences between the MB- and FB-TKAs were found in terms of mean and median patellar tilt in this study, which corresponds to Heinert's results in a cadaveric study [89]. The rate of lateral releases was reported by Ferguson [90]. Lateral release was performed when tilting or subluxation was observed using the "no thumb" technique. The rate of releases was equal between the MB and FB groups. In contrast significantly smaller intra-operative lateral tilts of the patella were reported by Sawaguchi [55]. The average maximum contact stress of the patella was also significantly smaller. Skwara et al. [56] performed in vitro measurements of the patella. The MB design TKA showed evidently lower patellofemoral contact stresses than the FB design. Recent meta-analyses [42, 81, 88] reported no significant differences in lateral tilt of the patella between the MB and FB design TKA.

Conclusion
No statistically significant difference was found between the FB and MB design PS-TKA in terms of patellofemoral pain and function at 5 years follow-up in this study.

Limitation of the study
There are a few limitations to the study. There was no postoperative analysis on CT scan for the rotational position of the femoral component since it has a great influence on the patellar tilt. The authors also see a ceiling effect in the scoring lists and the question is whether they are sensitive enough to arrive at conclusions.

Abbreviations
AKP: Anterior knee pain; CRPS: Complex regional pain syndrome; CT: Computer tomography; FB: Fixed-bearing; FU: Follow-up; KSS: Knee society score; MB: Mobile-bearing; PS: Posterior stabilized; RAND-36: Research

and development survey; ROM: Range of motion; SPSS (software): Statistical package for the social sciences; TEA: Transepicondylar line; TKA: total knee arthroplasty; VAS: Visual analogue scale; WOMAC: Western Ontario and McMaster Universities Arthritis Index

Acknowledgements

Not applicable.

Funding

All costs of the study which takes part of the Dutch standard medical care (admission, operation, standard follow-up, implant) was covered by the insurance of the participants. All costs of this study which does not belong to the Dutch standard medical care was financially supported by Stryker Corporation. Three hundred fifty euro per patient was paid for not standard, study related follow-up (3 months, 2 years, 5 years) and radiological examinations (5 times patella series). Three hundred thirty euro per patient was paid database management, administrative support, registration costs and statistical analyses. The study was initiated through the surgeons. During the period of the study Stryker was the supplier of hip and knee implants. All study data belong to Maasticht University Medical Centre. The statistics and the article was made without the influence of the sponsor.

Authors' contribution

FPZ collected data, wrote and submitted the paper. JLM participated in the design of the study and coordinated the study. vSMJ initiated the study, participated in the design of the study and performed the operations. DP participated in the design of the study, performed the operations and revised the manuscript. EPJ helped in the interpretation of the data and revised the manuscript. AJJ initiated the study, participated in the design of the study. All authors read and approved the final manuscript.

Consent for publication

Not applicable: the manuscript does not contain any form of person's data.

Competing interests

All authors declare that they have no competing interests.

Author details

[1]Department of Orthopaedic Surgery, CAPHRI Research School, Maastricht University Medical Centre, P. Debyelaan 25, 6229 HX Maastricht, the Netherlands. [2]Reynaert Private Hospital, Maastricht, the Netherlands. [3]Department of Orthopaedic Surgery, Zuyderland Hospital, Heerlen, the Netherlands.

References

1. Font-Rodriguez DE, Scuderi GR, Insall JN. Survivorship of cemented total knee arthroplasty. Clin Orthop Relat Res. 1997;345:79–86.
2. Callaghan JJ, O'Rourke MR, Iossi MF, Liu SS, Goetz DD, Vittetoe DA, Sullivan PM, Johnston RC. Cemented rotating-platform total knee replacement. A concise follow up, at a minimum of fifteen years, of a previous report. J Bone Joint Surg Am. 2005;87(9):1995–8.
3. Keating EM, Meding JB, Faris PM, Ritter MA. Long-term followup of nonmodular total knee replacements. Clin Orthop Relat Res. 2002;404:34–9.
4. Gill GS, Joshi AB. Long-term results of cemented, posterior cruciate ligament-retaining total knee arthroplasty in osteoarthritis. Am J Knee Surg. 2001;14(4):209–14.
5. Pavone V, Boettner F, Fickert S, Sculco TP. Total condylar knee arthroplasty: a long-term follow-up. Clin Orthop Relat Res. 2001;388:18–25.
6. Ritter MA, Faris PM, Keating EM, Meding JB. Postoperative alignment of total knee replacement. Its effect on survival. Clin Orthop Relat Res. 1994;299:153–6.
7. Rodriguez JA, Bhende H, Ranawat CS. Total condylar knee replacement: a 20-year follow-up study. Clin Orthop Relat Res. 2001;388:10–7.
8. Shan L, Shan B, Suzuki A, Nouh F, Saxena A. Intermediate and long-term quality of life after total knee replacement: a systematic review and meta-analysis. J Bone Joint Surg Am. 2015;97(2):156–68.
9. Popovic N, Lemaire R. Anterior knee pain with posterior-stabilized mobile-bearing knee prosthesis: the effect of femoral component design. J Arthroplast. 2003;18:396–400.
10. Waters TS, Bentley G. Patellar resurfacing in total knee arthroplasty: a prospective, randomized study. J Bone Joint Surg Am. 2003;85-A:212–7.
11. Breugem SJ, Sierevelt IN, Schafroth MU, Blankevoort L, Schaap GR, van Dijk CN. Less anterior knee pain with mobile-beraring prosthesis compared with fixed bearing prosthesis. Clin Orthop Relat Res. 2008;466(8):1959–65.
12. Petersen W, Rembitzki IV, Brüggemann GP, Ellermann A, Best R, Koppenburg AG, Liebau C. Anterior knee pain after total knee arthroplasty: a narrative review. Int Orthop. 2014;38(2):319–28.
13. Shervin D, Pratt K, Healey T, Nguyen S, Mihalko WM, El-Othmani MM, Saleh KJ. Anterior knee pain following primary total knee arthroplasty. World J Orthop. 2015;6(10):795–803.
14. Singh JA, Gabriel S, Lewallen D. The impact of gender, age and preoperative pain severity on pain after TKA. Clin Orthop Relat Res. 2008;466(11):2717–23.
15. Lavernia CJ, Alcerro JC, Contreras JS, Rossi MD. Ethnic and racial factors influencing well-being, perceived pain and physical function after primary joint arthroplasty. Clin Orthop Relat Res. 2011 Jul;469(7):1838–45.
16. Bonnin MP, Basiglini L, Archbold HA. What are the factors of residual pain after uncomplicated TKA? Knee Surg Sports Traumatol Arthrosc. 2011;19(9):1411–7.
17. Liu SS, Buvanendran A, Rathmell JP, Sawhney M, Bae JJ, Moric M, et al. Predictors of moderate to severe acute postoperative pain after total hip and knee replacement. Int Orthop. 2012;36(11):2261–7.
18. Forsythe ME, Dunbar MJ, Hennigar AW, Sullivan MJ, Gross M. Prospective relation between catastrophizing and residual pain following knee arthroplasty: two-year follow-up. Pain Res Manag. 2008;13(4):335–41.
19. Brander VA, Stulberg SD, Adams AD, Harden RN, Bruehl S, Stanos SP, Houle T. Predicting total kne replacement pain a prospective, observational study. Clin Orthop Relat Res. 2003;416:27–36.
20. van Jonbergen HP, Reuver JM, Mutsaerts EL, Poolman RW. Determinants of anterior knee pain following total knee replacement: a systematic review. Knee Surg Sports Traumatol Arthrosc. 2014;22(3):478–99.
21. Dajani KA, Stuart MJ, Dahm DL, Levy BA. Arthroscopic treatment of patellar clunk and synovial hyperplasia after total knee arthroplasty. J Arthroplast. 2010;25(1):97–103.
22. Maloney WJ, Schmidt R, Sculco TP. Femoral component design and patellar clunk syndrome. Clin Orthop Relat Res. 2003;410:199–202.
23. Fukunaga K, Kobayashi A, Minoda Y, Iwaki H, Hashimoto Y, Takaoka K. The incidence of the patellar clunk syndrome in a recently designed mobile-bearing posteriorly stabilised total knee replacement. J Bone Joint Surg Br. 2009;91(4):463–8.
24. Rodríguez-Merchán EC, Gómez-Cardero P. The outerbridge classification predicts the need for patellar resurfacing in TKA. Clin Orthop Relat Res. 2010;468(5):1254–7.
25. Banks SA, Harman MK, Hodge WA. Mechanism of anterior impingement damage in total knee arthroplasty. J Bone Joint Surg Am. 2002;84-A(Suppl 2):37–42.
26. Bonnin MP, Schmidt A, Basiglini L, Bossard N, Dantony E. Mediolateral oversizing influences pain, function and flexion after TKA. Knee Surg Sports Traumatol Arthrosc. 2013;21(10):2314–24.
27. Bellemans J, Carpentier K, Vandenneucker H, Vanlauwe J, Victor J. The John Insall award: both morphotype and gender influence the shape of the knee in patients undergoing TKA. Clin Orthop Relat Res. 2010;468(1):29–36.
28. Mahfouz M, Abdel Fatah EE, Bowers LS, Scuderi G. Three-dimensional morphology of the knee reveals ethnic differences. Clin Orthop Relat Res. 2012;470(1):172–85.
29. Hamilton DF, Burnett R, Patton JT, Howie CR, Moran M, Simpson AHRW, Gaston P. Implant design influences patient outcome after total knee arthroplasty. Bone Joint J. 2015;97-B(1):64–70.
30. van Jonbergen HP, Scholtes VA, Poolman RW. A randomised, controlled trial of circumpatellar electrocautery in total knee replacement without patellar resurfacing: a concise follow-up at a mean of 3.7 years. Bone Joint J. 2014;96-B(4):473–8.
31. Cheng T, Zhu C, Guo Y, Shi S, Chen D, Zhang X. Patellar denervation with electrocautery in total knee arthroplasty without patellar resurfacing: a meta-analysis. Knee Surg Sports Traumatol Arthrosc. 2014;22(11):2648–54.

32. Meneghini RM. Should the patella be resurfaced in primary total knee arthroplasty? An evidence-based analysis. J Arthroplast. 2008;23(7 Suppl):11–4.

33. Li S, Chen Y, Su W, Zhao J, He S, Luo X. Systematic review of patellar resurfacing in total knee arthroplasty. Int Orthop. 2011;35(3):305–16.

34. Pilling RW, Moulder E, Allgar V, Messner J, Sun Z, Mohsen A. Patellar resurfacing in primary total knee replacement: a meta-analysis. J Bone Joint Surg Am. 2012;94(24):2270–8.

35. Heegaard JH, Leyvraz PF, Hovey CB. A computer model to simulate patellar biomechanics following total knee replacement: the effects of femoral component alignment. Clin Biomech (Bristol, Avon). 2001;16(5):415–23.

36. Lee TQ, Morris G, Csintalan RP. The influence of tibial and femoral rotation on patellofemoral contact area and pressure. J Orthop Sports Phys Ther. 2003;33(11):686–93.

37. Hsu HC, Luo ZP, Rand JA, An KN. Influence of patellar thickness on patellar tracking and patellofemoral contact characteristics after total knee arthroplasty. J Arthroplast. 1996;11(1):69–80.

38. Berger RA, Crossett LS, Jacobs JJ, Rubash HE. Malrotation causing patellofemoral complications after total knee arthroplasty. Clin Orthop Relat Res. 1998;356:144–53.

39. Merican AM, Ghosh KM, Iranpour F, Deehan DJ, Amis AA. The effect of femoral component rotation on the kinematics of the tibiofemoral and patellofemoral joints after total knee arthroplasty. Knee Surg Sports Traumatol Arthrosc. 2011;19(9):1479–87.

40. Miller MC, Berger RA, Petrella AJ, Karmas A, Rubash HE. Optimizing femoral component rotation in total knee arthroplasty. Clin Orthop Relat Res. 2001;392:38–45.

41. Vertullo CJ, Easley ME, Scott WN, Insall JN. Mobile bearings in primary knee arthroplasty. J Am Acad Orthop Surg. 2001;9(6):355–64.

42. Bo ZD, Liao L, Zhao JM, Wei QJ, Ding XF, Yang B. Mobile bearing or fixed bearing? A meta-analysis of outcomes comparing mobile bearing and fixed bearing bilateral total knee replacements. Knee. 2014;21(2):374–81.

43. O'Connor JJ, Goodfellow JW. Theory and practice of meniscal knee replacement: designing against wear. Proc Inst Mech Eng H. 1996;210(3):217–22.

44. Menchetti PP, Walker PS. Mechanical evaluation of mobile bearing knees. Am J Knee Surg. 1997;10(2):73–81.

45. Callaghan JJ, Insall JN, Greenwald AS, Dennis DA, Komistek RD, Murray DW, Bourne RB, Rorabeck CH, Dorr LD. Mobile-bearing knee replacement: concepts and results. Instr Course Lect. 2001;50:431–49.

46. D'Lima DD, Trice M, Urquhart AG, Colwell CW Jr. Comparison between the kinematics of fixed and rotating bearing knee prostheses. Clin Orthop Relat Res. 2000;380:151–7.

47. Hofstede SN, Nouta KA, Jacobs W, van Hooff ML, Wymenga AB, Pijls BG, Nelissen RG, Marangvan de Mheen PJ. Mobile bearing vs fixed bearing prostheses for posterior cruciate retaining total knee arthroplasty for postoperative functional status in patients with osteoarthritis and rheumatoid arthritis. Cochrane Database Syst Rev. 2015;(2):CD003130.

48. Moskal JT, Capps SG. Rotating-platform TKA no different from fixed-bearing TKA regarding survivorship or performance: a meta-analysis. Clin Orthop Relat Res. 2014;472(7):2185–93.

49. van der Voort P, Pijls BG, Nouta KA, Valstar ER, Jacobs WC, Nelissen RG. A systematic review and meta-regression of mobile-bearing versus fixed-bearing total knee replacement in 41 studies. Bone Joint J. 2013;95-B(9):1209–16.

50. Li YL, Wu Q, Ning GZ, Feng SQ, Wu QL, Li Y, Hao Y. No difference in clinical outcome between fixed- and mobile-bearing TKA: a meta-analysis. Knee Surg Sports Traumatol Arthrosc. 2014;22(3):565–75.

51. Capella M, Dolfin M, Saccia F. Mobile bearing and fixed bearing total knee arthroplasty. Ann Transl Med. 2016;4(7):127.

52. Buechel FF, Pappas MJ. New Jersey low contact stress knee replacement system. Ten-year evaluation of meniscal bearings. Orthop Clin North Am. 1989;20(2):147–77.

53. Stiehl JB, Dennis DA, Komistek RD, Keblish PA. In vivo kinematic comparison of posterior cruciate ligament retention or sacrifice with a mobile bearing total knee arthroplasty. Am J Knee Surg. 2000;13(1):13–8.

54. Colwell CW Jr, Chen PC, D'Lima D. Extensor malalignment arising from femoral component malrotation in knee arthroplasty: effect of rotating-bearing. Clin Biomech (Bristol, Avon). 2011;26(1):52–7.

55. Sawaguchi N, Majima T, Ishigaki T, Mori N, Terashima T, Minami A. Mobile-bearing total knee arthroplasty improves patellar tracking and patellofemoral contact stress: in vivo measurements in the same patients. J Arthroplast. 2010;25(6):920–5.

56. Skwara A, Tibesku CO, Ostermeier S, Stukenborg-Colsman C, Fuchs-Winkelmann S. Differences in patellofemoral contact stresses between mobile-bearing and fixed-bearing total knee arthroplasties: a dynamic in vitro measurement. Arch Orthop Trauma Surg. 2009;129(7):901–7.

57. Wyatt MC, Frampton C, Horne JG, Devane P. Mobile- versus fixed-bearing modern total knee replacements- which is the more patella-friendly design?: the 11-year New Zealand joint registry study. Bone Joint Res. 2013;2(7):129–31.

58. Matsuda Y, Ishii Y, Noguchi H, Ishii R. Varus-valgus balance and range of movement after total knee arthroplasty. J Bone Joint Surg (Br). 2005;87-B:804–8.

59. Eisenhuth SA, Saleh KJ, Cui Q, Clark CR, Brown TE. Patellofemoral instability after total knee arthroplasty. Clin Orthop Relat Res. 2006;446:149–60.

60. Middleton FR, Palmer SH. How accurate is Whiteside's line as a reference axis in total knee arthroplasty? Knee. 2007;14(3):204–7.

61. Lützner J, Krummenauer F, Günther KP, Kirschner S. Rotational alignment of the tibial component in total knee arthroplasty is better at the medial third of tibial tuberosity than at the medial border. BMC Musculoskelet Disord. 2010;11:57.

62. Steinbrück A, Schröder C, Woiczinski M, Müller T, Müller PE, Jansson V, Fottner A. Influence of tibial rotation in total knee arthroplasty on knee kinematics and retropatellar pressure: an in vitro study. Knee Surg Sports Traumatol Arthrosc. 2016;24(8):2395–401.

63. Asano H, Hoshino A, Wilton TJ. Soft-tissue tension total knee arthroplasty. J Arthroplast. 2004;19(5):558–61.

64. Streiner DL, Norman GR. Chapter 4: scaling responses, in health measurement. Oxford: Oxford University Press; 1995. p. 32.

65. Nies F de, Fidler MW. Visual analog scale for the assessment of total hip arthroplasty. J Arthroplast 1997;12(4):416-419.

66. Jones SE, Kon SS, Canavan JL, Patel MS, Clark AL, Nolan CM, Polkey MI, Man WD. The five-repetition sit-to-stand test as a functional outcome measure in COPD. Thorax. 2013;68(11):1015–20.

67. Norkin CC, White DJ. Measurement of joint motion; a guide to goniometry. F.A. Davis Company; Philadelphia. 4 edition 2009. ISBN 0803665792.

68. Brosseau L, Tousignant M, Budd J, Chartier N, Duciaume L, Plamondon S, O'Sullivan JP, O'Donoghue S, Balmer S. Intratester reliability and intertester reliability and criterion validity of the parallelogram and universal goniometers for active knee flexion in healthy subjects. Physiother Res Int. 1997;2(3):150–66.

69. Lenssen AF, van Dam EM, Crijns YH, Verhey M, Geesink RJ, van den Brandt PA, de Bie RA. Reproducibility of goniometric measurement of the knee in the in-hospital phase following total knee arthroplasty. BMC Musculoskelet Disord. 2007;8:83.

70. Insall JN, Dorr LD, Scott RD, Scott WN. Rationale of the knee society clinical rating system. Clin Orthop Relat Res. 1989;248:13–4.

71. Hays RD, Sherbourne CD, Mazel RM, The RAND. 36-item health survey 1.0. Health Econ. 1993;2(3):217–27.

72. Hays RD, Morales LS. The RAND-36 measure of health-related quality of life. Ann Med. 2001 Jul;33(5):350–7.

73. Ewald FC. The knee society total knee arthroplasty roentgenographic evaluation and scoring system. Clin Orthop Relat Res. 1989;248:9–12.

74. Jacobs W, Anderson P, Limbeek J, Wymenga A. Mobile bearing vs fixed bearing prostheses for total knee arthroplasty for post-operative functional status in patients with osteoarthritis and rheumatoid arthritis. Cochrane Database Syst Rev. 2004;2:CD003130.

75. Price AJ, Rees JL, Beard D, Juszczak E, Carter S, White S, de Steiger R, Dodd CA, Gibbons M, McLardy-Smith P, Goodfellow JW, Murray DW. A mobile-bearing total knee prosthesis compared with a fixed-bearing prosthesis. A multicentre single-blind randomised controlled trial. J Bone Joint Surg Br. 2003;85(1):62–7.

76. Breugem SJ, van Ooij B, Haverkamp D, Sierevelt IN, van Dijk CN. No difference in anterior knee pain between a fixed and a mobile posterior stabilized total knee arthroplasty after 7.9 years. Knee Surg Sports Traumatol Arthrosc. 2014;22(3):509–16.

77. Beard DJ, Pandit H, Price AJ, Butler-Manuel PA, Dodd CA, Murray DW, Goodfellow JW. Introduction of a new mobile-bearing total knee prosthesis: minimum three year follow-up of an RCT comparing it with a fixed-bearing device. Knee. 2007;14(6):448–51.

78. Biau D, Mullins MM, Judet T, Piriou P. Mobile versus fixed-bearing total knee arthroplasty: mid-term comparative clinical results of 216 prostheses. Knee Surg Sports Traumatol Arthrosc. 2006;14(10):927–33.

79. Pais-Brito JL, Rafols-Urquiza B, Gonzalez-Massieu L, Herrera-Perez M, Aciego-De Mendoza M, De Bergua Domingo J. Reduced patellofemoral and walking pain with mobile-bearing vs. fixed-bearing total knee replacements:

a mid-term prospective analytic study. Acta Orthop Traumatol Turc. 2015;49(4):375–81.

80. Woolson ST, Northrop GD. Mobile- vs. fixed-bearing total knee arthroplasty: a clinical and radiologic study. J Arthroplast. 2004;19(2):135–40.

81. Smith H, Jan M, Mahomed NN, Davey JR, Gandhi R. Meta-analysis and systematic review of clinical outcomes comparing mobile bearing and fixed bearing total knee arthroplasty. J Arthroplast. 2011;26(8):1205–13.

82. Haas B, Dennis DA, Komistek RD, Brumley JT 2nd, Hammill C. Range of motion of posterior-cruciate-substituting total knee replacements: the effect of bearing mobility. J Bone Joint Surg Am. 2001;83-A Suppl 2(Pt 1):51–5.

83. Carothers JT, Kim RH, Dennis DA, Southworth C. Mobile-bearing total knee arthroplasty: a meta-analysis. J Arthroplast. 2011;26(4):537–42.

84. Aglietti P, Baldini A, Buzzi R, Lup D, De Luca L. Comparison of mobile-bearing and fixed-bearing total knee arthroplasty: a prospective randomized study. J Arthroplasty. 2005;20(2):145-53.

85. Kim YH, Kim JS, Choe JW, Kim HJ. Long-term comparison of fixed-bearing and mobile-bearing total knee replacements in patients younger than fifty-one years of age with osteoarthritis. J Bone Joint Surg Am. 2012;94(10):866–73.

86. Stiehl JB, Dennis DA, Komistek RD, Keblish PA. In vivo kinematics analysis of a mobile bearing total knee prosthesis. Clin Orthop Rel Res. 1997;345:60–6.

87. Hopley CD, Crossett LS, Chen AF. Long-term clinical outcomes and survivorship after total knee arthroplasty using a rotating platform knee prosthesis: a meta-analysis. J Arthroplast. 2013;28(1):68–77.

88. Wen Y, Liu D, Huang Y, Li B. A meta-analysis of the fixed-bearing and mobile-bearing prostheses in total knee arthroplasty. Arch Orthop Trauma Surg. 2011;131(10):1341–50.

89. Heinert G, Kendoff D, Preiss S, Gehrke T, Sussmann P. Patellofemoral kinematics in mobile-bearing and fixed-bearing posterior stabilised total knee replacements: a cadaveric study. Knee Surg Sports Traumatol Arthrosc. 2011;19(6):967–72.

90. Ferguson KB, Bailey O, Anthony I, Stother IG, Blyth MJ. A comparison of lateral release rates on fixed- versus mobile-bearing total knee arthroplasty. J Orthop Traumatol. 2015;16(2):87–90.

6

Risk factors for revision of total knee arthroplasty

L.L. Jasper[1], C. A. Jones[1]*, J. Mollins[2], S. L. Pohar[3] and L. A. Beaupre[1]

Abstract

Background: In spite of the increasing incidence of total knee arthroplasties (TKA), evidence is limited regarding risk factors for revision. The objective of this scoping review was to identify and assess demographic, surgical and health services factors that may increase the risk for revision surgery following TKA.

Methods: A scoping review was undertaken following an electronic search in MEDLINE (1990 to December 2013), CINAHL (to December 2013), EMBASE (1990 to December 2013) and Web of Science (1990 to December 2013).

Results: Of the 4460 articles screened, 42 were included of which 26 articles were based on registry data. Increased risk of revision was associated with demographic factors (younger age, African American), surgical factors related to the primary TKA (uncemented components, implant malalignment, increased surgery duration), and health services (low volume hospitals).

Conclusions: Identifying emerging trends in characteristics of those requiring revision following TKA can help identify those at risk and allocate appropriate resources. Further primary clinical articles on risk factors for revision of TKA are necessary to ensure maximal function and lifespan following TKAs.

Keywords: Total knee arthroplasty, Revision, Failure, Risk factor, Scoping review

Background

The effectiveness of total knee arthroplasty (TKA) in relieving pain and improving function has been well documented [1, 2]. TKA is considered a cost effective and efficacious treatment for patients with end stage knee osteoarthritis who experience severe pain, activity limitations and for whom conservative treatment is unsuccessful [3–5]. With more than 700 000 primary TKAs performed annually in the USA, estimates of TKA are projected to increase to 673 % by 2030 in the USA. The large demand for TKA is primarily related to the aging population, the obesity epidemic and technical advancement of the surgical procedure [6–8]. The longevity of implants is typically greater than 10 years with 32,700 revisions performed annually in the USA. Significant demand for primary TKA will correspond to a growing demand for revisions of TKA which are projected to increase by 601 % from 2005 to 2030 [6].

Revisions for TKA pose unique challenges as revision surgery is a more complex surgery than a primary TKA

with increased complication and mortality rates [9–11]. Identifying emerging trends in characteristics of those requiring revision following TKA can help identify those at risk and allocate appropriate resources. Several articles have identified risk factors for revision surgery of TKA yet, to our knowledge, the synthesis of these findings have not been documented. A more comprehensive understanding of the potential risk factors for revision of TKA will provide important knowledge for surgeons and patients. The objective of this scoping review was to identify and assess demographic, surgical and health services factors that lead to increased risk of revision surgery following TKA.

Methods

A scoping review of the literature was undertaken to identify and assess relevant evidence given the limited existing evidence on revisions of TKA. Inclusion criteria consisted of studies that comprised a) adult patients who received primary TKA and received a subsequent revision, b) comparative groups or risk-adjusted analyses, and c) at least 20 or more revision cases. Cohort and case control articles

* Correspondence: cajones@ualberta.ca
[1]Department of Physical Therapy, University of Alberta, Rm 2-50 Corbett Hall, Edmonton, AB T6G 2G4, Canada
Full list of author information is available at the end of the article

were included while descriptive studies and randomized controlled trials comparing specific interventions were excluded. Articles which included hemiarthroplasty, primary TKA used to stabilize a fracture or management of bone pathology or malignancy, simultaneous bilateral TKAs, and patellofemoral arthroplasty were excluded. Revisions for all reasons were included except revisions occurring in the first three months due to sepsis. Ethics was not obtained for this study as the study was a retrospective scoping review that did not involve any individual data or identifying information. In discussion with our Health Research Ethics Board at the University of Alberta, we do not require ethics for review.

Data sources and search strategies
A search strategy was developed and implemented by a health sciences librarian for 4 databases: Medline (1990-Dec 2013; includes in-process & other non-indexed citations), EMBASE (1990-Dec 2013), CINAHL (1990-Dec 2013), and Web of Science (1990-Nov 2012) (Additional file 1). Date (1990–2013) and language (English) restrictions were applied to the searches. The decision to restrict the search to English articles was based on findings from systematic research evidence that reported no empirical evidence of bias was seen if papers written in languages other than English (LOE) were excluded [12]. The search included an extensive list of subject headings and keyword terms for 3 concepts: 1) hip or knee arthroplasty, 2) revision surgery, and 3) prognosis (see Additional file 1). Total hip arthroplasty articles were included in the search because we did not want to inadvertently exclude articles that reported both total hip and total knee arthroplasties. Case articles or case reports were removed along with conference abstracts. This initial search yielded many non-relevant papers so an additional search string was added to increase the relevancy of the results (by including certain terms in either the title or marked as the most important subject headings). A "relevancy forcing search set" was performed to ensure that all relevant papers were captured. All duplicate citations were removed.

Study selection
To ensure consistency with screening of title and abstract, 20 citations were independently reviewed by both reviewers (LJ & SP) using a standardized form based on broad criteria including population intervention, comparison, outcome and study design. The remaining citations were then independently screened for relevance.

If a citation was selected by either reviewer, the full-text article was obtained for further review. Full-text articles were further screened for selection using a standard study

selection form, based upon the predetermined inclusion criteria. The study selection form was initially piloted on a sample of 20 articles to ensure that the selection criteria were applied consistently across reviewers. Relevant full-text articles were then reviewed by one of the two reviewers using standardized inclusion and exclusion criteria. Disagreement of article inclusion was resolved through consensus between reviewers or through third party adjudication if the reviewers did not arrive at consensus. Full-text papers were included only if consensus was achieved by reviewers. For those articles selected for full review, data were extracted by one reviewer (LJ) and verified by a second reviewer (LB or AJ). The first 20 full text articles reviewed by both reviewers had excellent agreement (Kappa value 0.96, $p < 0.0001$). All selected articles were included in data synthesis regardless of methodological quality. Inconclusive findings and gaps in the literature were identified. A narrative description of the included articles was completed and potential patterns identified in terms of targeted behaviors, study outcomes, and intervention effectiveness.

Quality assessment
The Oxford Level of Evidence was used to evaluate the quality of selected full-text articles [13], and has been recommended to determine a hierarchy of the best evidence [14]. SIGN guidelines were also used to assess study quality through completion of their cohort checklist including items such as subject selection, assessment, confounding and statistical analysis [15].

Results
Of the 4460 articles identified through the search strategies, 266 articles remained after the abstracts were screened for eligibility. After full text review, 42 articles met the inclusion criteria for the review (see Fig. 1). Twenty-six (62 %) articles were based on registry or insurance databases of which 12 were based on Nordic registries and 11 from American databases (see Additional file 2).

All articles were prognostic retrospective articles with level III quality except for one which was a level II prognostic prospective study [13, 16]. Using the SIGN guidelines, 31 articles were regarded of *acceptable* quality and 11 articles were deemed *poor* quality often due to incomplete reporting of multivariate analyses (see Additional file 2) [15].

Of the 34 (81 %) articles that reported mean follow-up from the primary TKA, six articles reported 10 year survival rates and two articles reported 20 year survival rates (see Table 1). While survival rates of the primary TKA were consistently high at 10 years ranging from

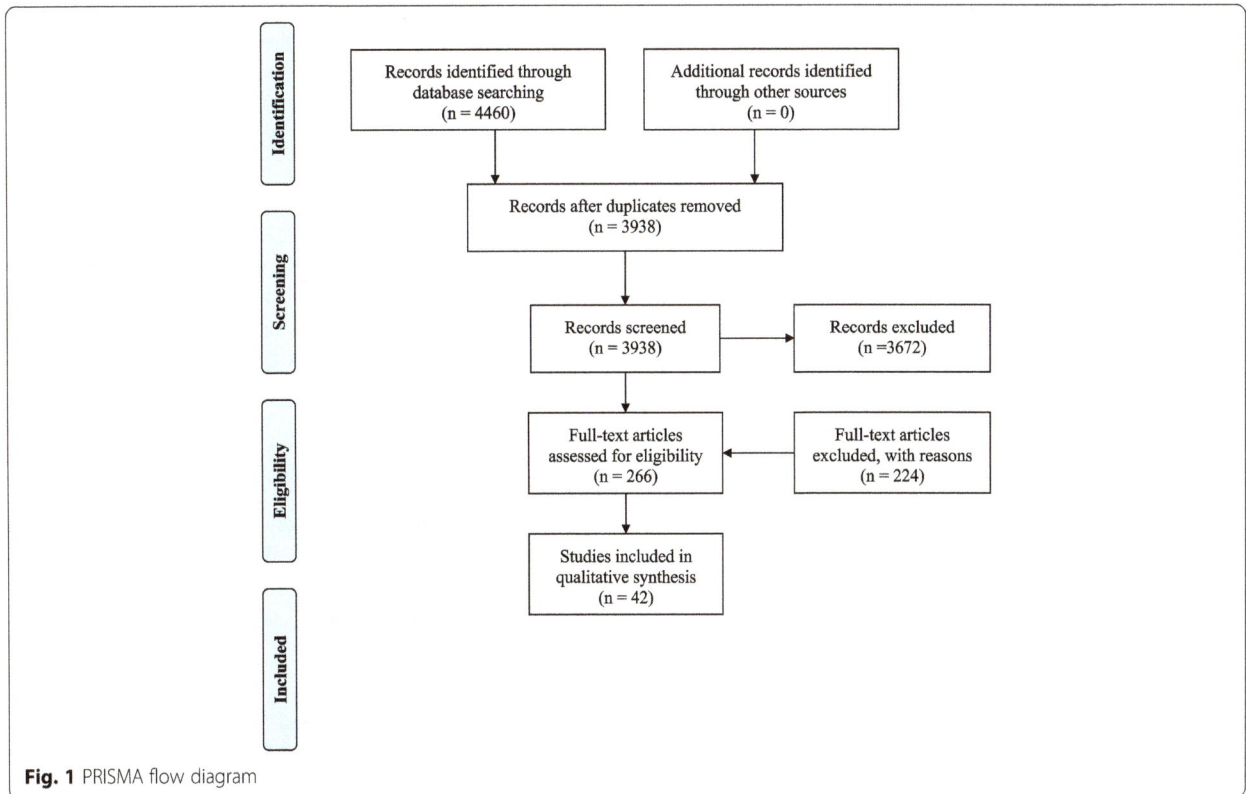

Fig. 1 PRISMA flow diagram

89.5 to 98.6 % [17–19, 20, 21, 42], 20 year survival rates were expectedly lower at 78–99 % [19, 23].

Demographic risk factors

Sex

While all articles reported sex, the association of sex and TKA revision was only examined in 10 articles (see Table 2).

Inconsistent findings were reported in that males had a higher risk of revision surgery than females in 5 articles (see Table 2), females had a higher risk of revision (HR 1.513, 95 % CI 1.116 to 2.051) in one article, based on American registry data, [24] and four articles, from different countries, did not find a significant association between sex and TKA revision [16, 18, 25–26].

Table 1 Survival rates at 10 and 20 Years[a]

Author(s), year	Duration of follow-up (yrs)	Index procedure (n)	Revision (n)	Survival rate (%, CI)
Badawy M. et al., 2013 [42]	10	26,698	1169	Low hospital volume[b]: 92.5 %, 95 % CI 91.5 to 93.4 High hospital volume: 95.5 %, 95 % CI 94.1 to 97.0
Gothesen, Ø. et al., 2013 [17]	10	17,782	NR	89.5 to 95.3 %, CI- NR
Himanen, A. et al., 2007 [20]	10	751	37	Prosthetic moulded component: 94.4 %, 95 % CI 90.4 to 96.7 Prosthetic modular component: 93.6 %, 95 % CI 89.7 to 96.0
Jämsen, E. et al., 2013 [21]	10	53,007	1919	94.5 %, 95 % CI 94.1 to 94.8
Rand, J. et al., 2003 [19]	10	11,606	NR	91 %, 95 % CI 90 to 91 %
Vessely, M. et al., 2006 [18]	10	1000	45	98.6 %, 95 % CI 97.8 to 99.4
Fang, D. et al., 2009 [23]	20	6070	51	99 %, CI - NR
Rand, J. et al., 2003 [19]	20	11,606	NR	78 %, 95 % CI 74 to 81 %

[a]See Additional file 2 for further detail. Not reported in publication, NR
[b]Low hospital volume is 1–24 TKA performed per year; High hospital volume is ≥150 TKA performed per year

Table 2 Sex and adjusted risk of revision[a]

Author(s)/year	Control	Hazard ratio (CI)
Blum, M. et al., 2013 [29]	Female	0.81, 95 % CI 0.71 - 0.92, $p < 0.01$
Fehring, T. et al., 2004 [52]	Male	2.771, 99 % CI 1.662 - 4.620, $p < 0.0001$
Harrysson, O. et al., 2004 [43]	Male	1.64, 95 % CI 1.23 - 2.18, $p = 0.0007$
Rand, J. et al., 2003 [19]	Male	1.6, 95 % CI 1.4 - 2.0, $p < 0.0001$
Schrama, J. et al., 2010 [30]	Female	0.67, 95 % C I 0.47 - 0.88
Stiehl, J. et al., 2006 [24]	Female	1.513, 95 % CI 1.116 - 2.051

[a]See Additional file 2 for further detail

Age
Among the 15 articles that examined age as a risk factor, 13 articles reported that revision rates decreased with older age (see Table 3).

Race
Race was examined in 3 American articles, of which 2 were based on the same registry [27, 28]. African American patients had a higher risk for revision than Caucasian patients (HR 1.73, 95 % CI 1.33 to 2.25, $p < 0.001$; HR 1.82, 95 % CI 1.33 to 2.48, $p < 0.001$; HR 1.39, 95 % CI 1.08 to 1.80, $p = 0.01$) and represented 5.5 and 8.4 % of the patient population reported in these registries. [27–29].

Medical risk factors
Primary diagnosis
Although the majority of patients undergoing TKA were diagnosed with osteoarthritis, 4 articles specifically examined diagnosis and its potential association with TKA revision with mixed results [19, 24, 25, 30]. Two large

Table 3 Age and adjusted risk of revision[a]

Author(s)/Year	Age	Hazard ratio (95 % CI)unless otherwise stated
Bini, S. et al., 2013 [31]	>55 years	0.43, 95 % CI 0.27 to 0.67, $p < 0.001$
Blum, M. et al., 2013 [29]	18–64 years vs. 65+ yrs	2.30, 95 % CI 1.96 to 2.69, $p < 0.0001$
Bordini, B. et al., 2009 [32]	Age at surgery (per year)	1.05, 95 % CI 1.03 to 1.06, $p = 0.0001$
Fehring, T. et al., 2004 [52]	Age at surgery (per year)	0.953, 99 % CI 0.932 to 0.975, $p < 0.0001$
Gioe, T. et al., 2004 [53]	Age <70 year	0.46, 95 % CI.0.33 to 0.64, $p < 0.001$
Harrysson, O. et al., 2004 [43]	Older patients (≥60 year) Revision Attributable to Any Reason Revision Attributable to Loosening of Components	0.49, 95 % CI 0.38 to 0.62, $p < 0.0001$ 0.41, 95 % CI 0.27 to 0.62, $p < 0.0001$
Julin, J. et al., 2010 [35]	Age ≤ 55 years: Revision for reasons other than infection Revision for any reason	2.9, 95 % CI 2.3 to 3.6 2.4, 95 % CI 2.0 to 3.0 Age 56–65 years
	Age 56–65 years: Revision for reasons other than infection Revision for any reason :	1.7 95 % CI 1.4 to 2.0 1.5, 95 % CI 1.3 to 1.7
Kreder, H. et al., 2003 [25]	Younger age per 10 year: At 1 year after revision At 3 years after revision	OR 0.77, 95 % CI 0.67 to 0.89 OR 0.70, 95 % CI 0.66 to 0.81
Lygre, S. et al., 2011 [37]	Age >70 year vs. <60 year	0.4, 95 % CI 0.3–0.4, 0 < 0.001
Namba, R. et al., 2013 [28]	Age (increasing 10 year increments)	0.62, 95 % CI 0.57 to 0.67, $p < 0.001$
Namba, R. et al., 2012 [27]	Age (increasing 10 year increments)	0.64, 95 % CI 0.58 to 0.70, $p < 0.001$
Rand, J. et al., 2003 [19]	Age 56–70 year vs. ≤55 years Age >70 year vs. ≤55 years	0.7, 95 % CI 0.5 to 0.9, $p < 0.01$ 0.5, 95 % CI 0.3 to 0.6, $p < 0.0001$
Stiehl, J. et al., 2006 [24]	Younger patients (for every yr increase)	0.979, 95 % CI 0.968 to 0.989

[a]See Additional file 2 for further detail

registry articles reported differing results with inflammatory arthritis having a greater and lesser risk for revisions than patients with osteoarthritis (HR 1.6, 95 % CI 1.06 to 2.38 and HR 0.5, 95 % CI 0.3 to 0.7, $p < 0.001$) [19, 30]. A clinical study of 4743 patients found that OA or post-traumatic arthritis had a greater risk of revision than RA (HR 1.51, 95 % CI 1.116 to 2.051) [24]. Further, in a clinical sample of 14352 patients, Kreder et al. reported no significant association between the diagnosis of OA and risk for revision [25].

Comorbidities

Eleven articles specifically looked at the effect of comorbidities examining both total number of conditions and specific conditions (see Additional file 2). Jamsen et al. found that risks increased if there were one or more of the comorbidities identified (HR 1.23, 95 % CI 1.16 to 1.30) [21]. Alternately, Kreder et al. did not find a significant association between the presence of comorbidities and revision following TKA [25].

When looking at comorbidities associated with OA, obesity, cardiac disease and diabetes were at high risk of revision. Two American TKA registries reported increased risk of revision for patients with a higher BMI (BMI 30–35 kg vs <30 kg HR 1.48, 95 % CI 1.00 to 2.19 and BMI ≥35 kg/m2 vs. <30 kg/m2 h 0.78, 95 % CI 0.63 to 0.96, $p = 0.020$) [28, 31]. However, 3 other articles did not find a significant relationship between BMI and risk for TKA revision [18, 20, 32].

The presence of cardiac conditions at time of the primary TKA increased the risk of revision including hypertension with early revision (0 – 5 years) (HR 1.14, 95 % CI 1.01 to 1.29), coronary disease (HR 1.27 95 % CI 1.07 to 1.50) and cardiovascular disease (HR 1.29, 95 % CI 1.14 to 1.45) [21, 33].

Three articles reported an increased risk of revision for the patients with diabetes. Jamsen et al. and Namba both found an association with diabetes and revision (HR 1.27, 95 % CI 1.08 to 1.50 and HR 1.21, 95 % CI 1.04 to 1.41, $p = 0.014$) although Jamsen et al. was examining early revisions [28, 21]. Similarly, King et al. also found the 46 to 55 years and 66 years + diabetic cohorts had increased risk of revision as compared to the non-diabetic cohort (HR 2.9 95 % CI 1.5 to 5.8, $p = 0.004$ and HR 1.5, $p = 0.0037$ respectively) although there was not a significant difference in the 56 to 65 years cohort [34].

Joint implant factors
Fixation
Two articles consisting of 9337 patients from the US found cemented primary TKAs had a protective effect on receiving revision as compared to cementless/hybrid TKAs [16, 19]. Hybrid fixation, in which the proximal component was cementless and the distal component was cemented, also demonstrated a higher risk for revision than cemented TKAs in both US and Norwegian studies [16, 35].

Cruciate retaining implants
Cruciate ligament status was reported in several articles with inconsistent findings (see Table 4) [16]. Two large American registry studies reported that posterior stabilized implants had increased risk of revision when compared to posterior cruciate-retaining implants (HR 2.6, 95 % CI 2.1 to 3.5, $p < 0.0001$ and HR = 2.0, 95 % CI 1.67 to 2.5, $p < 0.001$) [19, 36]. Conversely, an American registry study of 1047 patients found ligament status was not significant [16]. Further, Stiehl et al. found both posterior cruciate retaining arthroplasties and bicruciate retaining arthroplasties had increased risk of revision compared to rotating platform (HR 1.552, 95 % CI 1.157 to 2.081 and HR 2.188, 95 % CI 1.454 to 3.294) [24].

Patellar resurfacing
The articles that specifically examined patellar resurfacing had inconsistent findings. Three articles found that the risk of revision increased when the patella was resurfaced (patella not resurfaced HR 1.4, 95 % CI 1.2 to 1.7, patella resurfaced HR 0.84, 95 % CI: 0.071–1.0, $p = 0.052$, and patellar resurfaced HR 1.814, 95 % CI 1.320 to 2.558 respectively) [24, 35, 37]. Alternately, two articles found that the patellae not resurfaced patellae had higher risks of revision than resurfaced patellae (HR 2.09, 95 % CI 1.07 to 4.06, $p = 0.03$, HR 1.4, 95 % CI 1.2 to 1.7) [27, 35]. Two studies did not find an association between patellar resurfacing and revision significant [20, 38]. One study reported that metal-backed patella were more likely to be revised than all polyethylene patellar components (HR 2.4, 95 % CI 1.9 to 3.1, $p < 0.0001$) [19].

Alignment
Malalignment was reported to be a large risk factor for revisions (HR >2.7) in three studies with both varus and valgus malalignment having a greater risk of revision [23, 39, 40]. Two American studies reported an increased risk of revision with varus tibial malalignment (<90°) (HR 10.6, 95 % CI 5.4 to 20.6, $p < 0.0001$; OR 3.0, $p = 0.04$ respectively) [23, 39]. Valgus femoral malalignment also showed an increased risk with ≥8° of valgus (HR 5.1, 95 % CI 2.8 to 9.5, $p < 0.0001$) [40].

Bone quality
As bone stock is a key determinant of the type of implant used and possible peri-prosthetic fracture, bone quality is an important surgical consideration. Only one study examined bisphosphonate use and reported a

Table 4 Implant type/technique and adjusted risk of revision[a]

Author(s)/year	Implant type/technique	Reference	Hazard ratio (95 % CI) unless otherwise stated
Abdel, M. et al., 2011 [36]	Cruciate Status:		
	Posterior cruciate-retaining	Posterior cruciate-stabilizing	0.5, 95 % CI 0.4 - 0.6, $p < 0.001$
Rand, J. et al., 2003 [19]	Cruciate Status:		
	Posterior Stabilized	Posterior cruciate-retaining	2.6, 95 % CI 2.1 - 3.5, $p < 0.0001$
	Constrained condylar	Posterior cruciate-retaining	2.1, 95 % CI 0.9 - 4.9, $p = 0.08$
Stiehl J. et al., 2006 [24]	Cruciate Status		
	PCRs	Rotating platform	1.552, 95 % CI 1.157 - 2.081
	BCRs		2.188, 95 % CI 1.454 - 3.294
Gøthesen, O. et al., 2013 [17]	Implant Type:		
	Duracon	Profix	2.6, 95 % CI 1.9 - 3.4, $p < 0.001$
	LCS Classic HR		1.3, 95 % CI 1.0 - 1.6, $p = 0.017$
	LCS Complete		1.5, 95 % CI 1.1 - 1.9, $p = 0.002$
	AGC Universal		1.6, 95 % CI 1.3 - 2.0, $p < 0.001$
Lygre, S. et al., 2010 [37]	Implant Type:		Relative Risk =
	NR Tricon	NR AGC Universal	1.67, 95 % CI 1.24–2.24, $p = 0.001$,
	NR Genesis 1		1.43, 95 % CI 1.14–1.79, $p = 0.002$,
	NR Duracon		1.45, 95 % CI 1.05–1.99, $p = 002$.
	NR Profix		0.66, 95 % CI 0.52–0.82, $p < 0.001$,
	NR e.motion		0.09, 95 % CI 0.02–0.37, $p = 0.001$,
	NR AGC anatomic		0.66, 95 % CI 0.45–0.99, $p = 0.04$,
	PR AGC universal		0.48, 95 % CI 0.27–0.83, $p = 0.009$,
	PR NexGen		0.40, 95 % CI 0.22–0.74, $p = 0.004$.
Namba R. et al., 2013 [28]	Implant Type:		
	Rotate LCS	Fixed PS	2.07, 95 % CI 1.53 - 2.80, $p < 0.001$
	High flexion	Yes versus No	1.76, 95 % CI 1.29 - 2.41, $p < 0.001$
Namba R. et al., 2012 [27]	Implant Type:		
	LCS	Fixed	2.01, 95 % CI 1.41 - 2.86, $p < 0.001$
Inacio M. et al., 2013 [54]	Bearing or inserts:		
	CoCr-HXLPE	CoCr-CPE	NS 1.2, 95 % CI 0.9 - 1.5, $p > 0.05$
	OZ-CPE	COCr-CPE	NS 1.4, 95 % CI 0.3 - 5.9, $p > 0.05$

Abbreviations: RR relative risk, NS not significant, BCR bicruciate preservation, PCR posterior cruciate retention, (PR) patella resurfaced, (NR) patella non resurfaced, LCS low contact stress, OZ oxidized zirconium, CoCR cobalt chromium, CPE conventional polyethylene, HXLPE highly crosslinked polyethylene;
[a]See Additional file 2 for further detail

protective effect for risk for revision (HR 0.40, 95 % CI 0.15 to 1.07, $p = 0.068$) [41] recommending its use for those patients with the diagnosis of osteoarthritis.

Health services

Of the 3 articles that reported hospital volume in Canada, USA and Norway, low volume hospitals had an increased risk for revision of primary TKAs [25, 42, 22]. The definition of low volume, however, varied from less than 25 to less than 50 procedures annually. Further, Harrysson et al. found that the risk of revision decreased when comparing the year of surgery to the previous year

(HR 0.92, 95 % CI 0.89 to 0.96, $p < 0.0001$) over a 10 year time period [43].

Length of surgery for the primary TKA was also found to have a significant association with revision risk in TKA primary surgery >240 min (OR 1.34, 95 % CI 1.07 to 1.67, $p = 0.012$) as compared to <240 min, 150 to 180 min (OR 1.31, 95 % CI 1.09 to 1.57, $p = 0.004$) as compared to 120 to 150 min and <90 min (OR 1.47, 95 % CI 1.10–1.95, $p = 0.008$) as compared to 120 to 150 min [44].

Discussion

We identified 42 articles that reported risk factors for TKA revision using risk-adjusted analyses. Demographic, medical and implant factors were identified as risk factors for revision of TKA ranging from short-term (<5 years) to long-term follow-up (20+ years). Risk factors were derived largely from registry data, which inherently restricts the type of risk factors examined.

Primary TKA has been consistently identified as a successful surgery with high survival rates even at 10 and 20 years post-surgery. Others have reported rates of 1.26 revisions per 100 observed component years for TKA as compared to 1.29 revisions per 100 observed component years for total hip replacements and 3.29 revisions per 100 component years for total ankle replacements [45]. Given the success of the surgery, it has been suggested the focus of research should perhaps shift to patient selection for these procedures to optimize outcomes and health resources [46].

The trend of increasing revision rates will likely increase [46, 47]. This information was especially relevant given that the 45–64 year old cohort is one of the fastest growing demographics [48, 49]. Further, this age cohort demonstrated an increased use of TKA and will require a longer life expectancy for the TKA, an important consideration when planning for future allocation of resources [46, 49]. The increased risk for revision in the younger population must be further examined to determine if it is indeed age that is the risk factor or if age is a proxy for higher activity levels or increased expectations in this younger patient population.

Comorbidities such as diabetes, cardiovascular disease, hypertension, obesity, cancer and lung disease were found to increase the risk for revision. These findings are particularly meaningful given the increasing prevalence of multi-morbidity and the challenge of surgical management of patients with other chronic diseases [50, 51]. Further investigation of management programs of secondary chronic diseases such as hypertension, obesity and diabetes in patients with primary TKA is warranted.

Often heterogeneity was found among the reported results for other risk factors for TKA revision. For example, mixed results were reported regarding sex, primary diagnosis, BMI, patellar resurfacing and implant components suggesting a need for further investigation. Some consensus existed, however, regarding cemented prostheses which had a lower risk of revision than uncemented or hybrid in spite of an initial goal of uncemented fixation to decrease complications associated with aseptic loosening [16, 19, 35]. Increased surgery length and low hospital volumes were also found to negatively affect revision rates which is important information to consider in health resource allocation and planning.

In spite of a wide body of literature published on various surgical factors, many articles were of low quality and few included risk-adjusted analysis. The majority of included articles (41/42) were retrospective prognostic articles limiting the quality of the articles to an Oxford level III. Because the majority of data (26/42) was taken from registry data, the data were often limited to basic demographic information such as age, gender and BMI and did not evaluate pain and functional measures (see Additional file 2). An inherent limitation of these large, population-based registries is that demographic, surgical and health services data over decades have typically been evaluated and do not provide patient-reported outcomes or patient-reported experience measures which are central to clinical outcomes of TKA. Finally, findings were derived from two geographical populations, 26 in the USA and 11 in Nordic countries. External validity to other populations is uncertain because of different healthcare systems and potentially different prostheses.

In spite of an extensive search strategy and a strong systematic approach to undertaking this systematic review, identifying risk factors for revision was challenging because of low revision rates in the first 10 years following surgery. Most articles had follow-up periods of <10 years which reflected high survival rates of TKA. Due to these high survival rates, it can be a lengthy and costly process to undertake studies for the appropriate duration to acquire accurate information on revisions. Another consideration is that many early revisions occurring within 10 years are often related to surgical techniques and few articles made the distinction between early and later revisions. Finally, as TKAs are most often performed on an older population, the development of other chronic conditions and mortality poses a challenge to long-term follow-up.

Conclusions

Current literature suggests an increased risk for revision following TKA is associated with younger age, greater number of comorbidities, African American race, uncemented components, increased surgery duration, and lower volume hospitals. This scoping review allowed us to identify areas where consistent results were found but also highlight areas with heterogeneous results or insufficient data where further research is required. The findings also demonstrate the need for large scale and high quality investigations examining factors that increase the risk for revision following TKA including patient-reported outcomes and patient-reported experience measures. Given the increasing numbers of TKA procedures and revisions, information on risk factors for revisions following TKAs is necessary for appropriate interventions to be delivered in a timely manner and for the development of effective health care policy.

Competing interests
The authors declare that they have no competing interests.

Authors' contributions
All authors were involved in conception and design, analysis and interpretation of the data, drafting and revisions of the article and had final approval of the article.

Acknowledgments
Special gratitude is expressed to Liz Dennett, MLIS for her assistance with the extensive search.

Role of funding source
No funding was received for this work.

Author details
[1]Department of Physical Therapy, University of Alberta, Rm 2-50 Corbett Hall, Edmonton, AB T6G 2G4, Canada. [2]Alberta Health Services, Edmonton, Canada. [3]Canadian Agency for Drugs and Technologies in Health, Ottawa, Canada.

References
1. Ethgen O, Bruyere O, Richy F, Dardennes C, Reginster JY. Health-related quality of life in total hip and total knee arthroplasty. A qualitative and systematic review of the literature. J Bone Joint Surg Am. 2004;86-A:963–74.
2. Jones CA, Pohar S. Health-related quality of life after total joint arthroplasty: a scoping review. Clin Geriatr Med. 2012;28:395–429.
3. Losina E, Walensky RP, Kessler CL, Emrani PS, Reichmann WM, Wright EA, et al. Cost-effectiveness of total knee arthroplasty in the United States: patient risk and hospital volume. Arch Intern Med. 2009;169:1113–21.
4. Jenkins PJ, Clement ND, Hamilton DF, Gaston P, Patton JT, Howie CR. Predicting the cost-effectiveness of total hip and knee replacement: a health economic analysis. Bone Joint J. 2013;95-B:115–21.
5. Hawker G, Wright J, Coyte P, Paul J, Dittus R, Croxford R, et al. Health-related quality of life after knee replacement. J Bone Joint Surg Am. 1998;80:163–73.
6. Kurtz S, Ong K, Lau E, Mowat F, Halpern M. Projections of primary and revision hip and knee arthroplasty in the United States from 2005 to 2030. J Bone Joint Surg Am. 2007;89:780–5.
7. Martin KR, Kuh D, Harris TB, Guralnik JM, Coggon D, Wills AK. Body mass index, occupational activity, and leisure-time physical activity: an exploration of risk factors and modifiers for knee osteoarthritis in the 1946 British birth cohort. BMC Musculoskelet Disord. 2013;14:219.
8. Canadian Institute of Health Information. Hip and Knee Replacements in Canada: Canadian Joint Replacement Registry 2014 Annual Report. 2014. https://secure.cihi.ca/free_products/CJRR%202014%20Annual%20Report_EN-web.pdf. Accessed 10 May 2015.
9. Hamilton DF, Howie CR, Burnett R, Simpson AH, Patton JT. Dealing with the predicted increase in demand for revision total knee arthroplasty: challenges, risks and opportunities. Bone Joint J. 2015;97-B:723–8.
10. Liodakis E, Bergeron SG, Zukor DJ, Huk OL, Epure LM, Antoniou J. Perioperative complications and length of stay after revision total hip and knee arthroplasties: An analysis of the nsqip database. J Arthroplast. 2015;30:1868–71.
11. Dieterich JD, Fields AC, Moucha CS. Short term outcomes of revision total knee arthroplasty. J Arthroplast. 2014;29:2163–6.
12. Morrison A, Moulton K, Clark M, Polisena J, Fiander M, Mierzwinsjii-Urban. English-Language Restriction When Conducting Systematic Review-Based Meta-Analyses: Systematic Review of Published Studies. Canadian Agency for Drugs and Technologies in Health. 2009. https://www.cadth.ca/media/pdf/H0478_Language_Restriction_Systematic_Review_Pub_Studies_e.pdf. Accessed 11 May 2015.
13. OCEBM Levels of Evidence Working Group. The Oxford 2011 Levels of Evidence. Oxford. Centre for Evidence-Based Medicine. http://www.cebm.net/wp-content/uploads/2014/06/CEBM-Levels-of-Evidence-2.1.pdf. Accessed 10 May 2015.
14. Howick J, Chalmers I, Greenhalgh T, Heneghan C, Liberati A, Moschetti I et al. The 2011 Oxford CEBM Evidence Levels of Evidence (Introductory Document).
Oxford Centre for Evidence-Based Medicine. http://www.cebm.net/2011-oxford-cebm-levels-evidence-introductory-document/. Accessed 10 May 2015.
15. Scottish Intercollegiate Guidelines Network. SIGN Methodology Checklist 3: Cohort Studies. http://www.sign.ac.uk/methodology/checklists.html. Accessed 5 Jan 2014.
16. Gioe TJ, Novak C, Sinner P, Ma W, Mehle S. Knee arthroplasty in the young patient. Clin Orthop Rel Res. 2007;464:83–7.
17. Gothesen O, Espehaug B, Havelin L, Petursson G, Lygre S, Ellison P, et al. Survival rates and causes of revision in cemented primary total knee replacement: a report from the Norwegian Arthroplasty Register 1994–2009. Bone Joint J. 2013;95-B:636–42.
18. Vessely MB, Whaley AL, Harmsen WS, Schleck CD, Berry DJ. The Chitranjan Ranawat award: long-term survivorship and failure modes of 1000 cemented condylar total knee arthroplasties. Clin Orthop Rel Res. 2006;452:28–34.
19. Rand JA, Trousdale RT, Ilstrup DM, Harmsen WS. Factors affecting the durability of primary total knee prostheses. J Bone Joint Surg Am. 2003;85A:259–65.
20. Himanen AK, Belt EA, Lehto MU, Hamalainen MM. A comparison of survival of moulded monoblock and modular tibial components of 751 AGC total knee replacements in the treatment of rheumatoid arthritis. J Bone Joint Surg (Br). 2007;89B:609–14.
21. Jamsen E, Peltola M, Eskelinen A, Lehto MU. Comorbid diseases as predictors of survival of primary total hip and knee replacements: a nationwide register-based study of 96 754 operations on patients with primary osteoarthritis. Ann Rheum Dis. 2013;72:1975–82.
22. Manley M, Ong K, Lau E, Kurtz SM. Total knee arthroplasty survivorship in the United States Medicare population: effect of hospital and surgeon procedure volume. J Arthroplasty. 2009;24:1061–7.
23. Fang DM, Ritter MA, Davis KE. Coronal alignment in total knee arthroplasty: just how important is it? J Arthroplasty. 2009;24:39–43.
24. Stiehl JB, Hamelynck KJ, Voorhorst PE. International multi-centre survivorship analysis of mobile bearing total knee arthroplasty. Int Orthop. 2006;30:190–9.
25. Kreder HJ, Grosso P, Williams JI, Jaglal S, Axcell T, Wai EK, et al. Provider volume and other predictors of outcome after total knee arthroplasty: a population study in Ontario. Can J Surg. 2003;46:15–22.
26. Himanen AK, Belt E, Nevalainen J, Hamalainen M, Lehto M. Survival of the AGC total knee arthroplasty is similar for arthrosis and rheumatoid arthritis. Finnish Arthroplasty Register report on 8,467 operations carried out between 1985 and 1999. Acta Orthop. 2005;76:85–8.
27. Namba RS, Inacio MC, Paxton EW, Ake CF, Wang C, Gross TP, et al. Risk of revision for fixed versus mobile-bearing primary total knee replacements. J Bone Joint Surgery AM. 2012;94:1929–35.
28. Namba RS, Cafri G, Khatod M, Inacio MC, Brox TW, Paxton EW. Risk factors for total knee arthroplasty aseptic revision. J Arthroplasty. 2013;28:122–7.
29. Blum MA, Singh JA, Lee GC, Richardson D, Chen W, Ibrahim SA. Patient race and surgical outcomes after total knee arthroplasty: an analysis of a large regional database. Arthrit Care Res. 2013;65:414–20.
30. Schrama JC, Espehaug B, Hallan G, Engesaeter LB, Furnes O, Havelin LI, et al. Risk of revision for infection in primary total hip and knee arthroplasty in patients with rheumatoid arthritis compared with osteoarthritis: a prospective, population-based study on 108,786 hip and knee joint arthroplasties from the Norwegian Arthroplasty Register. Arthrit Care Res. 2010;62:473–9.
31. Bini SA, Chen Y, Khatod M, Paxton EW. Does pre-coating total knee tibial implants affect the risk of aseptic revision? Bone Joint J BR. 2013;95-B:367–70.
32. Bordini B, Stea S, Cremonini S, Viceconti M, De PR, Toni A. Relationship between obesity and early failure of total knee prostheses. BMC Musculoskelet Disord. 2009;10:29.
33. Peltola M, Malmivaara A, Paavola M. Introducing a knee endoprosthesis model increases risk of early revision surgery. Clin Orthop Related Res. 2012; 470:1711–7.
34. King KB, Findley TW, Williams AE, Bucknell AL. Veterans with diabetes receive arthroplasty more frequently and at a younger age. Clin Orthop Rel Res. 2013;471:3049–54.
35. Julin J, Jamsen E, Puolakka T, Konttinen YT, Moilanen T. Younger age increases the risk of early prosthesis failure following primary total knee replacement for osteoarthritis. A follow-up study of 32,019 total knee replacements in the Finnish Arthroplasty Register. Acta Orthop. 2010;81: 413–9.
36. Abdel MP, Morrey ME, Jensen MR, Morrey BE. Increased long-term survival of posterior cruciate-retaining versus posterior cruciate-stabilizing total knee replacements. J Bone Joint Surg Am. 2011;93A:2072–8.

37. Lygre SHL, Espehaug B, Havelin LI, Furnes O, Vollset SE. Pain and function in patients after primary unicompartmental and total knee arthroplasty. J Bone Joint Surg Am. 2010;92A:2890–7.

38. Robertsson O, Ranstam J. No bias of ignored bilaterality when analysing the revision risk of knee prostheses: analysis of a population based sample of 44,590 patients with 55,298 knee prostheses from the national Swedish Knee Arthroplasty Register. BMC Musculoskelet Disord. 2003;4:1.

39. Ritter MA, Davis KE, Meding JB, Pierson JL, Berend ME, Malinzak RA. The effect of alignment and BMI on failure of total knee replacement. J Bone Joint Surg Am. 2011;93A:1588–96.

40. Ritter MA, Davis KE, Davis P, Farris A, Malinzak RA, Berend ME, et al. Preoperative malalignment increases risk of failure after total knee arthroplasty. J Bone Joint Surg Am. 2013;95A:126–31.

41. Prieto-Alhambra D, Javaid MK, Judge A, Murray D, Carr A, Cooper C, et al. Association between bisphosphonate use and implant survival after primary total arthroplasty of the knee or hip: population based retrospective cohort study. BMJ. 2011;343:d7222.

42. Badawy M, Espehaug B, Indrekvam K, Engesaeter LB, Havelin LI, Furnes O. Influence of hospital volume on revision rate after total knee arthroplasty with cement. J Bone Joint Surg Am. 2013;95, e131.

43. Harrysson OL, Robertsson O, Nayfeh JF. Higher cumulative revision rate of knee arthroplasties in younger patients with osteoarthritis. Clin Orthop Rel Res. 2004;421:162–8.

44. Ong KL, Lau E, Manley M, Kurtz SM. Effect of procedure duration on total hip arthroplasty and total knee arthroplasty survivorship in the United States Medicare population. J Arthroplasty. 2008;23:127–32.

45. Labek G, Thaler M, Janda W, Agreiter M, Stockl B. Revision rates after total joint replacement: cumulative results from worldwide joint register datasets. J Bone Joint Surg (Br). 2011;93:293–7.

46. Carr AJ, Robertsson O, Graves S, Price AJ, Arden NK, Judge A, et al. Knee replacement. Lancet. 2012;379:1331–40.

47. Santaguida PL, Hawker GA, Hudak PL, Glazier R, Mahomed NN, Kreder HJ, et al. Patient characteristics affecting the prognosis of total hip and knee joint arthroplasty: a systematic review. Can J Surg. 2008;51:428–36.

48. Statistics Canada. Population Projections for Canada (2013 to 2063), Provinces and Territories (2013 to 2038). 2014. http://www.statcan.gc.ca/pub/91-520-x/91-520-x2014001-eng.htm. Accessed 8 January 2016.

49. Losina E, Thornhill TS, Rome BN, Wright J, Katz JN. The dramatic increase in total knee replacement utilization rates in the United States cannot be fully explained by growth in population size and the obesity epidemic. J Bone Joint Surg Am. 2012;94:201–7.

50. Public Health Agency of Canada. Preventing Chronic Disease Strategic Plan 2013–2016. 2013. http://publications.gc.ca/collections/collection_2014/aspc-phac/HP35-39-2013-eng.pdf. Accessed 13 January 2016.

51. Hung WW, Ross JS, Boockvar KS, Siu AL. Recent trends in chronic disease, impairment and disability among older adults in the United States. BMC Geriatr. 2011;11:47.

52. Fehring TK, Murphy JA, Hayes TD, Roberts DW, Pomeroy DL, Griffin WL. Factors influencing wear and osteolysis in press-fit condylar modular total knee replacements. Clin Orthop Rel Res. 2004;428:40–50.

53. Gioe TJ, Killeen KK, Grimm K, Mehle S, Scheltema K. Why are total knee replacements revised? analysis of early revision in a community knee implant registry. Clin Orthop Rel Res. 2004;428:100–6.

54. Inacio MC, Cafri G, Paxton EW, Kurtz SM, Namba RS. Alternative bearings in total knee arthroplasty: risk of early revision compared to traditional bearings: an analysis of 62,177 primary cases. Acta Orthop. 2013;84:145–52.

55. Adams AL, Paxton EW, Wang JQ, Johnson ES, Bayliss EA, Ferrara A, et al. Surgical outcomes of total knee replacement according to diabetes status and glycemic control, 2001 to 2009. J Bone Joint Surg Am. 2013;95:481–7.

56. Berend ME, Davis PJ, Ritter MA, Keating EM, Faris PM, Meding JB, et al. "Thicker" polyethylene bearings are associated with higher failure rates in primary total knee arthroplasty. J Arthroplasty. 2010;25:17–20.

57. Curtin B, Malkani A, Lau E, Kurtz S, Ong K. Revision after total knee arthroplasty and unicompartmental knee arthroplasty in the Medicare population. J Arthroplasty. 2012;27:1480–6.

58. Dy CJ, Wilkinson JD, Tamariz L, Scully SP. Influence of preoperative cardiovascular risk factor clusters on complications of total joint arthroplasty. Am J Orthop. 2011;40:560–5.

59. Furnes O, Espehaug B, Lie SA, Vollset SE, Engesaeter LB, Havelin LI. Early failures among 7,174 primary total knee replacements: a follow-up study from the Norwegian Arthroplasty Register 1994–2000. Acta Orthop Scand. 2002;73:117–29.

60. Gothesen O, Espehaug B, Havelin L, Petursson G, Furnes O. Short-term outcome of 1,465 computer-navigated primary total knee replacements 2005–2008. Acta Orthop. 2011;82:293–300.

61. Hooper GJ, Rothwell AG, Hooper NM, Frampton C. The relationship between the American Society of Anesthesiologists physical rating and outcome following total hip and knee arthroplasty an analysis of the New Zealand Joint Registry. J Bone Joint Surg Am. 2012;94A:1065–70.

62. Johnson TC, Tatman PJ, Mehle S, Gioe TJ. Revision surgery for patellofemoral problems: should we always resurface? Clin Orthop Rel Res. 2012;470:211–9.

63. McCleery MA, Leach WJ, Norwood T. Rates of infection and revision in patients with renal disease undergoing total knee replacement in Scotland. J Bone Joint Surg (Br). 2010;92:1535–9.

64. Parratte S, Pagnano MW, Trousdale RT, Berry DJ. Effect of postoperative mechanical axis alignment on the fifteen-year survival of modern, cemented total knee replacements. J Bone Joint Surg Am. 2010;92A:2143–9.

65. Robertsson O, Knutson K, Lewold S, Goodman S, Lidgren L. Knee arthroplasty in rheumatoid arthritis a report from the Swedish Knee Arthroplasty Register on 4,381 primary operations 1985–1995. Acta Orthop Scand. 1997;68:545–53.

7

The likelihood of total knee arthroplasty following arthroscopic surgery for osteoarthritis

Amelia R. Winter[1], Jamie E. Collins[1,3] and Jeffrey N. Katz[1,2,3,4*]

Abstract

Background: Arthroscopic surgery is a common treatment for knee osteoarthritis (OA), particularly for symptomatic meniscal tear. Many patients with knee OA who have arthroscopies go on to have total knee arthroplasty (TKA). Several individual studies have investigated the interval between knee arthroscopy and TKA. Our objective was to summarize published literature on the risk of TKA following knee arthroscopy, the duration between arthroscopy and TKA, and risk factors for TKA following knee arthroscopy.

Methods: We searched PubMed, Embase, and Web of Science for English language manuscripts reporting TKA following arthroscopy for knee OA. We identified 511 manuscripts, of which 20 met the inclusion criteria and were used for analysis. We compared the cumulative incidence of TKA following arthroscopy in each study arm, stratifying by type of data source (registry vs. clinical), and whether the study was limited to older patients (≥ 50) or those with more severe radiographic OA. We estimated cumulative incidence of TKA following arthroscopy by dividing the number of TKAs among persons who underwent arthroscopy by the number of persons who underwent arthroscopy. Annual incidence was calculated by dividing cumulative incidence by the mean years of follow-up.

Results: Overall, the annual incidence of TKA after arthroscopic surgery for OA was 2.62% (95% CI 1.73–3.51%). We calculated the annual incidence of TKA following arthroscopy in four separate groups defined by data source (registry vs. clinical cohort) and whether the sample was selected for disease progression (either age or OA severity). In unselected registry studies the annual TKA incidence was 1.99% (95% CI 1.03–2.96%), compared to 3.89% (95% CI 0.69–7.09%) in registry studies of older patients. In unselected clinical cohorts the annual incidence was 2.02% (95% CI 0.67–3.36%), while in clinical cohorts with more severe OA the annual incidence was 4.13% (95% CI 1.81–6.44%). The mean and median duration between arthroscopy and TKA (years) were 3.4 and 2.0 years.

Conclusions: Clinicians and patients considering knee arthroscopy should discuss the likelihood of subsequent TKA as they weigh risks and benefits of surgery. Patients who are older or have more severe OA are at particularly high risk of TKA.

Keywords: Osteoarthritis, Total knee arthroplasty, Arthroscopic partial meniscectomy, Arthroscopy

Background

Osteoarthritis (OA) is a debilitating disease, affecting over 40 million people in the United States [1, 2]. Of those affected, approximately 14 million have symptomatic knee OA [3], which presents with pain, loss of knee joint function, and loss of valued activities. In addition, about 90% of those with symptomatic knee OA have meniscal tears (MT) documented on magnetic resonance imaging (MRI) [4]. However, no available treatments modify the structural progression associated with OA. Symptoms are generally managed with conservative therapies (e.g., nonsteroidal anti-inflammatory drugs (NSAIDs), exercise, physical therapy). Patients and their physicians often turn to surgical treatments to address progressive pain and disability, including arthroscopy and total knee arthroplasty (TKA).

Over 600,000 arthroscopic partial meniscectomies (APM) are performed each year in the United States [5],

* Correspondence: jnkatz@partners.org
[1]Orthopaedic and Arthritis Center for Outcomes Research (OrACORe), Department of Orthopedic Surgery, Boston, MA, USA
[2]Division of Rheumatology, Immunology and Allergy, Brigham and Women's Hospital, 60 Fenwood St, Suite 5016, Boston, MA 02115, USA
Full list of author information is available at the end of the article

most commonly on persons over 45 with MT [5, 6]. The benefit of arthroscopic surgery in patients with OA is uncertain and debated. Moseley et al. showed that sham surgery and arthroscopic surgery for OA had similar pain relief and functional improvement up to 2 years post-surgery [7]. Kirkley and colleagues showed that arthroscopy and a conservative exercise regimen had similar symptomatic and functional outcomes in persons with knee OA [8]. With respect to MT in the setting of OA, several trials demonstrated that surgery was not superior to nonoperative therapy or sham surgery in intention to treat analyses [9–12], while one trial showed a benefit for surgery [13]. Thus, arthroscopic surgery is felt to be ineffective for OA per se, while the effectiveness of APM in persons with MT and concomitant OA is debated [14].

Often, people who undergo arthroscopic surgery for osteoarthritis progress to TKA. While some studies suggest that up to 20% of patients undergo TKA within one year of arthroscopy [15], other studies have shown TKA rates under 5% [16]. The various studies of the rate of TKA after arthroscopy have not been summarized, to our knowledge. Such a summary of the risk of TKA following arthroscopy and the duration between arthroscopy and TKA would be helpful for clinicians to better advise patients and their families on appropriate treatments plans. Surgery is expensive – about $2 billion dollars are spent on arthroscopy for OA [17] and over $10 billion dollars are spent on TKAs each year [18]. Therefore, improved knowledge of the risk for TKA following arthroscopy could also lead to better resource allocation for OA.

We performed a systematic review of the literature on the risk of TKA following arthroscopic surgeries for OA. We expected to see older patients and those with more severe OA, progress to TKA more quickly after surgery.

Methods
Definition of search terms
A search by title was performed on PubMed, Embase, and Web of Science using the major search terms: *osteoarthritis, knee; arthroscopy; and arthroplasty* (see Additional file 1: Table S1 for search strings). The search was performed in September 2016 and titles were downloaded to EndNote. One reviewer (ARW) manually screened titles for inclusion and exclusion criteria, arriving at a final list of titles. For these titles, the reviewer assessed abstracts for inclusion and exclusion criteria. For each abstract that was not excluded, the full manuscript was read to determine ultimate inclusion in the final analysis. A second reviewer confirmed that the final selected manuscripts met inclusion criteria.

Inclusion and exclusion criteria
We sought studies investigating the rate of arthroplasty after arthroscopic knee surgery for osteoarthritis. Therefore, inclusion criteria included: English language and human studies on the risk of TKA occurring following arthroscopic procedures for knee OA. Manuscripts were excluded if they were duplicates, written in a language other than English, or conducted on animals. Studies were also excluded if they examined only arthroscopy or arthroplasty rather than the risk of arthroplasty following arthroscopy. Case studies and studies with cohorts of mean age < 40 were also excluded. Confusion regarding inclusion of a study was resolved by consulting with the senior author (JNK).

Data abstraction
From the manuscripts, the reviewer (ARW) extracted the following information (if available): author, year, title, administrative data (e.g., clinical cohort or registry), country, patient selection criteria (e.g. age, KL grade), subgroup information, size of analysis group, mean age, analysis method (e.g., cumulative incidence), duration between arthroscopy and TKA, duration of follow-up, percentage of TKA, and study arm population description. Another reviewer abstracted key data (e.g., country, administrative data, patient selection criteria, follow-up years, analysis group, and total TKA numbers) from the included studies. The results from both abstractions were compared and found to be the same.

Categorization of studies
We examined the cumulative incidence of TKA following knee arthroscopy in specific patient subgroups. These included source of data (administrative data registries vs. clinical cohort studies), OA severity, older age (e.g., selection for population ≥ 50), and country. Some of the clinical cohort studies recruited patients with advanced OA, (i.e., KL grade ≥ 3 or Outerbridge score ≥ 2). We defined these study arms as "Clinical Cohort – More Severe OA." One study (Lyu et al., 2015) was included among the "Clinical Cohort – More Severe OA" group as its patient population was over 75% KL grade 3 or higher. Some registry studies were restricted to subjects with age greater than 50. We referred to these as "Registry – Older Age." We created a final categorization combining the source of data and selection criteria: "Registry – Unselected," "Registry – Older Age," "Clinical Cohort – Unselected," and "Clinical Cohort – More Severe OA." For countries, we combined England and Scotland as "U.K."

Quality assessment
We used the Quality Assessment Tool for Observational Cohort and Cross-Sectional Studies developed by investigators at the National Heartt, Lung and Blood Intitute (NHLBI), based upon work done at the Agency for Health Care Research and Quality. (https://www.nhlbi.nih.gov/health-pro/guidelines/in-develop/cardiovascular-risk-reduction/tools/cohort) [19]. This measure includes 14 items

relevant to the quality of cohort studies, with emphasis on explicit specification of sample characteristics, exposures, primary outcomes and potential confounders. Two authors performed the assessment independently and resolved any disagreements.

Analyses

For studies that did not provide cumulative incidence data, we calculated cumulative incidence using the number of TKAs divided by the number of arthroscopic patients included for follow-up analysis. We first examined the association between the type of data source – registry vs. cohort – and TKA rates. Then, we evaluated the association between study category ("Registry – Unselected," "Registry – Older Age," "Clinical Cohort – Unselected," and "Clinical Cohort – More Severe OA," as described above) and annual incidence. In secondary analyses, we evaluated the difference between TKA annual incidence in unselected study arms (clinical and registry) vs. selected study arms, regardless of registry status. We compared studies in which mean age of the study was >65 to those with mean age < 65.

We divided cumulative incidence of TKA by mean years of follow-up to obtain an annual incidence estimate. We computed exact confidence intervals for each yearly incidence value. We used a logistic random-effects model to create an overall combined estimate of annual TKA incidence across all studies and to evaluate the effect of study-level characteristics on TKA incidence. This approach allows for studies with zero cells (i.e., 0% incidence rate) without requiring an ad-hoc adjustment [20]. All analyses were conducted using SAS 9.4 (SAS Institute, Cary NC).

Results

Five hundred eleven unique articles were found using our search terms and three search engines. After screening the titles, we were left with 328 articles whose abstracts were subsequently reviewed. Over half of the articles excluded did not have arthroscopic surgery before TKA (36%) or did not report TKA (24%). Fifty-five articles underwent full article review. Thirty-five of the manuscripts were excluded from our analysis: 11 were not written in English, 2 did not report on arthroscopic procedures before TKA, 3 did not report on TKA, and 19 were excluded for other reasons, such as mixed cohort (e.g., OA and post-traumatic arthritis), secondary sources, or insufficient data on methodology.

These exclusions left 20 articles for the analysis (Fig. 1). The 20 studies contained 28 unique study arms (Table 1). The 28 study arms were reported from eight countries. The U.S.A. accounted for 15 of the 28, the U.K. for 5, Canada for 3, and Australia, Belgium, Italy, South Korea, and Taiwan for one each. The quality assessment documented relatively little variability in quality. Essentially

all the studies stated the research question clearly, specified the population and defined the exposure and outcome explicitly. Only one study provided a power calculation. Rates of participation among eligible subject and rates of follow up were generally high, particularly for administrative data studies in which participation and follow-up rates are typically 100%. Some of the quality items did not apply to the studies we reviewed because all subjects in our studies were 'exposed' (had arthroscopy).

Overall, the yearly incidence for TKA after arthroscopic surgery for OA was 2.62% (95% CI 1.73–3.51%). The mean and median duration between arthroscopy and TKA (years) were 3.4 and 2.0 years. From our 28 study arms, we identified sixteen clinical cohorts and twelve registry samples. The clinical cohort studies had a yearly TKA incidence of 2.94% (95% CI 1.54–4.33%), compared to the registry studies, which had an incidence of 2.36% (95% CI 1.26–3.46%) ($p = 0.5048$). We examined separately the risk of TKA in four distinct subgroups: "Registry – Unselected," "Registry – Older Age," "Clinical Cohort – Unselected," and "Clinical Cohort – More Severe OA." The four subgroups are shown in Fig. 2.

Registry - unselected

A total of nine study arms were unselected registries, with a median of 6972 (range 842–159,975) patients per study arm (Table 1). Of these, the average yearly incidence for TKA was 1.99% (95% CI 1.03 2.96%) (Fig. 2).

Registry – Older age

A total of three study arms were registries using data from patients ≥50 years old, with a median of 6212 (range 3033–40,804) patients per study arm (Table 1). Of these studies, the average yearly incidence for TKA was 3.89% (95% CI 0.69–7.09%) (Fig. 2).

Clinical cohort – Unselected

A total of seven study arms were unselected clinical cohorts, with a median of 42 (range 8–183) patients per study arm (Table 1). Of these studies, the average yearly incidence for TKA was 2.02% (95% CI 0.67–3.36%) (Fig. 2).

Clinical cohort – More severe OA

A total of nine study arms were clinical cohorts selecting for patients with more severe OA on the basis of KL grade or Outerbridge score, with a median of 69 (range 68–844) patients per study arm (Table 1). Of these studies, the average yearly incidence for TKA was 4.13% (95% CI 1.81–6.44%) (Fig. 2).

Comparisons: Age and OA severity

We evaluated the association between TKA incidence and study inclusion criteria using a logistic random-effects model. We found that selected studies - those

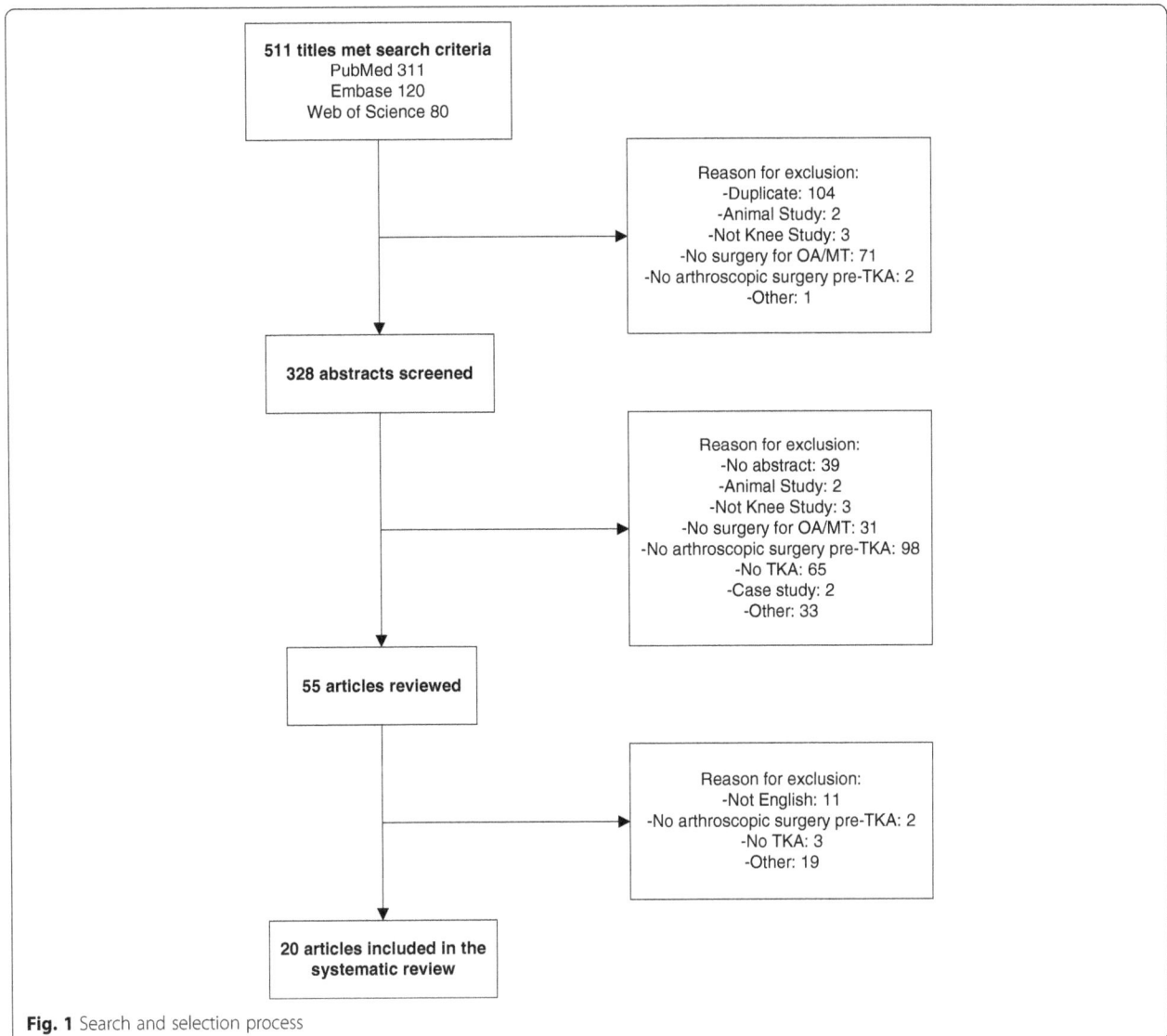

Fig. 1 Search and selection process

that selected subjects based on OA severity or age - were twice as likely to undergo TKA compared to unselected studies (4.05% compared to 2.00%; $p = 0.0243$). Studies of subject with a mean age of less than 65 had a yearly incidence of 1.87% (95% CI 1.16–2.57%) compared to 5.13% (95% CI 2.61–7.64%) for those with mean age over 65. This difference was statistically significant ($p = 0.0027$).

Discussion

We evaluated published literature on the risk of TKA in patients undergoing knee arthroscopy. A concern about the use of arthroscopic surgery in the setting of OA and OA with meniscal tear is that APM may lead to more rapid OA progression, leading to TKA more quickly [1, 15]. We found that on average the risk of TKA following arthroscopy was about 2% per year and that the mean and medican duration between arthroscopy and TKA were 3.4

and 2.0 years respectively. Further, study arms of patients who were older or had more advanced radiographic OA at the time of arthroscopy had two-fold higher risk of TKA than unselected study arms. These findings should be viewed in the context of other documented risk factors for OA progression including older age, female gender, varus and valgus malalignment and bone marrow lesions, among others [21].

Our findings are consistent with studies showing that OA severity and age are associated with TKA [22–32]. Indeed, surgeons may be reluctant to offer TKA to younger patients, because they face a risk of a revision TKA. Advanced OA is a typical indication for TKA, as embodied in guidelines such as those of the American Academy of Orthopaedic Surgeons [33].

Our study must be interpreted in the context of several limitations. The clinical cohort data provided insight into the KL grades and Outerbridge scores of patients

Table 1 Characteristics of included studies

			Author and Year	Country	Follow-Up (Years)	Mean Duration (years)	Analysis Group	Total TKA	Annual Incidence (%)	Lower 95% CI	Upper 95% CI
Clinical Cohort	Selected for More Severe OA	KL ≥ 3	Bernard et al. (2004) [22]	U.K.	5	Unknown	100	11	2.20%	1.10%	3.90%
		KL = 4	Bin et al. (2008) [34]	South Korea	4	4	68	4	1.36%	0.37%	3.43%
		Outerbridge ≥2	Koyonos et al. (2009)a [16]	U.S.A.	1	0.5	30	1	3.33%	0.08%	17.22%
					1	0	29	0	0.00%	0.00%	11.94%
		KL ≥ 3	Lyu et al. (2015) [35]	Taiwan	1	1	844	116	13.74%	11.49%	16.25%
		KL = 4	Pearse and Craig (2003) [36]	U.K.	4	4	126	39	7.14%	5.13%	9.64%
		KL ≥ 3	Rand et al. (1985) [37]	U.S.A.	2	0.5	87	2	1.15%	0.14%	4.09%
		Outerbridge ≥2	Skedros et al. (2014) [30]	U.S.A.	3	3	42	11	8.73%	4.44%	15.08%
		KL ≥ 3	Steadman et al. (2013) [31]	U.S.A.	10	4.4	69	43	6.23%	4.55%	8.30%
	Unselected		Jackson et al. (2003)a [25]	U.S.A.	5	2	8	0	0.00%	0.00%	8.81%
							32	0	0.00%	0.00%	2.28%
							39	3	1.54%	0.32%	4.43%
							42	12	5.71%	2.99%	9.77%
			McGinley et al. (1999) [27]	U.S.A.	13	7	91	30	2.50%	1.69%	3.55%
			Raaijmaakers et al. (2010) [28]	Belgium	3	1	183	40	6.83%	4.92%	9.18%
			Sansone et al. (2015) [29]	Italy	20	13.3	75	12	0.80%	0.41%	1.39%
Registry	Selected for Older Age	Age > 60	Dearing et al. (2010) [38]	U.K.	9	6	3033	800	2.93%	2.73%	3.14%
		Age > 65	Johanson et al. (2011) [26]	U.S.A.	10	9	40,804	13,261	3.25%	3.20%	3.30%
		Age > 50	Wai et al. (2002) [32]	Canada	3	3	6212	1146	6.15%	5.81%	6.50%
	Unselected		Adelani et al. (2016)a [39]	U.S.A.	4	2	6972	266	0.95%	0.84%	1.07%
							10,645	496	1.16%	1.06%	1.27%
			Fedorka et al. (2014) [23]	U.S.A.	5	Unknown	159,975	8319	1.04%	1.02%	1.06%
			Harris et al. (2013) [40]	Australia	8	2	121,115	9110	0.94%	0.92%	0.96%
				UK 1993		Unknown	6158	985	3.20%	3.00%	3.40%
			Hawker et al. (2008)a [24]	UK 1997	5		9048	1728	3.82%	3.64%	4.00%
				Canada 1993			3803	745	3.92%	3.65%	4.20%
				Canada 1997			3425	712	4.16%	3.86%	4.47%
			Zikria et al. (2016) [41]	U.S.A.	7	Unknown	842	131	2.22%	1.86%	2.63%

aStudies contain multiple unique study arms, which were separated for our analysis; Jackson rows: Severity stages I, II, III, IV

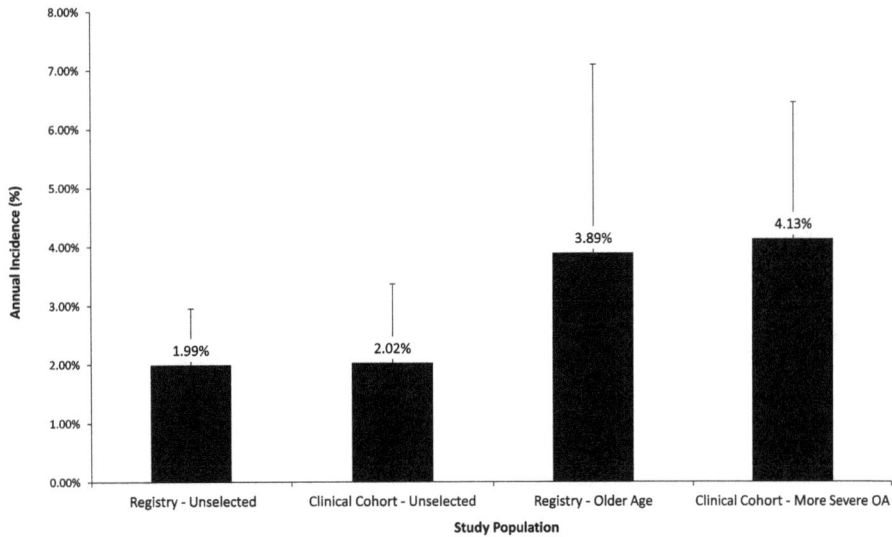

Fig. 2 Mean Annual Incidence of Registry – Unselected, Clinical Cohort – Unselected, Registry – Older Age, and Clinical Cohort – More Severe OA. Each bar represents the estimated yearly incidence of TKA from the logisitc random effects model. The vertical lines represent the 95% confidence intervals

whereas registry data included age but no information on OA severity nor on the details of surgery. The component studies did not perform analyses of subgroups that might be prognostically distinct, such as athletes and non-athletes, or males and females. Similarly, over half of the countries contributed just one cohort. This precludes meaningful analysis of between-country differences. While we performed replicate abstractions of all papers we did not repeat the screening of titles and abstracts in duplicate, creating the theoretical risk of our missing an eligible paper. As reflected in our quality assessment, the studies consistently defined the exposure and outcome explicitly. Since most of the larger studies used administrative data, the follow-up rates were generally 100%. We note as well that some patients with a medical 'need' for TKA (symptomatic, advanced OA) may not have received the procedure because of their own preferences or the practice styles of their physicians or still other reasons. When TKA is used as a health outcome, the role of these patient, physician and health system factors may attenuate the risk associated with specific variables such as prior arthroscopic surgery.

To the best of our knowledge, this is the first systematic review to analyze the yearly TKA incidence rate for those having undergone arthroscopic surgery for knee OA. Quality assessment of the studies generally reflected consistent specification of exposures, outcomes, and study samples and high rates of participation and follow-up. The findings suggest that OA patients undergoing arthroscopy and their physicians should anticipate an annual rate of TKA on the order of 2%, with higher rates among older patients and those with more advanced OA. These findings should be shared with patients when clinicians discuss the advantages and drawbacks of arthroscopy.

Conclusion

Clinicians and patients considering knee arthroscopy should discuss the likelihood of subsequent TKA as they weigh risks and benefits of surgery. Patients who are older or have more severe OA are at particularly high risk of TKA.

Abbreviations
KL: Kellgren-Lawrence; MRI: Magnetic resonance imaging; MT: Meniscal tear; NSAIDs: Nonsteroidal anti-inflammatory drugs; OA: Osteoarthritis; tka: Total knee arthroplasty

Acknowledgements
Not applicable.

Funding
National Institute of Arthritis, Musculoskeletal and Skin Diseases (National Institutes of Health) R01 AR 055557.

Authors' contributions
ARW and JNK developed final question and design of systematic review. ARW searched for and analyzed the included manuscripts, and was a major contributor to writing the manuscript. JEC performed the analysis in SAS, discussed the interpretation with the other authors and critically reviewed the manuscript. JNK consulted on final included manuscripts. All authors read, edited, and approved the final manuscript.

Consent for publication
Not applicable.

Competing interests
The authors declare they have no competing interests.

Author details
[1]Orthopaedic and Arthritis Center for Outcomes Research (OrACORe), Department of Orthopedic Surgery, Boston, MA, USA. [2]Division of Rheumatology, Immunology and Allergy, Brigham and Women's Hospital, 60 Fenwood St, Suite 5016, Boston, MA 02115, USA. [3]Harvard Medical School, Boston, MA, USA. [4]Departments of Epidemiology and Environmental Health, Harvard T. H. Chan School of Public Health, Boston, MA, USA.

References
1. Choong PF, Dowsey MM. Update in surgery for osteoarthritis of the knee. Int J Rheum Dis. 2011;14(2):167–74.
2. Dunlop DD, Manheim LM, Yelin EH, Song J, Chang RW. The costs of arthritis. Arthritis Rheum. 2003;49(1):101–13.
3. Deshpande BR, Katz JN, Solomon DH, Yelin EH, Hunter DJ, Messier SP, Suter LG, Losina E. Number of persons with symptomatic knee osteoarthritis in the US: impact of race and ethnicity, age, sex, and obesity. Arthritis Care Res. 2016;68(12):1743–50.
4. Bhattacharyya T, Gale D, Dewire P, Totterman S, Gale ME, McLaughlin S, Einhorn TA, Felson DT. The clinical importance of meniscal tears demonstrated by magnetic resonance imaging in osteoarthritis of the knee. J Bone Joint Surg Am. 2003;85-A(1):4–9.
5. Cullen KA, Hall MJ, Golosinskiy A. Ambulatory surgery in the United States. Natl Health Stat Rep. 2006;2009(11):1–25.
6. Kim S, Bosque J, Meehan JP, Jamali A, Marder R. Increase in outpatient knee arthroscopy in the United States: a comparison of National Surveys of Ambulatory Surgery, 1996 and 2006. J Bone Joint Surg Am. 2011;93(11):994–1000.
7. Moseley JB, O'Malley K, Petersen NJ, Menke TJ, Brody BA, Kuykendall DH, Hollingsworth JC, Ashton CM, Wray NP. A controlled trial of arthroscopic surgery for osteoarthritis of the knee. N Engl J Med. 2002;347(2):81–8.
8. Kirkley A, Birmingham TB, Litchfield RB, Giffin JR, Willits KR, Wong CJ, Feagan BG, Donner A, Griffin SH, D'Ascanio LM, et al. A randomized trial of arthroscopic surgery for osteoarthritis of the knee. N Engl J Med. 2008;359(11):1097–107.
9. Herrlin SV, Wange PO, Lapidus G, Hallander M, Werner S, Weidenhielm L. Is arthroscopic surgery beneficial in treating non-traumatic, degenerative medial meniscal tears? A five year follow-up. Knee Surg Sports Traumatol Arthrosc. 2013;21(2):358–64.
10. Katz JN, Brophy RH, Chaisson CE, de Chaves L, Cole BJ, Dahm DL, Donnell-Fink LA, Guermazi A, Haas AK, Jones MH, et al. Surgery versus physical therapy for a meniscal tear and osteoarthritis. N Engl J Med. 2013;368(18):1675–84.
11. Sihvonen R, Paavola M, Malmivaara A, Itala A, Joukainen A, Nurmi H, Kalske J, Jarvinen TL. Arthroscopic partial meniscectomy versus sham surgery for a degenerative meniscal tear. N Engl J Med. 2013;369(26):2515–24.
12. Yim JH, Seon JK, Song EK, Choi JI, Kim MC, Lee KB, Seo HY. A comparative study of meniscectomy and nonoperative treatment for degenerative horizontal tears of the medial meniscus. Am J Sports Med. 2013;41(7):1565–70.
13. Gauffin H, Tagesson S, Meunier A, Magnusson H, Kvist J. Knee arthroscopic surgery is beneficial to middle-aged patients with meniscal symptoms: a prospective, randomised, single-blinded study. Osteoarthr Cartil. 2014;22(11):1808–16.
14. Katz JN, Jones MH. Treatment of Meniscal Tear: the more we learn, the less we knowtreatment of meniscal tear: the more we learn, the less we know. Ann Intern Med. 2016;164(7):503–4.
15. Dervin GF, Stiell IG, Rody K, Grabowski J. Effect of arthroscopic debridement for osteoarthritis of the knee on health-related quality of life. J Bone Joint Surg Am. 2003;85-A(1):10–9.
16. Koyonos L, Yanke AB, McNickle AG, Kirk SS, Kang RW, Lewis PB, Cole BJ. A randomized, prospective, double-blind study to investigate the effectiveness of adding DepoMedrol to a local anesthetic injection in postmeniscectomy patients with osteoarthritis of the knee. Am J Sports Med. 2009;37(6):1077–82.
17. Losina E, Dervan EE, Paltiel AD, Dong Y, Wright RJ, Spindler KP, Mandl LA, Jones MH, Marx RG, Safran-Norton CE, et al. Defining the value of future research to identify the preferred treatment of meniscal tear in the presence of knee osteoarthritis. PLoS One. 2015;10(6):e0130256.
18. Healthcare Cost and Utilization Project. Nationwide Inpatient Sample. Rockville: Agency for Healthcare Research and Quality; 2014.
19. Quality Assessment Tool for Observational Cohort and Cross-Sectional Studies. [https://www.nhlbi.nih.gov/health-pro/guidelines/in-develop/cardiovascular-risk-reduction/tools/cohort]
20. Hamza TH, van Houwelingen HC, Stijnen T. The binomial distribution of meta-analysis was preferred to model within-study variability. J Clin Epidemiol. 2008;61(1):41–51.
21. Hunter DJ. Risk stratification for knee osteoarthritis progression: a narrative review. Osteoarthr Cartil. 2009;17(11):1402–7.
22. Bernard J, Lemon M, Patterson MH. Arthroscopic washout of the knee–a 5-year survival analysis. Knee. 2004;11(3):233–5.
23. Fedorka CJ, Cerynik DL, Tauberg B, Toossi N, Johanson NA. The relationship between knee arthroscopy and arthroplasty in patients under 65 years of age. J Arthroplast. 2014;29(2):335–8.
24. Hawker G, Guan J, Judge A, Dieppe P. Knee arthroscopy in England and Ontario: patterns of use, changes over time, and relationship to total knee replacement. J Bone Joint Surg Am. 2008;90(11):2337–45.
25. Jackson RW, Dieterichs C. The results of arthroscopic lavage and debridement of osteoarthritic knees based on the severity of degeneration: a 4- to 6-year symptomatic follow-up. Arthroscopy. 2003;19(1):13–20.
26. Johanson NA, Kleinbart FA, Cerynik DL, Brey JM, Ong KL, Kurtz SM. Temporal relationship between knee arthroscopy and arthroplasty. a quality measure for joint care? J Arthroplast. 2011;26(2):187–91.
27. McGinley BJ, Cushner FD, Scott WN: Debridement arthroscopy. 10-year followup. Clin Orthop Relat Res 1999(367):190-194.
28. Raaijmaakers M, Vanlauwe J, Vandenneucker H, Dujardin J, Bellemans J. Arthroscopy of the knee in elderly patients: cartilage lesions and their influence on short term outcome. A retrospective follow-up of 183 patients. Acta Orthop Belg. 2010;76(1):79–85.
29. Sansone V, de Girolamo L, Pascale W, Melato M, Pascale V. Long-term results of abrasion arthroplasty for full-thickness cartilage lesions of the medial femoral condyle. Arthroscopy. 2015;31(3):396–403.
30. Skedros JG, Knight AN, Thomas SC, Paluso AM, Bertin KC. Dilemma of high rate of conversion from knee arthroscopy to total knee arthroplasty. Am J Orthop (Belle Mead NJ). 2014;43(7):E153–8.
31. Steadman JR, Briggs KK, Matheny LM, Ellis HB. Ten-year survivorship after knee arthroscopy in patients with Kellgren-Lawrence grade 3 and grade 4 osteoarthritis of the knee. Arthroscopy. 2013;29(2):220–5.
32. Wai EK, Kreder HJ, Williams JI. Arthroscopic débridement of the knee for osteoarthritis in patients fifty years of age or older: Utilization and outcomes in the province of Ontario. Journal of Bone and Joint Surgery - Series A. 2002;84(1):17–22+Adv26.
33. Total Knee Replacement. American Academy of Orthopaedic Surgeons. 2015. http://orthoinfo.aaos.org/topic.cfm?topic=a00389. Accessed 4 April 2017.
34. Bin SI, Lee SH, Kim CW, Kim TH, Lee DH. Results of arthroscopic medial meniscectomy in patients with grade IV osteoarthritis of the medial compartment. Arthroscopy. 2008;24(3):264–8.
35. Lyu SR. Knee health promotion option for knee osteoarthritis: A preliminary report of a concept of multidisciplinary management. Healthy Aging Research. 2015;4
36. Pearse EO, Craig DM. Partial meniscectomy in the presence of severe osteoarthritis does not hasten the symptomatic progression of osteoarthritis. Arthroscopy. 2003;19(9):963–8.
37. Rand JA. Arthroscopic management of degenerative meniscus tears in patients with degenerative arthritis. Arthroscopy. 1985;1(4):253–8.
38. Dearing J, Brenkel IJ. Incidence of knee arthroscopy in patients over 60 years of age in Scotland. The surgeon : journal of the Royal Colleges of Surgeons of Edinburgh and Ireland. 2010;8(3):144–50.

8

Postoperative alignment of TKA in patients with severe preoperative varus or valgus deformity: is there a difference between surgical techniques?

Stefan Rahm[*], Roland S. Camenzind, Andreas Hingsammer, Christopher Lenz, David E. Bauer, Mazda Farshad and Sandro F. Fucentese

Abstract

Background: There have been conflicting studies published regarding the ability of various total knee arthroplasty (TKA) techniques to correct preoperative deformity. The purpose of this study was to compare the postoperative radiographic alignment in patients with severe preoperative coronal deformity ($\geq 10°$ varus/valgus) who underwent three different TKA techniques; manual instrumentation (MAN), computer navigated instrumentation (NAV) and patient specific instrumentation (PSI).

Methods: Patients, who received a TKA with a preoperative coronal deformity of $\geq 10°$ with available radiographs were included in this retrospective study. The groups were: MAN; $n = 54$, NAV; $n = 52$ and PSI; $n = 53$. The mechanical axis (varus / valgus) and the posterior tibial slope were measured and analysed using standing long leg- and lateral radiographs.

Results: The overall mean postoperative varus / valgus deformity was 2.8° (range, 0 to 9.9; SD 2.3) and 2.5° (range, 0 to 14.7; SD 2.3), respectively. The overall outliers (>3°) represented 30.2% (48 /159) of cases and were distributed as followed: MAN group: 31.5%, NAV group: 34.6%, PSI group: 24.4%. No significant statistical differences were found between these groups. The distribution of the severe outliers (>5°) was 14.8% in the MAN group, 23% in the NAV group and 5.6% in the PSI group. The PSI group had significantly ($p = 0.0108$) fewer severe outliers compared to the NAV group while all other pairs were not statistically significant.

Conclusions: In severe varus / valgus deformity the three surgical techniques demonstrated similar postoperative radiographic alignment. However, in reducing severe outliers (> 5°) and in achieving the planned posterior tibial slope the PSI technique for TKA may be superior to computer navigation and the conventional technique. Further prospective studies are needed to determine which technique is the best regarding reducing outliers in patients with severe preoperative coronal deformity.

Keywords: Outliers, Total knee arthroplasty, Severe coronal deformity, Patient specific instrumentation, Computer navigation, Manual instrumentation, Alignment, Measurement

* Correspondence: stefan_rahm@yahoo.com
Orthopaedic Department, Balgrist University Hospital, University of Zurich,
Forchstrasse 340, 8008 Zurich, CH, Switzerland

Background

The generally accepted radiographic goal in total knee arthroplasty (TKA) is the restoration of a neutral mechanical axis (zero degree +/– three degrees). An alignment, which lies beyond this range can lead to premature implant failure [1], abnormal wear [2, 3] and patello-femoral pain [4, 5]. Furthermore, the goal to achieve a neutral mechanical axis has been supported in biomechanical and clinical studies and therefore most authors agree on this concept [1, 5–7].

To date, the three most commonly used techniques for TKA are: 1) the conventional technique with manual instrumentation (MAN) using intramedullary and/or extramedullary jigs to position the cutting blocks; 2) computer navigated instrumentation (NAV) using either an optical or, recently introduced, an electromagnetic wireless system to intraoperatively position the cutting jigs correctly and 3) patient specific instrumentation technique (PSI) using individualized cutting jigs designed from 3D images from the patient's anatomy (based on a preoperative computer tomography (CT) scan or magnetic resonance imaging (MRI)).

The conventional technique has shown that outliers (>3°) may be produced at a rate of up to 32% [8, 9], encouraging more predictable techniques to be developed. The introduction of computer navigation has been associated with fewer outliers [8], but on the other hand, there is conflicting data regarding the radiographic accuracy in the coronal alignment. Some studies have shown that computer navigation provides no significant decrease in outlier incidence [10, 11] and in some cases, may even increase the proportion of outliers [12–14]. Overall, the majority of orthopaedic surgeons have not been convinced of computer navigation due to the uncertainty of a true benefit and potential downsides such as longer operating times, issues with bicortical tibial and femoral pins (iatrogenic fractures, infection) and higher costs [15–17].

An increasingly popular development in TKA is patient specific instrumentation (PSI), based on preoperative CT or MRI. Potential benefits include increased efficiency and accuracy with no additional intramedullary canal violation and less blood loss. However, there are also conflicting results concerning radiographic accuracy compared to the two other techniques [18–24].

It is well known that the severity of the preoperative coronal alignment is associated with a worse postoperative result independent of the surgical technique [25, 26]. There are no studies published, which analyse the postoperative radiographic accuracy regarding the three previously mentioned instrumentation techniques with respect to severe preoperative coronal deformity. Therefore, the rational of the present study is to retrospectively analyse the postoperative radiographic alignment of the three different techniques in patients with severe coronal deformity (≥ 10° varus or valgus).

The hypothesis was that computer navigation or PSI technique would provide better radiological accuracy than the conventional technique.

Methods

The study was approved by the Cantonal Ethics Committee of Canton Zurich (KEK-Zurich) (Institutional review board (IRB) No. 2015–0560). This was a retrospective study with retrospective data collection. We identified patients who had undergone primary TKA for osteoarthritis in the time period from 2004 until 2012. Overall 1063 primary TKAs were identified including 269 SAL UC; Self Aligning Ultra Congruent (Zimmer Inc., Warsaw, IN, USA) and 466 NexGen Legacy Posterior Stabilized Flex (Zimmer Inc., Warsaw, IN, USA) and 328 GMK; Global Medacta Knee (Medacta International S.A., Castel San Pietro, Switzerland).

The charts and radiographs of these patients were analysed and grouped into either manual instrumentation (MAN) using an intramedullary rod for the femoral and an extramedullary guide for the tibial cut, computer-navigation (NAV) (Navitrack surgical navigation system, Zimmer, Warsaw, IN, USA) or CT based patient specific instrumentation (MyKnee, Medacta International S.A., Castel San Pietro, Switzerland) [19]. Patients in the PSI group underwent preoperative CT scan including the hip and the ankle. The goal in all cases was to achieve a neutral coronal alignment.

Inclusion criteria included a complete pre- and postoperative radiograph set with a preoperative varus or valgus of 10 ° or more. Primary TKA using a semi-constrained or constrained type of TKA were excluded.

The three groups were analysed and compared to each other. Furthermore, a subgroup analysis regarding surgeon's experience and implant used was performed. In Table 1 the distribution of each group regarding the number of patients, surgeon experience, implant and varus/ valgus deformity is shown.

Radiographs

The preoperative radiographic assessment consisted of X-rays of the knee (ap / lateral / patella axial view) and a standing long-leg radiograph for assessment of the correct coronal alignment. For the PSI group an additional CT scan was performed according to a special protocol, which included the hip and ankle. Between 6 weeks and 3 months postoperatively, standard radiographs with long-standing X-ray were routinely performed in our outpatient clinic.

In 6 patients there was no standing long-leg radiograph available between 6 weeks and 3 months. Therefore in these 6 patients the postoperative standing long-

Table 1 The preoperative characteristics are depicted in this table. The *p*-value shows the homogeneity of the three groups regarding age, BMI, gender and preoperative coronal deformity and significant difference regarding surgeons experience and used implant

	All	Group MAN	Group NAV	Group PSI	$p =$ *
n=	159	54	52	53	n.a.
age (years mean (SD))	70 (10.1)	71 (9.1)	69 (10.)5	69 (10.6)	0.56
BMI (kg/m²; mean (SD))	30 (5.8)	30 (5.8)	31 (5.3)	29 (6.2)	0.482
Gender (n = f/m)	98/61	34/20	33/19	31/22	0.632
Varus n=	118	36	41	41	0.292
Varus degrees mean (SD)	13.0 (2.8)	12.6 (2.1)	13.0 (3.0)	13.8 (2.9)	0.13
Valgus n=	41	18	11	12	0.292
Valgus degrees mean (SD)	−13.0 (2.9)	−13.3 (3.6)	−12.8 (2.2)	−11.3 (1.7)	0.13
Surgeon's experience >100 TKA	104	30	24	50	<0.001
Surgeon's experience 50 to 100 TKA	55	24	28	3	<0.001
Zimmer NexGen n=	88	39	49	0	<0.001
Zimmer SAL n=	15	15	0	0	< 0.001
Global Medacta Knee n=	56	0	3	53	<0.001

SD standard deviation
∗ The Kruskal-Wallis test was applied to compare the distribution of continuous variables among groups and the Chi-square test was employed to compare the distribution of nominal variables among groups

leg radiograph were performed between 6 and 18 months postoperatively.

All measurements were performed by two senior orthopaedic residents (A.H. and C.L.) and the inter-rater reliability was calculated. The mechanical axis of the lower extremity in the frontal plane was measured in the pre- and postoperative standing long-leg radiographs. The measurement was from the centre of femoral head to the intercondylar notch of the distal femur, and the centre of the proximal tibia to the centre of the ankle.

The posterior tibial slope was measured in the lateral postoperative X-rays according to Faschingbauer et al. [27].

Outliers

A neutral postoperative mechanical alignment was defined within ±3°. An outlier was defined as a mechanical axis with more than 3° varus or valgus. The target posterior tibial slope varied between manufacturer designs. Therefore an outlier was defined as 3° or more than the targeted posterior tibial slope.

Statistics

Statistical analyses were performed with PRISM 5 Graphpad for MAC OS. Normally distributed variables are reported as mean with standard deviations (SD). The distribution of outlier between groups was analysed using fishers exact test. The unpaired and paired students-t-test as well as the Chi-square test, ANOVA (analysis of variance) or ANOVA by ranks as appropriate for comparison between more than two groups were employed for intergroup and Intra-group comparison,

respectively. The interrater reliability of continuous variables (varus/valgus/slope) was determined using interclass correlations (ICC) derived from 2-way mixed-effects ANOVA (average measures). Ninety-five percent confidence intervals (CI) are reported for ICC. The criteria of Landis and Koch were used for the magnitude of the reliability coefficient: 0 to 0.2 = poor, 0.21 to 0.4 = fair, 0.41 to 0.6 = moderate, 0.61 to 0.8 = substantial, 0.81 to 1.0 = excellent agreement. Statistical level of significance was defined with a $p < 0.05$.

Results

Pre- and postoperative measurement of varus and valgus and sagittal alignment had excellent agreement between both readers (varus: ICC: .995, CI: .993–.996, valgus: ICC: .988, CI: .983–991, sagittal alignment: ICC: 0.955 CI: 0.922–0.974). We therefore decided to use the mean of the two readers (A.H. and C.L.).

Coronal alignment

The overall mean postoperative varus / valgus deformity was 2.8° (range, 0 to 9.9°; SD 2.3) / 2.5° (range, 0 to 14.7°; SD 2.3), respectively. The postoperative results are summarized completely in Fig. 1 and show the larger variability in the MAN and the NAV group compared to the PSI group. In Fig. 2 the pre- to postoperative results are depicted of the patients with a preoperative varus deformity and in Fig. 3 with a preoperative valgus deformity, respectively. There are no significant differences found between the groups pre- or postoperatively. Further, the pre-to postoperative correlation did not reach

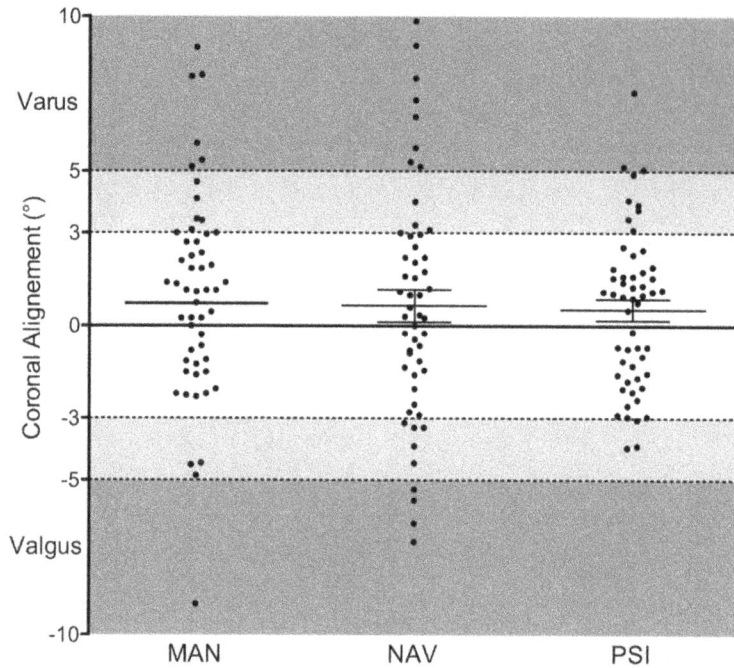

Fig. 1 Here are all patients' coronal alignment depicted with a dot and the distribution is visualized. The PSI group has the smallest variability

significance in any of the three groups. Group MAN r = 0.219, group NAV r = 0.102, group PSI r = 0.104. This means that a preoperative varus or valgus deformity did not influence the postoperative result regarding varus or valgus deformity significantly.

The overall coronal outliers defined as >3° reached 30.2% (48 /159). Table 2 shows the main results with the statistical significance. The PSI group showed the fewest number of severe outliers (>5°) compared to the other groups and showed statistical significance between PSI and NAV group; p = 0.011. The PSI group, including only the patients with preoperative varus deformity

again showed fewer severe outliers >5° compared to the NAV group; p = 0.026. The complete results regarding the separate preoperative varus and valgus groups are depicted in Figs. 4 and 5.

Subgroup analysis

The three groups were analysed separately after excluding the patients who had been operated by an attending with 50 to 100 TKA ending up with three homogenous groups regarding the surgeon's experience. There were no statistical differences found in the postoperative coronal outcome between the three subgroups and

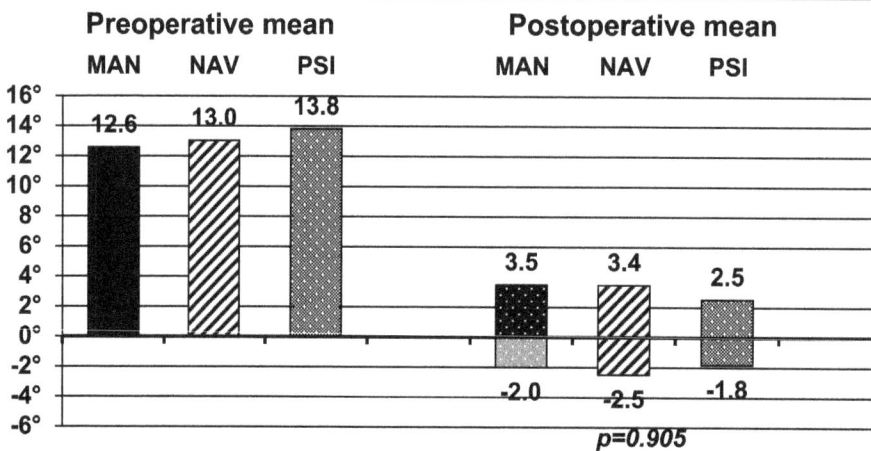

Fig. 2 The mean postoperative results of all patients with a preoperative <u>varus</u> deformity are depicted. There were no significant differences shown between the three groups.

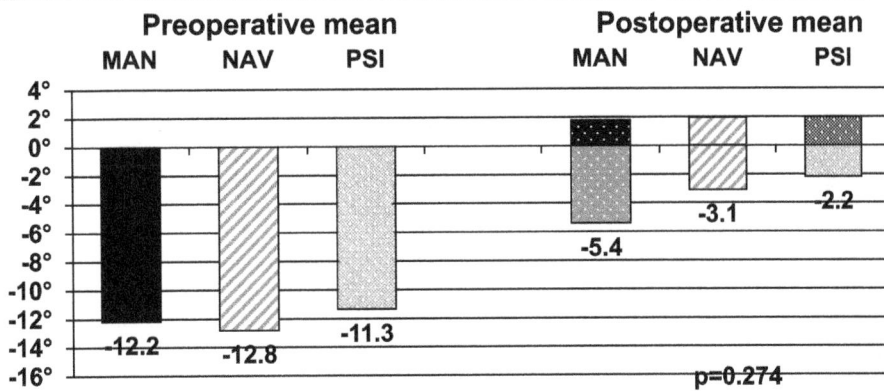

Fig. 3 The mean postoperative results of all patients with a preoperative valgus deformity are depicted. Again, there were no significant differences seen between the three groups

therefore no statistical differences compared to the complete group.

The three groups were analysed separately after excluding the different types of TKA ending up with three homogenous groups regarding the TKA type. These results showed no significant differences compared to the result of the three complete groups.

Sagittal alignment

The outliers defined as >3° off the planned posterior tibial slope are shown in Table 3. Two pairs show statistical significance; MAN / NAV: p = 0.007, MAN / PSI: p = 0.006.

Discussion

The most significant finding of the present study is that the overall outlier rate is rather high at 30.2% (48 /159), in patients with a severe preoperative varus or valgus deformity of 10° or more regardless of the surgical technique. Between the three groups there

was no significant difference regarding postoperative coronal accuracy. Therefore our hypothesis has to be rejected. However, in this study the preoperative coronal deformity did not correlate with the postoperative result regarding outliers or radiographic accuracy in varus or valgus. This can be well explained since the patients with less than 10° coronal deformities were excluded. Several authors have identified that a severe, preoperative deformity is associated with a relatively poor postoperative alignment and therefore also a worse clinical long-term outcome [25, 26, 28, 29]. Comparing our results to the literature, the overall outlier range is higher in the patient population with a severe preoperative coronal deformity. The overall outliers (>3°) reached 30.2% (48 /159), which is over the value of most of the studies found in literature regardless of the surgical technique. This is a very important finding that a higher outlier rate occurs in severe deformity and this information maybe should be shared with our patients.

Table 2 Overall results showing the postoperative outliers in the coronal plane

Group	Total n	Outliers (>3°) n	Outliers (>3°) %	Outliers (>5°) n	Outliers (>5°) %
MAN	54	17	31.5	8	14.8
NAV	52	18	34.6	12	23
PSI	53	13	24.4	3	5.6

	Significance			Significance	
	MAN / NAV	p=0.885		MAN / NAV	p=0.277
	MAN / PSI	p=0.229		MAN / PSI	p=0.119
	NAV / PSI	p=0.181		NAV / PSI	p=0.011

Statistical significance was calculated by Fisher Exact Test. Gray shaded = significant

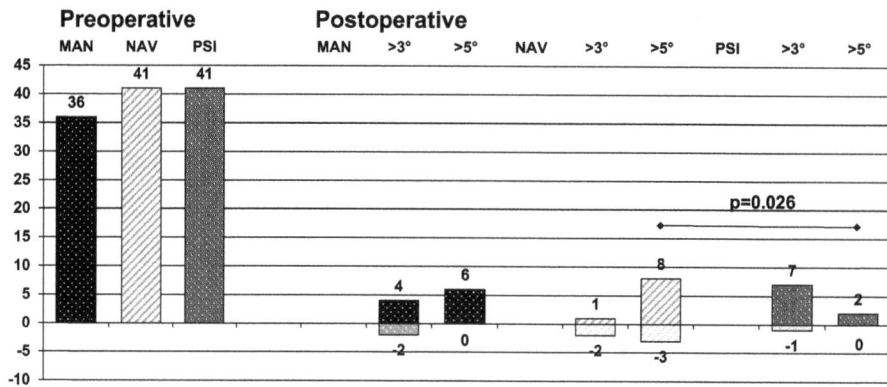

Fig. 4 The results summarized of all the patients with a preoperative varus deformity showing postoperative outliers (>3°) and severe outliers (>5°). The PSI group shows significantly less outliers than the NAV group

The PSI group had the fewest proportion of outliers (>3° for the frontal mechanical axis) with 24.4% compared to 31.5% in the MAN group and 34.6% in the NAV group. Although not statistically significant, there was a trend towards a benefit in the PSI group. When using a threshold value of >5°, defined to be severe outliers, the results showed larger differences reaching statistical significance with a $p = 0.011$ between the PSI and the NAV group. Further, the accuracy reaching the planned posterior tibial slope was statistically worse in the MAN group with 48.1% outliers (>3° of the planned value) compared to the PSI group with 22.6% ($p = 0.006$) and to the NAV group with 23.1% ($p = 0.007$).

The PSI group has significantly fewer severe outliers due to the precise preoperative planning and accurate cutting guides which should result in a 0° mechanical axis. In our hands this technique seems to be the most accurate in this patient group. On the other hand a preoperative CT scan is necessary in all the patients who received a PSI TKA and therefore this is a potential appreciable downside. However, the outlier range of

24.4% is still too high when comparing the results with a study performed in our hospital with the same TKA and PSI technique. In this group with less severe coronal deformity the outlier group represented 12% [19]. Two other studies using the same PSI system showed outliers of 10% [18] and 37% [30]. The relatively high outlier proportion in the study of Ensini et al. [30] may be explained by a small study population and the associated issues with learning a new PSI technique. Therefore, this huge variability of the different studies is explained. The accuracy regarding the posterior tibial slope is similar in the PSI and the NAV group but interestingly here the MAN group was significantly worse than the other two.

Our findings suggest that the computer navigation did not improve accuracy in this study population. This is in contrast to other authors reporting fewer outliers with computer navigation [8]. The reasons are multifactorial and not fully understood. One potential reason for this discrepancy may be due to the varied experience between the surgeons. Less experienced surgeons who performed fewer than 100 represented 28 of the 52 cases with computerized navigation.

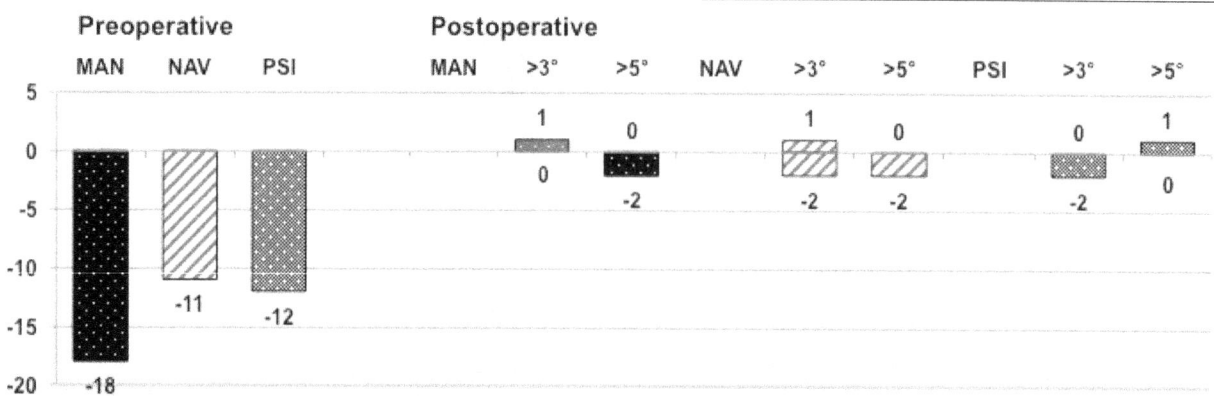

Fig. 5 The results summarized, similar to Fig. 4, all the patients with a preoperative valgus deformity showing postoperative outliers and severe outliers. No significant differences were detected

Table 3 Overall results showing the postoperative outliers in the sagittal plane regarding the posterior tibial slope. An outlier was defined when more than 3° difference to the planned posterior tibial slope

Group	Total n	Outliers (>3°) n	Outliers (>3°) %
MAN	54	26	48.1
NAV	52	12	23.1
PSI	53	12	22.6
Significance			
MAN / NAV		p=0.007	
MAN / PSI		p=0.006	
NAV / PSI		p=0.958	

Statistical significance was calculated by Fisher Exact Test. Gray shaded = significant

In a study performed by Carli et al. [31] comparing two different computer navigation systems, the results showed a significant difference. However, in both study groups there were rather high numbers of outliers, 24 and 32%, respectively.

In the study of Willcox et al. [32] the intraoperative alignment according to the navigation differed from the alignment measured using a standing long-leg radiograph.

There are considerable limitations to this study. First, the standing long-leg radiograph can mimic a false coronal deformity if the patient does not fully extend their knee and/or a rotational malalignment is present [33, 34]. We do not believe that it is justified to perform a postoperative CT scan in order to address this concern. Secondly the groups are not in all aspects homogenous. However, the subgroup analysis did not change the main conclusion and we therefore believe that this limitation is negligible.

Conclusion

In severe varus / valgus deformity the three surgical techniques demonstrated similar postoperative radiographic alignment. However, in reducing severe outliers (> 5°) and in achieving the planned posterior tibial slope the PSI technique for TKA may be superior to computer navigation and the conventional technique. Further prospective studies are needed to determine which technique is the best regarding reducing outliers in patients with severe preoperative coronal deformity.

Abbreviations
CI: Confidence intervals; CT: Computer tomography; GMK: Global medacta knee; ICC: Interclass correlations; IRB: Institutional review board; MAN: Manual instrumentation; MRI: Magnetic resonance imaging; NAV: Computer navigated instrumentation; PSI: Patient specific instrumentation; SAL UC: Self aligning ultra congruent; TKA: Total knee arthroplasty

Funding
No fundings.

Authors' contributions
All authors have made substantial contributions to this study; SR was involved in conception and design, analysis and interpretation of data and in drafting the manuscript. RC was involved in conception and design, acquisition and interpretation of data. AH, CL and DB were involved in conception and the acquisition of data, analysis and interpretation of data. MF was involved in conception, analysis and statistics. SF was involved in conception, analysis and interpretation of data and revising the manuscript critically for important intellectual content. All authors read and approved the final manuscript.

Competing interests
The authors declare that they have no competing interests.

Consent for publication
All participants gave their written consent to this study.

References

1. Green GV, Berend KR, Berend ME, Glisson RR, Vail TP. The effects of varus tibial alignment on proximal tibial surface strain in total knee arthroplasty: The posteromedial hot spot. J Arthroplast. 2002;17:1033–9.
2. Liau JJ, Cheng CK, Huang CH, Lo WH. The effect of malalignment on stresses in polyethylene component of total knee prostheses–a finite element analysis. Clin Biomech (Bristol, Avon). 2002;17:140–6.
3. Werner FW, Ayers DC, Maletsky LP, Rullkoetter PJ. The effect of valgus/varus malalignment on load distribution in total knee replacements. J Biomech. 2005;38:349–55.
4. Choong PF, Stoney JD. Does accurate anatomical alignment result in better function and quality of life? comparing conventional and computer-assisted total knee arthroplasty. J Arthroplast. 2009;24:560–9. Elsevier Inc.
5. Figgie HE, Goldberg VM, Figgie MP, Inglis AE, Kelly M, Sobel M. The effect of alignment of the implant on fractures of the patella after condylar total knee arthroplasty. J Bone Joint Surg Am. 1989;71:1031–9.
6. Huang NFR, Dowsey MM, Ee E, Stoney JD, Babazadeh S, Choong PF. Coronal alignment correlates with outcome after total knee arthroplasty: five-year follow-up of a randomized controlled trial. J Arthroplast. 2012;27:1737–41.
7. Wasielewski RC, Galante JO, Leighty RM, Natarajan RN, Rosenberg AG. Wear patterns on retrieved polyethylene tibial inserts and their relationship to technical considerations during total knee arthroplasty. Clin Orthop Relat Res. 1994;229:31–43.
8. Hetaimish BM, Khan MM, Simunovic N, Al-Harbi HH, Bhandari M, Zalzal PK. Meta-analysis of navigation vs conventional total knee arthroplasty. J Arthroplast. 2012;27:1177–82.
9. Mason JB, Fehring TK, Estok R, Banel D, Fahrbach K. Meta-analysis of alignment outcomes in computer-assisted total knee arthroplasty surgery. J Arthroplast. 2007;22:1097–106.
10. Yau WP, Chiu KY, Zuo JL, Tang WM, Ng TP. Computer navigation did not improve alignment in a lower-volume total knee practice. Clin Orthop Relat Res. 2008;466:935–45.
11. Kim Y-H, Kim J-S, Choi Y, Kwon O-R. Computer-assisted surgical navigation does not improve the alignment and orientation of the components in total knee arthroplasty. J Bone Joint Surg Am. 2009;91:14–9.
12. Chauhan SK, Clark GW, Lloyd S, Scott RG, Breidahl W, Sikorski JM. Computer-assisted total knee replacement. A controlled cadaver study using a multi-parameter quantitative CT assessment of alignment (the Perth CT Protocol). J Bone Joint Surg Br. 2004;86:818–23.
13. Gøthesen O, Espehaug B, Havelin LI, Petursson G, Hallan G, Strøm E, et al. Functional outcome and alignment in computer-assisted and conventionally operated total knee replacements: a multicentre parallel-group randomised controlled trial. Bone Joint J. 2014;96-B:609–18.
14. Jenny J-Y, Clemens U, Kohler S, Kiefer H, Konermann W, Miehlke RK. Consistency of implantation of a total knee arthroplasty with a non-image-based navigation system: a case-control study of 235 cases compared with 235 conventionally implanted prostheses. J Arthroplast. 2005;20:832–9.
15. Blakeney WG, Khan RJK, Wall SJ. Computer-assisted techniques versus conventional guides for component alignment in total knee arthroplasty: a randomized controlled trial. J Bone Joint Surg Am. 2011;93:1377–84.
16. Bauwens K, Matthes G, Wich M, Gebhard F, Hanson B, Ekkernkamp A, et al. Navigated total knee replacement. A meta-analysis. J Bone Joint Surg Am. 2007;89:261–9.
17. Desai AS, Dramis A, Kendoff D, Board TN. Critical review of the current practice for computer-assisted navigation in total knee replacement surgery: cost-effectiveness and clinical outcome. Curr Rev Musculoskelet Med. 2010;4:11–5.
18. Anderl W, Pauzenberger L, Kölblinger R, Kiesselbach G, Brandl G, Laky B, et al. Patient-specific instrumentation improved mechanical alignment, while early clinical outcome was comparable to conventional instrumentation in TKA. Knee Surg Sports Traumatol Arthrosc. 2014;
19. Koch PP, Müller D, Pisan M, Fucentese SF. Radiographic accuracy in TKA with a CT-based patient-specific cutting block technique. Knee Surg Sports Traumatol Arthrosc. 2013;21:2200–5.
20. MacDessi SJ, Jang B, Harris IA, Wheatley E, Bryant C, Chen DB. A comparison of alignment using patient specific guides, computer navigation and conventional instrumentation in total knee arthroplasty. Knee. 2014;21:406–9. Elsevier B.V
21. Yan CH, Chiu KY, Ng FY, Chan PK, Fang CX. Comparison between patient-specific instruments and conventional instruments and computer navigation in total knee arthroplasty: a randomized controlled trial. Knee Surg Sports Traumatol Arthrosc. 2014;
22. Mannan A, Smith TO, Sagar C, London NJ, Molitor PJA. No demonstrable benefit for coronal alignment outcomes in PSI knee arthroplasty: a systematic review and meta-analysis. Orthop Traumatol Surg Res. 2015;101:461–8.
23. Chen JY, Yeo SJ, Yew AKS, Tay DKJ, Chia S-L, Lo NN, et al. The radiological outcomes of patient-specific instrumentation versus conventional total knee arthroplasty. Knee Surg Sports Traumatol Arthrosc. 2014;22:630–5.
24. Ng VY, DeClaire JH, Berend KR, Gulick BC, Lombardi AV. Improved accuracy of alignment with patient-specific positioning guides compared with manual instrumentation in TKA. Clin Orthop Relat Res. 2011;470:99–107.
25. Ritter MA, Davis KE, Davis P, Farris A, Malinzak RA, Berend ME, et al. Preoperative malalignment increases risk of failure after total knee arthroplasty. J Bone Joint Surg Am [Internet]. 2013;95:126–31. Available from: http://eutils.ncbi.nlm.nih.gov/entrez/eutils/elink.fcgi?dbfrom=pubmed&id=23324959&retmode=ref&cmd=prlinks.
26. Sorrells RB, Murphy JA, Sheridan KC, Wasielewski RC. The effect of varus and valgus deformity on results of cementless mobile bearing TKA. Knee. 2007;14:284–8.
27. Faschingbauer M, Sgroi M, Juchems M, Reichel H, Kappe T. Can the tibial slope be measured on lateral knee radiographs? Knee Surg Sports Traumatol Arthrosc. 2014;22:3163–7.
28. Karachalios T, Sarangi PP, Newman JH. Severe varus and valgus deformities treated by total knee arthroplasty. J Bone Joint Surg Br. 1994;76:938–42.
29. Chandler JT, Moskal JT. Evaluation of knee and hindfoot alignment before and after total knee arthroplasty: a prospective analysis. J Arthroplast. 2004;19:211–6.
30. Ensini A, Timoncini A, Cenni F, Belvedere C, Fusai F, Leardini A, et al. Intra- and post-operative accuracy assessments of two different patient-specific instrumentation systems for total knee replacement. Knee Surg Sports Traumatol Arthrosc. 2013;22:621–9.
31. Carli A, Aoude A, Reuven A, Matache B, Antoniou J, Zukor D. Inconsistencies between navigation data and radiographs in total knee arthroplasty are system-dependent and affect coronal alignment. Can J Surg. 2014;57:305–13.
32. Willcox NMJ, Clarke JV, Smith BRK, Deakin AH, Deep K. A comparison of radiological and computer navigation measurements of lower limb coronal alignment before and after total knee replacement. J Bone Joint Surg Br. 2012;94:1234–40.
33. Lonner JH, Laird MT, Stuchin SA. Effect of rotation and knee flexion on radiographic alignment in total knee arthroplasties. Clin Orthop Relat Res. 1996;102–6.
34. Krackow KA, Pepe CL, Galloway EJ. A mathematical analysis of the effect of flexion and rotation on apparent varus/valgus alignment at the knee. Orthopedics. 1990;13:861–8.

9

Knee arthrodesis versus above-the-knee amputation after septic failure of revision total knee arthroplasty: comparison of functional outcome and complication rates

Sven Hungerer[1,2]* iD, Martin Kiechle[1], Christian von Rüden[1,2], Matthias Militz[1], Knut Beitzel[3] and Mario Morgenstern[1,2,4]

Abstract

Background: After septic failure of total knee arthroplasty (TKA) and multiple revision operations resulting in impaired function, bone and/or soft-tissue damage a reconstruction with a revision arthroplasty might be impossible. Salvage procedures to regain mobility and quality of life are an above-the-knee amputation or knee arthrodesis. The decision process for the patient and surgeon is difficult and data comparing arthrodesis versus amputation in terms of function and quality of life are scarce. The purpose of this study was to analyse and compare the specific complications, functional outcome and quality of life of above-the-knee amputation (AKA) and modular knee-arthrodesis (MKA) after septic failure of total knee arthroplasty.

Methods: Eighty-one patients treated with MKA and 32 patients treated with AKA after septic failure of TKA between 2003 and 2012 were included in this cohort study. Demographic data, comorbidities, pathogens and complications such as re-infection, implant-failure or revision surgeries were recorded in 55MKA and 20AKA patients. Functional outcome with use of the Lower-Extremity-Functional-Score (LEFS) and the patients reported general health status (SF-12-questionnaire) was recorded after a mean interval of 55 months.

Results: A major complication occurred in more than one-third of the cases after MKA and AKA, whereas recurrence of infection was with 22% after MKA and 35% after AKA the most common complication. Patients with AKA and MKA showed a comparable functional outcome with a mean LEFS score of 37 and 28 respectively ($p = 0.181$). Correspondingly, a comparable physical quality of life with a mean physical SF-12 of 36 for AKA patients and a mean score of 30 for MKA patients was observed ($p = 0.080$). Notably, ten AKA patients that could be fitted with a microprocessor-controlled-knee-joint demonstrated with a mean LEFS of 56 a significantly better functional outcome than other amputee patients ($p < 0.01$) or MKA patients ($p < 0.01$).

Conclusion: Naturally, the decision process for the treatment of desolate situations of septic failures following revision knee arthroplasty is depending on various factors. Nevertheless, the amputation should be considered as an option in patients with a good physical and mental condition.

Keywords: Prosthetic joint infection, Revision total knee arthroplasty, Knee-arthrodesis, Above-the-knee amputation

* Correspondence: sven.hungerer@bgu-murnau.de
[1]BG Unfallklinik Murnau, Prof. Küntscher Str. 8, Murnau 82418, Germany
[2]Institute of Biomechanics, Paracelsus Medical University Salzburg and BG Unfallklinik Murnau, Prof. Küntscher Str. 8, Murnau 82418, Germany
Full list of author information is available at the end of the article

Background

Prosthetic joint infections (PJI) following total knee arthroplasty (TKA) pose a devastating complication, since eradication of infection and restoration of functionality present a significant challenge to both patients and surgeons [1, 2]. Despite tremendous efforts and targeted therapy, infection reoccurs in up to 14 to 28% after revision TKA and causes severe morbidity as well as substantial treatment costs [3, 4]. If infection cannot be eradicated or if multiple revision TKAs led to loss of soft-tissue, extreme bone defects or instability as well as deficiency of the extensor apparatus successful reconstruction or control of infection using revision TKA may no longer be possible [5, 6]. In these cases knee-arthrodesis or above-the-knee amputation (AKA) are beside resection arthroplasty often the only treatment options [2, 5]. Wu et al. performed a systematic review on treatment options in persistent infection after failed revision TKA and concluded that arthrodesis should strongly be considered in this case to control infection and to maximize function [7]. In contrast, Rohner et al. recently reported an infection persistence of 50%, substantially impaired quality of life and pain after knee-arthrodesis. They concluded that bone fusion following septic failure of revision TKA should be regarded with scepticism [2]. On the other hand, poor functional outcome and high complication rates of more than 30% are also described for AKA after TKA [8–10]. There are scant data on directly comparing functionality and complication rates of AKA and knee-arthrodesis performed after septic failure of TKA. Solely, one retrospective study compared the functional outcome of bone fusion and AKA after PJI in small numbers [11]. There is no study comparing AKA with access to modern orthotics and modular knee arthrodesis (MKA) in this situation. Knee-arthrodesis with modular endoprosthesis provides advantages over bone fusion including immediate fixation and weight bearing as well as modularity, which allows the reconstruction of segmental deficits [12].

Therefore the central aims of our study was to analyse the clinical course, complications, functionality and quality of life of AKA and MKA after septic failure of TKA. We hypothesize that neither AKA nor MKA after septic failure of TKA is superior in terms of functional outcome and complication rates and that the treatment decision process should be judged individually according to the patients` overall condition and the local bone and soft-tissue status.

Methods

All patients treated in our department over a ten-years time period (2003–2012) with MKA or AKA after septic failure of revision TKA were included in this retrospective cohort study. Additional inclusion criteria were: minimum follow-up interval of 12-month, a sufficient patient data set and complete radiographic imaging studies. A PJI was diagnosed according to the American Academy of Orthopaedic Surgeons clinical practice guideline [13].

Demographic data was collected and the overall medical condition of the patient was evaluated using the Charlson comorbidity index (CCI) [14]. The initial infecting pathogens detected in the underlying PJI were documented. Patients were seen in regular visits (minimum visits after surgery: 6 weeks, 6 months, 1 year) and underwent physical and radiographic examination.

In patients with KA the following items were documented: implant positioning and leg length discrepancy. Distance arthrodesis was performed with a modular system (Peter Brehm GmbH, Weisendorf, Germany). Major complications after arthrodesis such as re-infection, implant-failure /–loosening or fracture were documented and surgical revisions like implant exchange, debridement or amputation were quoted. A recurrence or persistent infection was defined when local and/ or systemic signs of infection or one of the mentioned diagnosis criteria for PJI were present [13]. Loosening was defined as migration of the implant and the presence of a radiolucent liner larger than 2 mm [2]. Survival of the implant or arthrodesis was deemed to be the absence of above-mentioned complications or surgical revisions.

In patients with AKA the following was documented: level of amputation, fitted with a functional prosthesis and type of prosthesis (mechanic and microprocessor-controlled-knee-joint). Major complications after amputation such as stump healing disorder, recurrence of infection and revision amputation were recorded.

In 58 patients functional outcome was assessed with use of the Lower Extremity Functional Scale (LEFS) [15] and the SF-12 [16]. According to previous validation studies the SF-12 is comparable to the SF-36 for assessing patients` physical (Physical Component Summary; PCS) and emotional quality of life (Mental Component summary; MCS) [17]. The LEFS describes the functionality of the lower extremity (maximum score of 80 equates to the best functional outcome) [15]. Patients, in which amputation was performed after MKA, were excluded from analysis of functional outcome.

Statistical analysis

Statistical analysis was performed using SPSS® Statistics for Windows 19.0 (IBM Corp., Armonk, New York, U.S.A.). Results in this study are presented as mean values with standard deviation. Significance for categorical data was calculated using the Pearson's chi-squared test. Analysis of variance was used to detect differences between the groups. Numeric data were tested for normal distribution with the Kolmogorov Smirnov Test. Assuming parametric data, statistical differences were tested using the paired T-test for independent variables. A result was considered to be statistically significant with p-value <0.05. Implant survival was calculated by Kaplan-Meier survival plot. The functional outcome, assessed with the LEFS was defined the primary aim. The complication rate, as well as the patients' physical (PCS) and emotional quality of life (MCS) were defined secondary aims.

Results

Overview – Patient cohorts

In the time period between 2003 and 2012 we treated 127 patients with knee-arthrodesis and 157 patients with AKA due to various indications. Patients undergoing knee-arthrodesis or AKA due to other indication than PJI were excluded from this study. In total in 32 patients AKA and in 81 MKA was performed after septic failure of revision TKA and therefore patients were included in the current study. In six patients knee-arthrodesis after PJI was performed by bone fusion using an external fixator, plates or an intramedullary nail and they were excluded from this investigation (Fig. 1).

Modular knee arthrodesis – Clinical course and complications

Demographic data and infection characteristics of MKA patients are summarized in Table 1. After MKA, three patients (4%) died postoperatively and death was related to the underlying infection or a serious postoperative complication. Six patients reportedly died in the first year after arthrodesis. In total, 17 patients with MKA were lost to follow-up examination, leaving 55 patients for analysis.

During the follow-up period loosening occurred after eight (15%) arthrodeses. A peri-implant fracture was seen in four patients (7%) and a technical implant failure in one patient (2%). Re-infection was observed in 12 cases (22%). An amputation had to be performed due to persisting or recurrent infection in six patients (11%) (Table 2). In nine patients at least one re-arthrodesis had to be performed due to periprosthetic fracture, implant loosening or re-infection. This was leading to a total number of 93 arthrodeses in 81 patients. An overall survival rate for all 93 modular arthrodeses was after one year 86%, after five years 71% and after ten years 61% (Table 1).

Above-the-knee amputations –clinical course and complications

Demographic data and infection characteristics of amputee patients are summarized in Table 3. After AKA four patients (13%) died postoperatively and death was related to the underlying disease or a serious postoperative complication. Two patients reportedly died in the first year after in AKA. In total, five patients (16%) with AKA were lost to follow-up examination, leaving 20 patients for analysis (Table 3). At follow-up 80% of the patients were fitted with a functional prosthesis ($n = 16$), six of them with a mechanic knee joint (30%) and ten with a

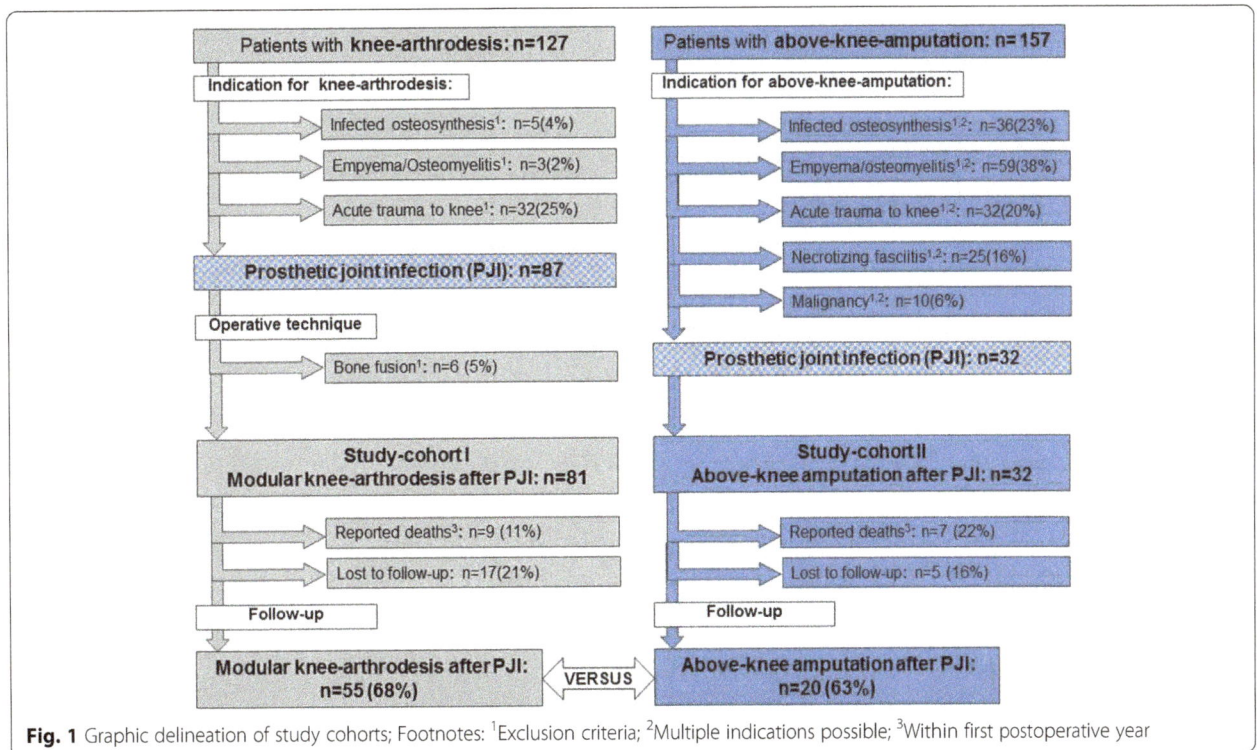

Fig. 1 Graphic delineation of study cohorts; Footnotes: [1]Exclusion criteria; [2]Multiple indications possible; [3]Within first postoperative year

Table 1 Modular knee-arthrodesis (MKA) after prosthetic joint infection (PJI): demographic and clinical data, implant survival rate

Characteristic	MKA after PJI
Number of patients, n	81
Demographic data	
Mean age (in years), mean (sd; Min - Max)	68.6 (11.2; 29–85)
Male sex, n (%)	43 (53.1)
Charlson Comorbidity Index, mean (sd)	4.8 (2.0)
Death within 1st year, n (%)	9 (11.1)
Lost to follow-up, n (%)	17 (21.0)
Patients with min. Follow-up, n (%)	55 (67.9)
Disease causing pathogens[a]	
S. aureus, n (%)	25 (30.9)
S. epidermidis, n (%)	31 (38.3)
Others[2], n (%)	25 (30.9)
Leg length discrepancy after MKA in cm, mean (sd)	1.8 (1.4)
Survival rate (SR) for MKA after PJI	
One – year SR	85.6%
Five – years SR	71.1%
Ten – years SR	60.9%

[a]Disease causing pathogen isolated in PJI leading MKA

microprocessor-controlled-knee-joint (50%). After initial AKA a revision surgery with irrigation and debridement was required due to non-healing stumps or recurrent infections in seven patients (35%). Re-amputation had to be performed in four cases (20%) (Table 2).

Comparison of complications and functional outcome of MKA and AKA

Patients with AKA showed a tendency towards a higher postoperative death rate with 13% when compared with patients with MKA (4%) ($p = 0.081$). Major complications, which required surgical revision, were seen in both cohorts equally, in 36% after MKA ($n = 20$) and in 35% after AKA ($n = 7$) ($p = 0.91$). Recurrence of in infection was the most common complication and occurred within follow-up interval in 22% after MKA ($n = 12$) and in 35% after AKA ($n = 7$) ($p = 0.25$). Due to this, amputation had to be performed in six cases after MKA (11%) and re-amputation was necessary in four (20%) after AKA ($p = 0.31$).

The functional outcome and quality of life, which were assessed in average 53 months after MKA and 62 months after AKA showed now significant differences between both procedures. Patients after amputation reached an average LEFS of 37 points and a mean PCS of 36, whereas after arthrodesis a mean LEFS of 28 points ($p = 0.181$) and a PCS of 30 ($p = 0.080$) could be observed. In both cohorts a comparable mental quality of life could be observed with a mean MCS for AKA and MKA of 47 and 46, respectively ($p = 0.755$) (Table 2). In total ten AKA patients could be fitted

Table 2 Modular knee-arthrodesis (MKA) versus Above-the-knee amputation (AKA) after prosthetic joint infection (PJI): clinical course, complications, functional outcome and quality of life

Characteristic	MKA after PJI	p-value	AKA after PJI
Patients with min. Follow-up (12 month), n (%)	55 (67.9)		20 (62.5)
Follow-up interval in month			
• Mean (sd)	53 (26)		62 (40)
• Min-Max	12–119		12–112
Complications			
Patients with major complication, n (%)	20 (36.4)	0.91	7 (35.0)
Recurrence of infection, n (%)	12 (21.8)	0.25	7 (35.0)
(Re-) Amputation, n (%)	6 (10.9)	0.31	4 (20.0)
MKA Loosening, n (%)	8 (14.5)	n/a	–
MKA Implant failure, n (%)	1 (1.8)	n/a	–
Peri-implant fracture, n (%)	4 (7.3)	n/a	–
Patients with functional follow up, n (%)	48 (59.3%)		10 (31.3%)
Functional follow-up examination			
LEFS[a], mean (sd)	28 (13.7)	0.181	37 (26.4)
Physical SF-12, mean (PCS) (sd)	30 (9.1)	0.080	36 (14.5)
Mental SF-12, mean (MCS) (sd)	46 (11.2)	0.755	47 (12.0)

[a]LEFS = Lower Extremity Functional Scale. A maximum score of 80 equates to the best functional outcome

Table 3 Above-the-knee amputation (AKA) after prosthetic joint infection (PJI): demographic and clinical data, level of AKA and orthotics

Characteristic	AKA after PJI
Number of patients, n	32
Demographic data	
Mean age (in years), mean (sd; Min – Max)	63.4 (14.4; 29–85)
Male sex, n (%)	17 (53.1)
Charlson Comorbidity Index, mean (sd)	5.5 (2.1)
Death within 1st year, n (%)	7 (21.8)
Lost to follow-up, n (%)	5 (15.6)
Patients with min. Follow-up, n (%)	20 (62.5)
Disease causing pathogens[a]	
S. aureus, n (%)	11 (34.4)
S. epidermidis, n (%)	9 (28.1)
Others, n (%)	12 (37.5)
Level of AKA	
Proximal, n (%)	5 (15.6)
Midshaft, n (%)	11 (34.4)
Distal, n (%)	16 (50.0)
Fitted with functional prosthesis[b], n (%)	16 (80.0)
Mechanic knee joint, n (%)	6 (30.0)
Microprocessor knee joint, n (%)	10 (50.0)

[a]Disease causing pathogen isolated in PJI leading to AKA
[b]Out of 20 patients, which were available for FUP

with a modern microprocessor-controlled-knee-joint. This sub-group showed a significantly better functional outcome with a mean LEFS of 56, compared to patients with a mechanic knee joint (mean LEFS: 20, $p < 0.01$) or those who received an arthrodesis ($p < 0.01$). Four patients that couldn't be fitted with prosthesis had with a mean LEFS of 14 a significantly compromised outcome when compared with MKA patients ($p < 0.01$).

In amputee patients age at surgical amputation was associated with a significantly lower functional outcome and quality of life at final follow-up examination ($p < 0.01$). Patients aged less than 60 years could all be fitted with prosthesis and reached a mean LEFS of 56, patients aged 60 to 69 years showed a mean LEFS of 36 and those who were aged between 70 and 79 years had a mean LEFS of just 14. All patients aged older than 80 years at amputation were lost to follow-up. In contrast, in patients receiving arthrodesis age did not significantly influence the functional outcome, since the age groups of below 60 years, 60 to 69 years, 70 to 79 years and more than 80 years showed a comparable LEFS value of 28, 30, 28 and 27 respectively.

Discussion

If infection after septic failure of TKA cannot be controlled or multiple revisions led to extensive bone or soft-tissue damage, salvage of a failed TKA remains difficult and the only alternatives to regain mobility and quality of life for the patient are AKA or KA [7, 10, 18–20]. Previous research does not provide a proper answer, if knee-arthrodesis or AKA with proper orthotic care is superior in terms of functional outcome, quality of life and postoperative complications. Therefore we compared these parameters in patients with AKA and knee-arthrodesis after PJI and revealed that as well AKA as knee-arthrodesis patients suffered an equally high rate of major complications of around 35%. Correspondingly, patients with AKA and knee-arthrodesis after septic failure of revision TKA showed a comparably compromised functional outcome and physical quality of life, whereas AKA patients that were fitted with a microprocessor-controlled-knee-joint reached a significantly better functional outcome, compared to all other amputee patients or those who received arthrodesis. Therefore, patients with a proper physical and mental state that will be able to mobilize with proper orthotics may benefit from an AKA. In amputee patients increasing age was associated with a lower functional outcome and decreasing number of patients fitted with prosthesis. In contrast, in arthrodesis patients age did not influence the functional outcome.

In literature a comparable complication rate of 31–32% after AKA [10, 21] and 30–50% after knee-arthrodesis is reported [2, 11]. Recurrence of infection was the most common complication in our study populations, which surprisingly occurred with 35% more frequently after AKA, than after MKA (22%). It is astonishing that reinfection is less common after MKA, despite a huge implant is present. Infection in MKA led in 15% to implant loosening and in 50% of these cases no re-arthrodesis was possible and amputation had to be performed. The implant survival rate of MKA was after one year 86%, after five years 71% and after ten years 61%. These results are considerably higher than literature data, which showed survivorship of MKA of 50% and 25% at five and ten years, respectively [12].

Death, which was related to the underlying disease or a serious postoperative complication, occurred in 4% after MKA and in 13% after AKA. This and the higher re-infection rate may be explained that patients with AKA had a more compromised overall health status and that the underlying infection was more often caused by a more virulent pathogen, such as S. aureus. It is widely accepted that in uncontrolled and occasionally life-threatening infections amputation is the preferred treatment option.

In literature on knee-arthrodesis after PJI, contrary results about functional outcome and quality of life as well as high complication rates are reported [2, 7, 11, 18, 22]. It has to be noted that in several above-cited studies knee-arthrodesis was performed with bone fusion using external fixator or intramedullary nail. A specific problem of multiple revision TKAs is an increasing bone defect and therefore a direct bony fusion would result in a leg length discrepancy of more than 5 cm. Such a leg length discrepancy, is known as a major factor to reduce the functional outcome and quality of life [5, 7]. In our cohort we performed arthrodesis with modular endoprostheses. This technique provides above-mentioned advantages over bone fusion and allows the reconstruction of segmental deficits and consequently adaption of a leg length discrepancy [12, 23].

Conway et al. concluded in a literature review on knee-arthrodesis, that a patient with successful knee-arthrodesis may be able to walk effectively, particularly in comparison to AKA [18]. Further studies reported a very poor functional outcome after amputation above septic failure of TKA [8–10]. But, the listed studies and the studies cited by Conway et al. analysed amputations which were mainly performed in the 1970's until the 1990's. Functional results of this era are meanwhile obsolete and can't be compared with nowadays. Meanwhile considerable engineering process with development of microprocessor-controlled knee-joints improved functional outcome and quality of life after AKA [24]. Our AKA cohort was fitted in 80% with prosthesis and mainly with a microprocessor-controlled -knee-joint, which may explain the deviating functional results compared to previous studies. In contrast, in the study of Sierra et al., who reported a poor functional outcome for AKA, just 36% of the patients were fitted with prosthesis [10]. Chen et al. stated a worse functional outcome for AKA when comparing with knee-arthrodesis after PJI. But in their AKA cohort also just 30% were fitted with prosthesis and no details are provided on the type of prosthesis.

The good functional outcome of our AKA population may also be explained by the fact that they showed a lower mean age with 63 years when compared to the MKA cohort (69 years). The age at amputation is significantly influencing the later functional outcome, as proven by our results.

The major limitation of the current study is that the patients are not prospectively randomized to one cohort. However, a randomization is ethically not acceptable. The decision process is depended on a multitude of factors such as soft tissue and bony situation, infection parameters, overall medical condition and the patients` preference. Nevertheless, the knowledge of the prognosis and what the individual patient has to expect from a MKA or an AKA in terms of quality of life or complication rates are important aspects in this decision process. Both cohorts were not matched in terms of age and gender, because AKA and MKA are rare procedures and matched cohorts with a representative sample-size are

only feasible in a multi-center study. Further limitation is a lack of the pre-operative documentation of functional status and quality of life and ta functional outcome score. However, a pre-operative functional status has a limited value, because at this stage most of the patients are bedridden due to the underlying PJI. Furthermore the aim of the study was to compare the functional outcome between the two surgical procedures and not within one cohort. Another limitations are the inhomogeneous follow-up intervals and the high lost to follow-up rate of 32% after MKA and 37% after AKA. The inhomogeneous follow-up intervals are a consequence of the retrospective study design. The high drop out rate is explained by the advanced age of a part of patients at inclusion and is consequently accounting for a limited number of patients available for follow-up examination. At follow-up, the mean LEFS was 37 for AKA patients and 28 for MKA patients, but statistical analysis could not show any significant difference. The missing significance may be explained by the limited power of the study. Nevertheless, the current data provide basic information for a proper sample size calculation for a multicentre study. A multicentre study is needed for more reliable outcome data and the indications for AKA or MKA after septic failure of revision arthroplasty are rare and drop out rates in this cohort are high.

Conclusion

Patients treated with AKA and MKA after septic failure of revision TKA showed a comparable functional outcome, quality of life and postoperative complication rate. Younger amputee patients, that could be fitted with microprocessor-controlled-knee-joint presented a significantly better functional outcome than MKA patients. If AKA patients could not be fitted with a prosthesis functional outcome was devastating. In unsalvageable situations of septic failure after TKA the treatment decision process is depending on the patients' expectations, overall medical condition, physical strength, severity of infection and soft-tissue envelope. Taking these factors into account each case has to be evaluated carefully to determine which treatment option might lead to the best achievable outcome. For the daily clinical routine these data should be considered in the decision-making amputation vs. modular arthrodesis: Younger patients in a proper physical and mental state may benefit from an AKA with proper orthotics, whereas in physically compromised older patients arthrodesis seems to be the superior treatment.

Abbreviations
AKA: Above the knee amputation; CCI: Charlson comorbidity index; LEFS: Lower Extremity Functional Scale; MCS: Mental component summary; MKA: Modular knee prosthesis; PCS: Physical component summary; PJI: Prosthetic joint infection; TKA: Total knee arthroplasty

Acknowledgements
Not applicable.

Funding
This study was not funded.

Authors' contributions
MM₁, MK, CVR, KB and SH searched literature, drafted the manuscript, participated in conception, design and coordination. MM₂, MK and SH contributed to acquisition of data, analysis and interpretation of data. SH supervised the whole study. All authors read and approved the final manuscript.

Consent for publication
Not applicable.

Competing interests
The authors declare that they have no competing interests.

Author details
[1]BG Unfallklinik Murnau, Prof. Küntscher Str. 8, Murnau 82418, Germany. [2]Institute of Biomechanics, Paracelsus Medical University Salzburg and BG Unfallklinik Murnau, Prof. Küntscher Str. 8, Murnau 82418, Germany. [3]Department of Orthopedic Sports Medicine, Technische Universität München, Isamningerstr. 22, 81675 Munich, Germany. [4]Department of Orthopaedic Surgery and Traumatology, University Hospital Basel, Spitalstr. 21, 4031 Basel, Switzerland.

References
1. Matar WY, Jafari SM, Restrepo C, Austin M, Purtill JJ, Parvizi J. Preventing infection in total joint arthroplasty. The Journal of bone and joint surgery American volume. 2010;92(Suppl 2):36–46.
2. Rohner E, Windisch C, Nuetzmann K, Rau M, Arnhold M, Matziolis G. Unsatisfactory outcome of arthrodesis performed after septic failure of revision total knee arthroplasty. The Journal of bone and joint surgery American volume. 2015;97(4):298–301.
3. Mittal Y, Fehring TK, Hanssen A, Marculescu C, Odum SM, Osmon D. Two-stage reimplantation for periprosthetic knee infection involving resistant organisms. The Journal of bone and joint surgery American volume. 2007; 89(6):1227–31.
4. Mortazavi SM, Vegari D, Ho A, Zmistowski B, Parvizi J. Two-stage exchange arthroplasty for infected total knee arthroplasty: predictors of failure. Clin Orthop Relat Res. 2011;469(11):3049–54.
5. Jones RE, Russell RD, Huo MH. Alternatives to revision total knee arthroplasty. The Journal of bone and joint surgery British volume. 2012;94(11 Suppl A):137–40.
6. Gottfriedsen TB, Schroder HM, Odgaard A. Knee arthrodesis after failure of knee Arthroplasty: a Nationwide register-based study. The Journal of bone and joint surgery American volume. 2016;98(16):1370–7.
7. CH W, Gray CF, Lee GC. Arthrodesis should be strongly considered after failed two-stage reimplantation TKA. Clin Orthop Relat Res. 2014;472(11): 3295–304.
8. Isiklar ZU, Landon GC, Tullos HS. Amputation after failed total knee arthroplasty. Clin Orthop Relat Res. 1994;299:173–8.
9. Pring DJ, Marks L, Angel JC. Mobility after amputation for failed knee replacement. The Journal of bone and joint surgery British volume. 1988; 70(5):770–1.
10. Sierra RJ, Trousdale RT, Pagnano MW. Above-the-knee amputation after a total knee replacement: prevalence, etiology, and functional outcome. J Bone Joint Surg Am. 2003;85-A(6):1000–4.
11. Chen AF, Kinback NC, Heyl AE, McClain EJ, Klatt BA. Better function for fusions versus above-the-knee amputations for recurrent periprosthetic knee infection. Clin Orthop Relat Res. 2012;470(10):2737–45.
12. Angelini A, Henderson E, Trovarelli G, Ruggieri P. Is there a role for knee arthrodesis with modular endoprostheses for tumor and revision of failed endoprostheses? Clin Orthop Relat Res. 2013;471(10):3326–35.
13. Della Valle C, Parvizi J, Bauer TW, DiCesare PE, Evans RP, Segreti J, Spangehl M, Watters WC, 3rd, Keith M, Turkelson CM et al: American Academy of Orthopaedic surgeons clinical practice guideline on: the diagnosis of periprosthetic joint infections of the hip and knee. The Journal of bone and joint surgery American volume 2011, 93(14):1355–1357.
14. Charlson ME, Pompei P, Ales KL, MacKenzie CR. A new method of classifying prognostic comorbidity in longitudinal studies: development and validation. J Chronic Dis. 1987;40(5):373–83.
15. Binkley JM, Stratford PW, Lott SA, Riddle DL. The lower extremity functional scale (LEFS): scale development, measurement properties, and clinical application. North American Orthopaedic rehabilitation research network. Phys Ther. 1999;79(4):371–83.
16. Ware J Jr, Kosinski M, Keller SD. A 12-item short-form health survey: construction of scales and preliminary tests of reliability and validity. Med Care. 1996;34(3):220–33.
17. Jenkinson C, Layte R, Jenkinson D, Lawrence K, Petersen S, Paice C, Stradling J. A shorter form health survey: can the SF-12 replicate results from the SF-36 in longitudinal studies? J Public Health Med. 1997;19(2):179–86.
18. Conway JD, Mont MA, Bezwada HP. Arthrodesis of the knee. J Bone Joint Surg Am. 2004;86-A(4):835–48.
19. Rao N, Crossett LS, Sinha RK, Le Frock JL. Long-term suppression of infection in total joint arthroplasty. Clin Orthop Relat Res. 2003;414:55–60.
20. Thornhill TS, Dalziel RW, Sledge CB. Alternatives to arthrodesis for the failed total knee arthroplasty. Clin Orthop Relat Res. 1982;170:131–40.
21. Fedorka CJ, Chen AF, McGarry WM, Parvizi J, Klatt BA. Functional ability after above-the-knee amputation for infected total knee arthroplasty. Clin Orthop Relat Res. 2011;469(4):1024–32.
22. Bargiotas K, Wohlrab D, Sewecke JJ, Lavinge G, Demeo PJ, Sotereanos NG. Arthrodesis of the knee with a long intramedullary nail following the failure of a total knee arthroplasty as the result of infection. The Journal of bone and joint surgery American volume. 2006;88(3):553–8.
23. Somayaji HS, Tsaggerides P, Ware HE, Dowd GS. Knee arthrodesis–a review. Knee. 2008;15(4):247–54.
24. Bellmann M, Schmalz T, Blumentritt S. Comparative biomechanical analysis of current microprocessor-controlled prosthetic knee joints. Arch Phys Med Rehabil. 2010;91(4):644–52.

10

The importance of informational, clinical and personal support in patient experience with total knee replacement: a qualitative investigation

Laurie J. Goldsmith[1*], Nitya Suryaprakash[2], Ellen Randall[2,3], Jessica Shum[2,4], Valerie MacDonald[5], Richard Sawatzky[6,7], Samar Hejazi[8], Jennifer C. Davis[9,10], Patrick McAllister[11] and Stirling Bryan[2,3]

Abstract

Background: Total knee arthroplasty (TKA) is the most frequently performed joint replacement surgery in North America. Patient perspectives on TKA have been investigated in various ways, including finding as many as 20% of TKA patients are dissatisfied with their surgical outcomes. Understanding the patient experience with TKA broadly and in relation to patient satisfaction is a key gap in existing literature.

Methods: We report on the qualitative component of a mixed methods prospective cohort study examining patient experience and satisfaction post-TKA for adults in British Columbia, Canada. Data collection consisted of 45 in-depth interviews about individuals' knee surgery experiences conducted eight months after surgery. Analysis consisted of thematic coding by multiple coders.

Results: Participants' descriptions of their TKA experiences were primarily concerned with support, or the provision of aid and assistance. Support was insufficient when their expectations of support were not met; unmet support expectations led to an overall negative TKA experience. Support operated in three key domains: (1) informational support, (2) clinical support, and (3) personal support. Key sources of informational and clinical support included pre-optimisation clinics, surgeons, and physiotherapists. Key topics for informational support included pain, pain management, and recovery trajectories. Personal support was provided by family, friends, other TKA patients, employers, and themselves.

Conclusions: Patient needs and expectations for support are shaped both before and after TKA surgery. Patients with an overall positive TKA experience had improvement in their knee pain, stiffness or functioning post-TKA, had their major expectations and needs for support met during their TKA recovery, and believed that any significant future expectations or needs for ongoing support would be adequately met. In contrast, patients with an overall negative TKA experience had at least one major expectation or need for support not met during their TKA recovery, even in cases where they had good TKA outcomes. Suggested interventions to improve the experience of persons receiving TKA include an expanded patient navigator model, revised pre-surgery educational materials, particularly around pain expectations and management, and comprehensive sharing of other patients' TKA experience.

Keywords: Total knee arthroplasty, Qualitative research, Patient experience, Patient-centred care, Support

* Correspondence: laurie_goldsmith@sfu.ca
[1]Faculty of Health Sciences, Simon Fraser University, Blusson Hall 10506, 8888 University Drive, Burnaby, BC V5A 1S6, Canada
Full list of author information is available at the end of the article

Background

Total knee arthroplasty (TKA) is the most frequently performed joint replacement surgery in North America, with age and sex-standardized rates of TKA increasing over time [1, 2]. Various aspects of TKA have been studied to improve clinical outcomes and reduce costs, including reducing surgical wait times and hospital length of stay [3–5]. More recently, researchers have investigated patient perspectives on TKA, reflecting the current interest in patient-centred care [6–8]. Paying attention to the patient perspective—in this case, focusing on improving the patient experience of care—is also a key aspect of the Institute for Healthcare Improvement's Triple Aim framework. This framework explicitly states that it is possible to design health care interventions that improve the patient experience while also simultaneously reducing per capita health care costs and improving the health of populations [9]. In other words, improving the patient experience does not have to come at the expense of, and can even augment, other cost and quality goals.

Research on the patient perspective on TKA employs two major approaches. The first major approach quantitatively evaluates patient satisfaction after TKA, finding that as many as 20% of TKA patients are dissatisfied with their surgical outcomes [10, 11]. Factors found to influence patient satisfaction include knee pain, stiffness, and functioning before and after TKA, postoperative complications, and patient characteristics including expectations, social support, age, gender, and ethnicity [10–15]. The second major approach qualitatively investigates particular aspects of the patient experience before and after TKA surgery, including deciding to have or not have surgery [16, 17], waiting for surgery [18, 19], pre-surgery pain [20], pre-surgery education [21, 22], post-surgery pain [23], the hospital experience [24], rehabilitative practices [25], managing recovery [26, 27], and returning to physical activity [28, 29]. While it is helpful that these two approaches to patient perspective research exist, it is difficult to integrate and more deeply understand their results. The existing quantitative work on patient satisfaction does not usually take patient experience into account and the existing qualitative work on patient experience does not usually take patient satisfaction into account. The qualitative work on patient experience also tends to focus on specific aspects of the TKA experience rather than examining the patient experience broadly. New qualitative and mixed methods research can build from this knowledge base through allowing for a fuller account of the patient experience and investigating both patient satisfaction and patient experience without fully constraining either focus by preconceived variables and topics. Including a qualitative approach can also provide rich data on patient meanings

and preferences [30, 31] and help strengthen decision-making around system resource use and design [32].

We conducted a multiphase mixed-methods study [33] to improve our understanding of patient experience and patient satisfaction following TKA surgery. This paper reports on the foundational qualitative work from our mixed-methods study investigating patient experience and satisfaction with TKA. Our qualitative investigation asked patients to reflect on their TKA experience broadly, across a variety of aspects of their knee replacement experience, and in relation to their self-reported satisfaction after TKA surgery.

Methods

The qualitative work reported here is embedded within a mixed-methods, prospective cohort study investigating patient experience and satisfaction with TKA. We recruited 515 adults aged 19 years or older with a primary or secondary diagnosis of osteoarthritis scheduled to undergo primary TKA in British Columbia between April 2012 and August 2013. Study participants were recruited from the mandatory pre-surgical total joint replacement education sessions at six sites across the province, including at least one site in each of the five geographic health regions. Ethics approval was obtained from relevant universities and health regions. For the quantitative component of the study (not reported here), each participant completed a pre-surgery, paper-based, self-administered, English-language, questionnaire and most completed additional surveys at 6 and 12 months post-surgery (91 and 88% of baseline, respectively). Questionnaires included demographics and patient-reported outcome measures about pre- and post-surgery pain, stiffness and functioning, health status, expectations, and satisfaction. For the qualitative portion of the overall study, we conducted 70 semi-structured, in-depth interviews with 57 purposefully selected individuals either once or twice at 8 and 14 months post surgery ($n = 45$ persons interviewed at 8 months, $n = 25$ persons interviewed at 14 months, with 12 of the 25 persons interviewed for the first time at 14 months). The number of possible interviews overall and at each time-point was established prior to collecting data due to resource planning constraints. We anticipated this sample size, which included 8–10 participants per health region (both urban and rural), would be necessary for reaching informational redundancy on key themes and key TKA outcomes and experiences, and for achieving maximum patient variation [34, 35].

This paper focuses on the 45 individuals interviewed about their TKA experience 8 months post-surgery. Our qualitative data are rich and multi-faceted; restricting our initial analytic focus to first-time interviews at 8 months post-surgery allowed us to deeply understand major issues in patients' initial post TKA-experience. Additional analysis of the qualitative and mixed methods data will build off of the foundation established in this paper—including understanding the effects of time on patients' post-TKA experience and satisfaction—and will be reported elsewhere.

Sample selection and data collection

To create the qualitative sample from the quantitative cohort, we considered all cohort participants for inclusion other than 6-month survey non-respondents and those having survey completion assistance. We interviewed in every provincial region multiple times and interviewed as many persons as possible who reported dissatisfaction with their TKA results on their 6-monthpost-surgery questionnaire. We further purposefully sampled for maximum variation on other key characteristics from our survey data and associated literature, including sex, ethnicity, employment status, self-rated health, and various pain, functioning, and emotional health measures. Those purposefully selected were approached by letter followed by telephone call to schedule an interview. Interviews took place where convenient for the participant, including participants' homes and medical clinics. Interviews were conducted in English by experienced interviewers. The semi-structured interview guide was designed to understand the individual's knee surgery experience and outcomes. Interviewee-specific probes were also created based on their answers to the baseline and 6-month surveys. Interviews generally lasted 45–65 min. Participants received an honorarium at interview completion. After leaving the participant, the interviewer completed a standardized interview debrief on the key information learned and suggested interview guide revisions. The interviews and debriefs were digitally recorded and transcribed.

Data analysis

All transcripts and debriefs were thematically coded using NVivo software (NVivo qualitative data analysis software; QSR International Pty Ltd. Version 10, 2012). The coding scheme was initially developed through two coders (NS, ER) independently coding the same transcripts and debriefs and constructing a thematic coding framework through consensus and input from a third coder (LJG). Remaining transcripts and debriefs were coded by one of four coders (LJG, NS, ER, JS) with new codes created when needed to reflect new concepts. Coders met on a regular basis to discuss analysis with key decisions. Text coded at key codes was also regularly reviewed and discussed by other team members to further develop the analysis and provide a check on coding consistency and construct validity. Once all the transcripts were coded with the initial coding scheme,

combinations of up to five team members (LJG, NS, ER, JS, SH) met on multiple occasions to discuss key themes and their relationships with the goal of arriving at a higher abstraction of key themes. Individual coders then reviewed text coded at key codes to further develop relationships between key themes and identify representative quotations with results further discussed in larger team meetings. Reflective memos were constructed throughout. Our analysis approach meant that key codes and significant portions of interview transcripts were reviewed in multiple ways by multiple team members. This multi-step coding process helped to ensure the rigor of our analysis [34, 36].[1]

Results

We purposefully sampled 65 participants from the overall cohort to obtain the 45 persons interviewed approximately 8 months after their TKA surgery. Thirteen persons declined participation due to worsening health or other reasons and 7 were not contactable. Post-surgery interview timing varied based on scheduling, averaging 7.9 months (minimum 6.6, maximum 9.4 months). Each health region was represented by an average of 9 persons (minimum 7, maximum 11). Demographics and other key details of the 45 participants are provided in Table 1. Given our focus on understanding patient dissatisfaction, we oversampled from the 15% of those who reported TKA dissatisfaction in their 6-month survey, resulting in 58% of the 45 qualitative interviewees having reported dissatisfaction (i.e., reporting neutral, dissatisfied, or very dissatisfied on the 5-point dissatisfaction scale). We secondarily oversampled those who indicated that they were uncertain or would not be willing to have their TKA surgery again if they could go back in time (44% of the 45 qualitative interviewees vs. 12% of the quantitative cohort). Our qualitative sample otherwise roughly mirrors key distributions in the overall cohort, with over half of the sample being women, having married or common-law status, a household income below $60,000, or North American or European ethnicity. Over half of both our qualitative and cohort sample also were experiencing their first knee surgery or had waited more than 12 months from the onset of their knee symptoms and first seeing their TKA surgeon.

Participants' descriptions and sense-making of their TKA experiences were primarily concerned with the provision of aid and assistance, a concept we label "support." Support was deemed to be insufficient when their expectations of support were not met; unmet support expectations often led to an overall negative TKA experience. Support expectations were both formed in advance of surgery and in response to emergent needs after surgery. TKA patients' experiences in this study primarily operated in three key domains: (1)

Table 1 Participants' Descriptive Details (n = 45)

		Count
Age, average	65 years	
Sex	Female	30
	Male	15
Marital status	Married or common-law	34
	Widowed	3
	Single, divorced or separated	8
Household income	< $40,000	12
	$40,000 to < $60,000	10
	$60,000 to < $80,000	10
	$80,000 or more	10
	Missing	3
Education	High school or less	19
	College/technical school	12
	Undergraduate degree	3
	Graduate degree	8
	Other	2
	Missing	1
Ethnicity	North American	33
	European	8
	South Asian	2
	Central/South American	1
	Other	1
Received TKA surgery on first or second knee	First knee	32
	Second knee	12
	Missing	1
Time between knee symptoms and first time seeing surgeon	<6 months	9
	≥6 to < 12 months	9
	≥12 months	25
	Do not remember	2
Satisfaction with TKA surgery results, self-evaluated 6 months post-surgery[a]	Very satisfied	8
	Satisfied	10
	Neutral	15
	Dissatisfied	9
	Very dissatisfied	2
	Missing	1
Willing to have TKA surgery again, self-evaluated 6 months post-surgery	Yes	25
	Uncertain	12
	No	8

[a]The 5-point satisfaction scale can also be reduced to a 2-point satisfaction scale where satisfied is composed of those who answered "very satisfied" or "satisfied" on the 5-point scale and dissatisfied is composed of those who answered "neutral," "dissatisfied" or "very dissatisfied" on the 5-point scale

informational support, (2) clinical support, and (3) personal support. These domains interact with each other (Fig. 1) and a deficiency in one domain can sometimes be compensated for by another domain, as explained below and through illustrative quotations from varied participants (Tables 2, 3 and 4).

Informational support

All participants noted the importance of information about TKA preparation and recovery. Patients received information through formal clinical sources, such as pre-surgical education sessions and health care providers, and informal personal sources, such as friends and family, the internet, and, when applicable, their experience with having already received TKA on their other knee.

Each participant identified the pre-surgical education sessions as a key form of informational support from a clinical source. The provided information was often also described as insufficient—many participants wanted more information than routinely provided at the sessions to be better prepared for TKA recovery and to actively participate in their own care. Some participants further said that their education session information was not meaningful as it was difficult to understand or remember the instructions or it was difficult to reconcile the different messages they received from different presenters. This information was further complicated by having hip-replacement patients at the same education session as knee-replacement patients. Participants also reflected on how they were overwhelmed, anxious, or scared before the surgery, which made it challenging to retain information from the education session.

Surgeons were both expected and actual key clinical sources of information about TKA preparation and recovery, although many participants wanted more information from their surgeon than they received. Multiple patients described their visits to the surgeon as too "matter of fact," emphasizing checking physical functioning. Participants described surgeons as not readily providing wanted information and not having or making time to answer questions. This situation was exacerbated by patients feeling overwhelmed by their visit to the surgeon, which often led to patients not asking their prepared questions. Participants noted and appreciated when a surgeon took time to provide sufficient and helpful information. A few participants recounted that even though their TKA outcome was not as good as they expected, the time and information provided by their surgeon both before and after the surgery improved their TKA experience. Regardless of the surgeon's ability to provide information support, patients typically saw their surgeon a few times following their surgery which

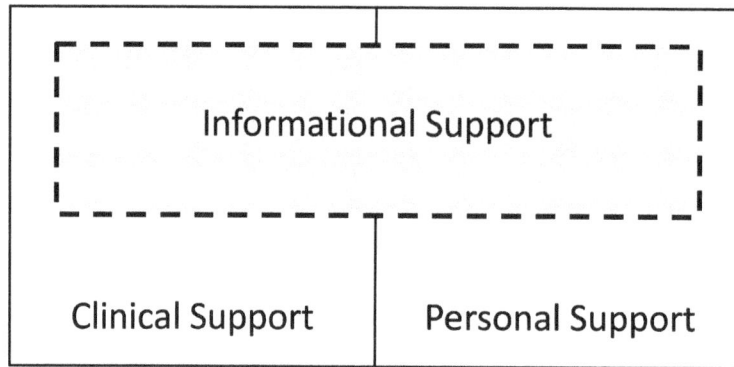

Fig. 1 Key domains of support in patient experience of total knee arthroplasty

restricted patients' ability to use the surgeon as an information source.

Other health care providers could be valuable sources of information post-TKA but were inconsistent sources of information support. Many participants recounted that their family doctor was no longer involved once the decision to have TKA had been made. Some sought advice from their family doctor after their TKA surgery if their surgeon was unavailable but found that their family doctor provided no or limited information. Physiotherapists provided information about post-TKA exercise and recovery and often interacted with participants multiple times after the surgery, but some participants still felt that the exercise information was not comprehensive enough. One hospital had physiotherapists make home visits to TKA patients after their surgery which participants found helpful for understanding their recovery in their home context.

Talking to other TKA patients was another form of informational support. Although a few participants expressed a preference for dealing with things on their own, the majority of participants stressed the importance of talking to other patients with previous TKA experience. Patients shared information about surgeons, types of treatment, exercises, and healing and recovery strategies and trajectories. Such information sharing was sometimes a response to insufficient information from clinical sources.

The most frequent type of informational support identified as needing improvement was information on pain expectations. Many participants expected that the surgery would alleviate their pain and were surprised and unhappy when they experienced intense pain after their surgery, particularly when pain was long-lasting. A few people thought that when the arthritis was "taken out" of their knee with the surgery that their pain would be completely gone. Some participants said that their pre-surgery education session did not tell them they would experience post-TKA pain; others said that while their education session did provide information about pain,

not enough information was provided. Participants on their second knee TKA experience illustrated the empowering nature of this knowledge, recounting that they knew this time around to expect significant pain and to exercise through it. Despite their interest in having more information about pain in advance of their surgery, some participants felt that fully forewarning others might stop them from having surgery.

Participants also expressed concern about inadequate information regarding pain management. Pain management education was sometimes offered by physiotherapists during rehabilitation. Some family doctors provided assurance about pain medication addiction concerns and home care nurses provided education about icing techniques. Despite the existence of these forms of assistance, inadequate pain management information support was a frequent issue for participants. When reflecting on how they could have better learned about pain and pain management, many participants suggested that TKA patients should have access to a "go to" clinical person to answer patient questions. The clinical expertise of this person was left unspecified, although many participants also expressed that surgeons should be more available to patients to discuss pain and other recovery concerns.

Multiple participants wanted to understand the variety of TKA recovery trajectories so they could be assured they were on some sort of a track to recovery, even if it was not the ideal track or an ideal recovery. To supplement the inadequate recovery trajectory information, many participants compared themselves to other TKA patients they knew. When their recovery experience was worse than others' experiences, participants did not know how to make sense of this mismatch and wanted clinical support in understanding their problems. Many participants suggested that a formal patient buddy program would be helpful, where patients could be paired with a former TKA patient to normalize the recovery experience. Some participants had already started doing that for others in an informal way.

Table 2 Informational support illustrative quotes

(1) Pre-surgical education session as a source of informational support

"The [education session] is really informative….They prepare you for everything. If I went to the hospital without this program and woke up with my leg looking and feeling the way it did, I think I might have wanted a new limb."

"I went to all the pre-surgery meetings…But nobody ever really said, 'This is not a real knee. This is not going to be the same as your other knee was. There will be limitations.'… I did read all the literature but nowhere did I see that said."

"The [education session] was pretty good but not good enough. I don't think we really got enough warning about how much assistance you need afterwards…But maybe they can't tell you what to expect because there's so many differences in people too—it would take forever and maybe scare some people needlessly."

"I still don't think that they explained how painful exercises are going to be at the pre-op session. You are told, but it doesn't sink in. I think that should really be pushed. It is going to be painful but you can't do any damage. Like, once the knee is in place, you can't really harm it."

(2) Surgeons as a source of informational support

"The one you really want to rely on is of course the surgeon. [You want to ask] 'What did you do to me?' or 'What are you going to do to me?'"

"They are always in a hurry,… [My surgeon] showed me the x-ray. 'And this is fine. It's fine. You're going to be fine.'…You are just a number and you just go and it's quick, quick, quick."

"I think the hardest thing was [my surgeon]'s so hard to talk to…I think that probably was a lot of my problem, not feeling like I was given enough information."

"I only saw [my surgeon] a few times…a very nice person, very friendly to me. I wish I could see him more to get more information…but they have so many patients, [the visit is] so very fast."

"The surgeon, when I first met him, I thought, 'Boy, that guy's got no personality.' When I got to know him I realized he does, but he's a busy man. They are very busy. He's willing to answer any questions but if you don't have the questions to ask, how can they answer them?"

"I wanted to know why I was so numb in my knee and [the surgeon] didn't answer me. He just said 'You're going to have to give it time.'"

"You have to be really prepared and aware what you want to ask. You got to go in prepared because you get a little nervous. You get intimidated by these guys."

"[My surgeon] walked us step by step. He showed me what the surgery would do and what it would look like and then he showed me the x-rays of my knee and he explained everything that was going on…I can't praise him enough."

(3) Other health care providers as a source of informational support

"My family doctor is fine but he—perhaps because of the little bit more complexities in this case, he really didn't have any opinions of his own about things. He really deferred everything to the surgeon."

"When I went for physio, the therapist kept on saying, 'It's going to be a year.' And so that gave me hope too because when I first went there, I thought I'd be better already. I would have thought 'A month has gone. What's wrong here?'"

"The [physiotherapists] here tell you to get on with the exercises and don't back off on that. They did point out quite emphatically that if you have pain, use the medication. Don't back off on the exercise because of pain. If the knee hurts, take a pill. Don't stop bending it."

Table 2 Informational support illustrative quotes *(Continued)*

"The physiotherapists set you up with a program. You're only allowed to go for three visits. So you are cramming in three visits all these exercises which you are supposed to do. And rather than following up, people just go back to their old patterns because no one is checking up."

(4) Other TKA patients as a source of informational support

"We are all comparing scars [saying] 'Oh, your scar is so much nicer than mine.'"

"If I had met [another TKA patient] who would have told me the honest truth—'This could happen' or 'I had this happen' or 'There's quite a bit of pain at first,' you know, this sort of thing. I might have had more questions to ask [the surgeon]."

"My girlfriend is getting it done so she was asking me different things… I did tell her to go to all the physio…. I said that through other people that were in physio, I did hear that [her surgeon] was a good doctor."

"I think seeing where other people are at [physiotherapy] gives you incentive too and makes you say, 'I should be able to do this.' Or 'I should be working at it harder.'"

(5) Informational support for pain expectations

"I don't think it's stressed enough and I don't think I ever read or heard before I had the surgery that the pain is not going to go away for a year. I thought [it would go away] in a month"

"I thought it would be better than it is…The twisting pain I'm hoping will get less but it's still pretty severe…I thought my knee wouldn't hurt when I walked down the stairs, and maybe it won't, given some more time. I am constantly told 'Wait, wait, wait.' so, I'm waiting. I just expected less discomfort after this period of time."

"The meeting at the hospital before you went in for surgery where they were explaining kind of what is going to happen. And they kept saying, 'Oh, yes, you'll have a little pain.' I wish they had been a little bit more honest as to *the amount of pain.*"

"I got mixed messages particularly when I went to physio. One person would say to me 'Oh well, don't do it if it hurts.' Another person would say 'Well, that's the way it is.'…It's a bit confusing."

"[After my first knee replacement] I was afraid to push it too hard because I didn't know if I was going to do damage because of the pain. This time [for my second knee replacement] I knew I couldn't really do any harm…I think probably for a lot of people the pain with the exercises, they are not prepared for it."

(6) Informational support for pain management

"I'm frustrated [by the pain]… I've been back to my GP a few times saying, 'Come on, there's got to be something.' 'No, you are doing great.' I go to physiotherapy. He says, 'Oh, look at the movement in your leg. You are doing terrific.' Okay, I am doing terrific but it hurts."

"The physiotherapist said it's breaking down scar tissue which tends to form. You have to break it down to get the range of motion. And that gets uncomfortable. So bear with it. Use the pain killers as necessary but don't let pain restrict your recovery."

"I kept on talking to [my family] doctor saying, 'I don't want to get [addicted].' They say, 'Take the pain medication, the pain medication. Manage it so you can move it.' And I said, 'Well, I don't want to get addicted to it.' 'Oh, don't worry about that, don't worry about that.' But I did worry about it."

"I think that if I'd had somebody I could call, even a couple of times like now and say, okay, it's seven months, I'm in pain, the swelling is really bad today, what the hell do I do?"

Table 2 Informational support illustrative quotes *(Continued)*

"There is nobody to talk to. You call the surgeon and unless there is like a major problem they don't want to hear it from you because all they care about is what the x-ray shows and the x-ray shows perfect. It's fine. The GPs, they didn't do the surgery so it's more pain control—like, 'Do you want stronger pain pills?' And I said no. I don't want to just cover up the symptoms. I need to know what is going on. So you can get on the internet and check things, but there is nobody to really talk to about the pain, the swelling."

(7) Informational support about recovery trajectories

"Unless I'm the exception. I don't know if everybody has [these problems]. ….It would be nice for them to say, 'Okay. This is the scenario. Some people may get full movement back but some people may not,' you know. If they could let you know those options but they didn't.

"My brother had both of his [knees] done two years previous and a friend of mine had hers done and the neighbour across the street had hers done with the same doctor that I got it done with so I kind of knew what to expect."

"I should have sat down with [my neighbour] longer because he's had his knees done…I'd like to have a phone-a-buddy, to phone somebody that's had an knee operation the same time I did and ask 'How's your recovery going?'"

(8) Informational support about other post-surgery issues

"Nobody said anything about the clicking…It kind of [worried me] because I was wondering if there was something wrong, that it shouldn't be like that. And, of course, I got told it was quite normal. Everybody's knee pretty much does it. And he explained why, which was good. Once I got the information and I understood that it wasn't a big deal, it was fine."

"[The surgeon should] take some time to really explain to somebody what's really going to happen, like, what your expectations should be. You may not have the pain you had before but this knee is going to make noise when you walk. This knee is going to feel like it's crunching inside your leg. You're going to have quite an ugly scar. You're knee won't be shaped the same as your other knee anymore."

"This [part of my knee] is still numb. I asked about that. [My surgeon] said, 'Oh, it may never come back.' It looks very different than my other knee. I know I've got ugly knees but it's small. This is smaller. It gets warm still and that's something the physio said is not good… [My knee is] a lot better than it was but it's certainly not as good as I would like it to be."

Italics indicate word was emphasized by participant

Other areas participants identified as needing additional information support included post-surgery issues like knee clicking, infection and scarring; post-surgery exercise and functioning; and alternative and supplementary rehabilitative options.

Clinical support

Patients expected that surgeons would be key helpers for making sense of their TKA experience but few participants were provided with this clinical support. Many participants wanted more personal and higher quality interactions with surgeons where ideal interaction examples consisted of both emotional support and support with their health needs, including information support. Most patients wanted a surgeon who was both a skilled

technician and an empathetic individual, yet participants often described surgeons as mainly providing surgery specific support, with little to no effort at building rapport or making the patient feel like an individual. A lack of personal interaction often impeded patient reassurance and many participants had a hard time understanding why their questions and concerns were unanswered or diminished.

Patient sense-making was further challenged by mismatches between the patient's and surgeon's perspectives. The first type of mismatch was where the surgeon lacked empathy for the patient's experience, including times that patients learned for the first time post-surgery that their knee should have been replaced much sooner than it was and their post-surgery pain indicated a longer recovery timeline. Another type of mismatch was demonstrated when the surgeon did not appear to be seriously investigating the patient's unresolved post-surgery problems, which often left the patient frustrated and confused. The lack of availability of the surgeon post-surgery was a third mismatch and was sometimes interpreted by the patient as the surgeon not caring about or not believing the patient. Some participants reported that mismatches resulted in losing trust in the surgeon and expecting that future interactions would be as unsatisfying as in the past. Participants sometimes attributed mismatches to the power imbalance between the surgeon and patient, describing the surgeon as condescending or arrogant.

Physiotherapists and physiotherapy services provided key clinical support. Physiotherapy helped patients regain mobility and resume their regular activities. Many participants felt that a "good physiotherapist" was critical to properly recovering from surgery. Good physiotherapists had effective communication skills, treated each patient as a person, had time for patients, and tailored the services to the patient's needs, including extending the number of sessions provided to the patient. Hospital-based physiotherapists were valuable due to their proximity to the surgeon, although some private-practice physiotherapists were valued for their flexible schedules. Physiotherapy was also a place where patients could share information, interact with others, and benchmark their recovery with other TKA patients.

A few patients received inadequate physiotherapy support, usually resulting from not getting scheduled for physiotherapy until long after their surgery. Most of these examples were from patients having their surgery outside of their local catchment area and then trying to receive outpatient physiotherapy close to home, although a few participants were not scheduled for outpatient physiotherapy even when their surgery was at their local hospital. Some of these unscheduled patients were assisted by persons within the health care system

Table 3 Clinical support illustrative quotes

(1) Surgeons as a source of clinical support

"[My surgeon] has a good reputation. The hospital thinks the world of him…So I went to visit him and it was just a great match. He covers all the bases and tells you everything. There's no secrets, no big surprises. He said if everything goes well, I'd only be in the hospital three days. That's what it was."

"[My surgeon was] not really reassuring or anything. Very matter of fact…very 'It'll be this way. If that doesn't happen, this will happen and we'll do it that way.' And basically that was it…he wasn't very personable…It wasn't any kind of conversation. It was very quick."

"[The surgeon] said, 'I just wish I had more patients that were like you, that were healing quicker.'…I felt good because he did a good job and I felt good because I'd done a good job doing my exercises and everything. It was a win for both of us."

"[My surgeon] is so caring…even when I am crying he is like, 'Oh, we'll do this. We'll get through it.'…I knew that he was going to help me."

"I think the minute he heard or saw my psychiatric file, I think he probably thought this person isn't worthy of a knee replacement."

"The surgeon is useless to get information out of…6 weeks [after the surgery] I went in there and he said to me something which I didn't understand and I'm sorry I never pursued it."

"I'd saved up these questions. I wanted to know if it was cement or screwed in. I wanted to know if the scar was the way it should be, if the numbness should be there. He answered my questions but in a very different way than I would have assumed he'd answer them. I would think that rather than make it sound so ordinary—this isn't an ordinary thing."

(2) Physiotherapists and physiotherapy as a source of clinical support

"Physiotherapy is the one thing you can count on."

"I went to physio twice a week and each week I could tell, getting in and out of the vehicle and walking into the hospital, I could feel that it was getting stronger."

"[The physiotherapist's] attitude was all help. If you needed help, she helped. Very positive, saying things like 'Work through the pain, you're doing great, just push a little harder.'"

"I went to rehab at the hospital and I could have done it as long as I wanted. They were fantastic. And it was all covered. I never got asked to pay for anything, it was all covered."

"One of the things they worked on [in physiotherapy] that I found very helpful, so did other people, was they developed a camaraderie, this big family get-together type of thing, to talk to people, compare notes and get a little encouragement from patient to patient. So it wasn't just an isolated one-on-one therapist to patient. There was a lot of dialogue between patients."

"They were sending in a referral to [hospital name] for physio. I was given a phone number to call. So the first week home I called and they said there is nothing available yet…I was getting very desperate and in about the fourth week I started calling other hospitals… I was almost in tears. I was at my wits end, didn't know what to do. And the woman in reception there said, 'This isn't acceptable, I'm going to talk to the physio and I'm going to call you back. I'm sure we will fit you in.' She phoned back the next day…Without them—if they would have taken the same attitude as everybody else—I probably still wouldn't be able to bend my knee."

(3) Family doctors as a source of clinical support

"I have a GP who has been with me through the whole pain medication process, to the reduction of opiates, to the pre-surgery consult through the referral. He took my staples out at the end of the

Table 3 Clinical support illustrative quotes (Continued)

surgery. He followed me along through the recovery process post-surgery to make sure there was no infection. He followed along with the physiotherapist's recommendations."

"I think my GP does know [that I still have unresolved pain in my knee]. I think he does. He knows I am under a lot of stress, a combination of the pain and being a caregiver. But there is nothing he can do. He can only give me so many Prozac and so many painkillers."

"I did go to the GP about my knee and asking him for advice on what I can do because the system isn't doing it. And he suggested Aquafit."

"I don't talk to my family doctor about it because he's not interested. That's the surgeon's problem. [My family doctor] doesn't want to get involved."

to eventually get physiotherapy, although the patients had to first advocate for themselves to multiple points in the system before finding an advocate in the system.

Although they played a minor role in post-TKA clinical support, family doctors sometimes assisted with pain medication or provided additional recovery advice, such as suggesting other rehabilitative activities like massage therapy and water exercises. Other family doctors were reluctant to provide information; participants perceived this was because the family doctor did not want to get involved in the "surgeon's business."

Personal support

Family and friends were important sources of personal support for a variety of activities. Participants recounted needing much assistance with activities of daily living after TKA surgery. When first sent home from the hospital, participants described needing assistance turning over in bed, bathing, using the bathroom, and using stairs. Participants were initially unable to drive after surgery; some had family or friends drive them to health care appointments while others relied on public transportation. Family and friends also went grocery shopping and prepared meals. Some family members—male spouses/partners in particular––and some friends were not capable of providing personal physical support. Reasons for this lack of capability included: being anxious, feeling unskilled, not understanding what support was needed, their own physical impairment, and being busy in their own lives.

The physical support provided by family and friends often also helped patients feel emotionally supported. Participants also described explicit emotional support provided by family and friends through visiting and going out for meals or social activities. Other TKA patients also provided key emotional support through validating participants' feelings and providing encouragement about recovery.

Table 4 Personal support illustrative quotes

(1) Family and friends as a source of personal support

"My son has been very helpful. He'd do the shopping or the laundry and cleaning or drive me places to my appointments."

"My wife and daughter were trying this idea of one on each side and then three people abreast across can't go up the staircase. But our nurse friend knew how to negotiate all that."

"There are people here in the co-op. They were only a phone call away if I needed anything. They'd phone, 'I'm going grocery shopping. Do you need anything?'"

"I needed to get to a physio…I didn't want to impose on [my friends] to drive me over there and sit for an hour. But I couldn't really trust my husband because he's got dementia."

"The whole surgery thing made [my husband] very anxious. So his daughter had come to stay with us for a couple of days…and once I had the surgery she left. So I had to get back on my feet almost immediately and I was driving within 10 days, you know, could just barely move my foot but I could move it enough, to drive the car."

"[My friend] said, "Well, we can't go walking or do anything because you're an invalid. You can't walk.' So my social life has gone downhill."

"Our church family was so supportive too…It's incredible, the cards, the phone calls, the meals I would get…it shows they care. I think that is such a huge part of recovery."

(2) Other TKA patients as a source of personal support

"[My friends who had knee surgery] knew what it was all about and they told me how important it is. 'Do your exercises. Don't put them off.' And when I could see how well they were doing, it encouraged me."

"I talked to more people that are waiting to have [their knee replacement] done to encourage them. I find that a lot of people are scared and I try to encourage them because I say you just won't believe how you feel the day after your surgery to have that pain anymore."

"I spoke to about half a dozen people that had it and they were all walking around, they were fine, they were back to playing sports and doing whatever."

(3) Self as a source of personal support

"I was prepared and knew you need to have a toilet riser, you need to have a cane, you need to have a walker… I even went to the Red Cross and got everything there."

"One of the things I learned [before surgery was] change your life before [surgery] and you'll heal better. Which I did. I stopped drinking. I'm not a big drinker but I totally stopped alcohol."

"I was very good about doing all my exercises every single day, twice a day as they told me. I went to physio on my own after I ran out of physio at the hospital, which I have no coverage for so that was another three hundred and fifty bucks [out of my pocket.]"

"I was also an active participant in the process which I think has got to be one of the keys to it. You can't be a passive person and let them kind of do things to you because ultimately you have to be responsible for your own rehabilitation and recovery, be involved in it right from the very beginning."

(4) Employers as a source of personal support

"The union is supportive. The company is supportive… People try to be as accommodating as they can if somebody needs help."

Table 4 Personal support illustrative quotes *(Continued)*

"So I postponed going to work for that month, plus I work for a doctor and she knows what is involved, and she said, 'No, definitely take another month off, take the time that you need.'"

"I am not at full time yet. I am working five hours a day. I hoped to increase that but my knee would keep flaring up and I couldn't attend at all. Work has agreed to rent a recliner. Sometimes my knee is swollen and I need to keep it up. That's the difficult part."

"We have a really good extended health care program. They covered everything….I had to get a pool pass. He just said, 'Just send us a receipt. We'll cover you.'"

"I've had some issues with my employment, about getting back to work and its very aggravating and its very stressful…after two months they were phoning me, 'You can come back to work.'… But then I said I also have physio. There's where they have a fine line: you go to physio and now you're on sick time again."

"I went back to work and did full time for three months and I just crashed. I couldn't do it anymore… My manager was… unsympathetic."

Participants further recounted the importance of self support. Many undertook pre-surgery preparation of their home for post-surgery safety and convenience. Many felt highly responsible for their own healing and recovery and expressed this responsibility through creating pre- and post-surgery exercise routines, undertaking lifestyle changes such as dieting and losing weight, maintaining hobbies, and keeping a positive attitude despite post-surgery challenges. Self-support was also expressed through advocating for better treatment or extra attention from providers and specifying from whom they received care.

Employers could be additional sources of personal support for working participants. Many working participants described their employers as supportive and understanding of their situation, including allowing them to work at home. Some participants also had insurance through their employer that covered all or some of their health care expenses, such as extra physiotherapy. Other working participants had negative experiences with their employers, including being unable to take enough sick days for recovery and having to return to work with minimal physical accommodation.

Discussion

We found that patient experience of TKA can be conceptualized in terms of patient needs for informational, clinical and personal support, where patient expectations for support is shaped both before and after TKA surgery. Patients with an overall positive TKA experience had improvement in their knee pain, stiffness or functioning post-TKA, had their major expectations and needs for support met during their TKA recovery, and believed that any significant future expectations or needs for ongoing support would be adequately met. In contrast, patients with an overall negative TKA experience had at least one major expectation or need for support not met during their TKA recovery, even in cases where they had good TKA outcomes. Patients with overall negative TKA experiences sometimes also believed that any significant future expectations or needs for ongoing support would not be met in an adequate way, usually based on having already experienced multiple instances of inadequate support.

Having appropriate support could help address post-TKA pain, functioning or stiffness problems, which were identified as significant challenges by several participants. In all cases where our study participants reported having post-TKA knee issues, having caring and informative clinical input, especially from the surgeon, made the participant more likely to report positive experiences than would be expected given her or his knee problem. Participants were clearly comfortable with knowing that recovery would take time, that not everything would work out perfectly, and that they had a role to play in having a good TKA experience. In other words, participants were very comfortable with taking on their part to support a positive TKA outcome, even without perfect knowledge of all that would be expected of them. Along with assuming their own responsibility, participants expected health care providers and the health care system to support them to achieve positive TKA outcomes across a variety of patient experiences, including difficult, challenging, or unusual patient experiences. Where health care providers did not support this approach—such as telling the patient that everything is fine with their knee when the patient thinks their knee is far from fine—our study participants challenged this thinking, suggesting that clinicians and the system needed to expand the boundary of when they end their support for the patient.

Participants in our study were clearly asking for clinicians and the health care system to adopt a more patient-centred approach across their surgery and recovery experience. Improving patient-centredness is the responsibility of all involved in the health care system [6, 8, 37]; surgeons are neither the sole problem nor the sole solution, even though surgeons played a key role in participants' narratives. The current system structure positions the surgeon as one of few resources the TKA patient can turn to for problem-solving, which carries with it all of the limitations and vulnerabilities of single node systems, including bottlenecks [38]. This does not need to be the system structure of the future. Orthopedic clinics and hospitals could offer additional options for patient problem-solving. One intervention that could fill this gap would be an expanded patient navigator for TKA patients, where the patient navigator role is held by a clinician such as a nurse practitioner who can provide patient care and education and liaison with surgeons, physiotherapists, primary

care, home care, and social services. Other possible gap-filling interventions could expand the offered support beyond the health care system, such as implementing the "TKA buddy" program advocated by participants in our study, where current TKA patients are paired up with another current or previous TKA patient to provide a venue for informational and social support. Our study participants also suggested that pre-surgery educational materials could be improved, including sharing the recovery stories of multiple TKA patients to illustrate the variety of TKA patient trajectories and provide another form of informational support, particularly around benchmarking and normalizing individual situations and experiences.

Our results resemble other qualitative studies showing that a mismatch between patient expectations and TKA outcomes are associated with negative patient experiences and patient dissatisfaction with knee replacement [24, 26, 27, 39–42]. One quantitative review also came to the same conclusion [14] but a second quantitative review found that no such relationship after adjustment for confounders [43]. Although these two quantitative reviews used a different set of studies, we suggest their different conclusions result more from the inadequate conceptualization of patient expectations, particularly around post-surgery care. Our study showed that patient expectations around TKA outcomes were not always related to the knee itself. Patient expectations, particularly post-surgery, were also related to receiving clinical support for resolving knee problems. Participants in our study who reported problems with their knee and yet were told by their surgeon that their knee was fine did not have their expectations of clinical support met. Similarly, managing patient expectations is in part about providing appropriate and sufficient information to the patient throughout the TKA process [44]. Our study participants' comments about how more advance knowledge about pain expectations and management would have more positively shaped their experience is one example where information support can lead to good management of patient expectations. Information support can also lead to shared decision-making, or active participation by both patients and clinicians in care decisions, which has a variety of positive outcomes, including improved patient experience, satisfaction, and other outcomes [22, 45, 46].

Our results also resemble other qualitative studies in documenting and specifying the importance of a variety of types of support, although our study differs from previous literature by enhancing, elaborating and unifying a variety of expressions of support as conceptualized in other patient experience studies in joint replacement and osteoarthritis. For instance, Westby and Bachman's investigation of rehabilitation practices and outcomes from the perspectives of hip and knee replacement patients and providers found that "[rehabilitation] takes all kinds of support." Although they did not specify categories of support within the "all kinds" description, they did provide examples that directly map onto our study's informational, clinical and personal support categories [25]. Another qualitative study found that communication about multiple aspects of the care process was a key factor in the patient's hospital experience with knee and hip replacement [24]. A third qualitative study found both patients and clinicians identified that clinicians needed to provide more consistent clinical attention and improved information to improve care of people with osteoarthritis [47]. Other qualitative and quantitative studies of knee and hip replacement experiences identify the importance of patient education, care continuity, pain management and other physical, psychological and social aspects of the patient experience [48, 49]. Rather than replicating the existing literature's current approach of listing themes and categories within a single study, future work could use our study's support framework as an impetus for a deeper understanding of the kinds of support important to patients and the interrelationships between these types of support.

Using a qualitative approach means that our study is limited in its ability to generalize to populations as qualitative research can only be generalized to theory rather than populations [34]. However, having interviewed people from across the province, with purposeful sampling guided by advance knowledge of the variation across our large cohort sample, means that our ability to theorize is rich and varied [50]. Our results contribute relevant insights in understanding the patient experience and the related needs for different types of support for a variety of TKA patients.

This study interviewed participants 8 months postsurgery; different information and perspectives may have arisen had we interviewed people closer to their surgery. However many participants described their TKA experience across time, including shortly after surgery. We only explored patient experience with TKA for those patients who can read English and were well enough to participate in an in-depth interview. Our overall study and the qualitative portion included few persons from racial and ethnic minority groups. We are unable to say whether our results apply to patients more marginalized or challenged in their TKA experience through language or racial or minority status [51, 52]. These results do not explore the experiences of those who never receive TKA surgery in the first place, either by their decision to not have surgery or by being less likely to be offered surgery [53]. Nevertheless, our study's results provide insight into a wide variety of experiences and the importance of various types of support in TKA patient experience.

Conclusions

The three domains of support identified in this study—informational support, clinical support, and personal support—can provide guidance for clinicians and other health care system decision makers on areas needing improvement for patient experience and satisfaction with TKA surgery. Clinicians and other decision makers should also keep in mind that patient needs and expectations for support are shaped both before and after TKA surgery. With attention to patient-centred care and a better understanding of the existence and needs of these three domains of support, clinicians and other decision makers can take appropriate actions that could potentially improve the overall patient experience and satisfaction with TKA.

Endnotes

[1]Our research team was highly interdisciplinary; as such our analysis for this paper was informed by persons trained in at least one of the following disciplines: health services and policy research, population and public health, health economics, psychology, epidemiology, political science, nursing, and orthopedic surgery.

Abbreviations
TKA: Total knee arthroplasty

Acknowledgements
We thank the TKA patients who participated in this research study, and acknowledge the data collection contributions from Faith Furlong, Heidi Howay, Christine Morrison, Valerie Oglov and Christina Parkin. Study guidance was provided by our collaborators and advisory team members, including Ramin Mehin, Susann Camus, Susan Chunick, Alison Dormuth, Denise Dunton, Vivian Giglio, Charlie Goldsmith, David Nelson, Cindy Roberts, Magdelena Newman, Joan Vyner, Mike Wasdell, Robert Bourne, and many others.

Funding
The study "Why are so many patients dissatisfied with knee replacement surgery? Exploring variations of the patient experience" was funded through support from the Canadian Institutes of Health Research Partnerships for Health System Improvement (CIHR PHSI) operating grant (number 114106), the Michael Smith Foundation for Health Research (MSFHR; number PJ HSP 00004(10–1)), and the BC Rural & Remote Health Research Network. Funding and in-kind support were received from Vancouver Coastal Health Authority and Fraser Health Authority. Dr. Sawatzky holds a Canada Research Chair (CRC) in Patient-Reported Outcomes from the Government of Canada CRC program. Dr. Davis held postdoctoral funding from CIHR and MSFHR during this study. Assistance with the pre-funding study design was provided through in-kind support from the Fraser Health Authority. Otherwise, no funder of this study was involved in the design of the study and collection, analysis and interpretation of data and in writing the manuscript.

Authors' contributions
LJG led and participated in the design, conduct and analysis of this study and the drafting of this manuscript. NS and ER participated in the design, conduct and analysis of the study and helped draft the manuscript. JS, VM, RS, SH, JD, PM, and SB participated in the design, conduct and analysis of the study and revised the manuscript critically for important intellectual

content. SB also led the overall mixed methods study within which this qualitative study was embedded. All authors read and approved the final manuscript.

Competing interests
The authors declare that they have no competing interests.

Consent for publication
All study participants provided written informed consent for the information collected to be used for publication where no information that disclosed their identity was released or published.

Author details
[1]Faculty of Health Sciences, Simon Fraser University, Blusson Hall 10506, 8888 University Drive, Burnaby, BC V5A 1S6, Canada. [2]Centre for Clinical Epidemiology and Evaluation, Vancouver Coastal Health Research Institute, 7th floor, 828 West 10th Avenue, Vancouver, BC V5Z 1M9, Canada. [3]School of Population and Public Health, University of British Columbia, 2206 East Mall, Vancouver, BC V6T 1Z3, Canada. [4]Department of Experimental Medicine, Faculty of Medicine, University of British Columbia, 10th Floor, 2775 Laurel Street, Vancouver, BC V5Z 1M9, Canada. [5]Burnaby Hospital & Surgical Network, Fraser Health, 3935 Kincaid Street, Burnaby, BC V5K 2X6, Canada. [6]School of Nursing, Trinity Western University, 7600 Glover Road, Langley, BC V2Y 1Y1, Canada. [7]Centre for Health Evaluation and Outcome Sciences, Providence Health Care Research Institute, St. Paul's Hospital, 588-1081 Burrard Street, Vancouver, BC V6Z 1Y6, Canada. [8]Department of Evaluation and Research Service, Fraser Health, Suite 400, Central City Tower, 13450 102 Avenue, Surrey, BC V3T 0H1, Canada. [9]Department of Physical Therapy, Faculty of Medicine, University of British Columbia, 212 Friedman Building, 2177 Wesbrook Mall, Vancouver, BC V6T 1Z3, Canada. [10]Aging, Mobility, and Cognitive Neurosciences Lab, University of British Columbia, Djavad Mowafaghian Centre for Brain Health, 2215 Wesbrook Mall, Vancouver, BC V6T 1Z3, Canada. [11]Rebalance MD, 104-3551 Blanshard Street, Victoria, BC V8Z 0B9, Canada.

References
1. CIHI. Increase in hip and knee replacements over past 5 years. Ottawa: CIHI; 2014.
2. Slover J, Zuckerman JD. Increasing use of total knee replacement and revision surgery. JAMA. 2012;308:1266–8.
3. Husni ME, Losina E, Fossel AH, Solomon DH, Mahomed NN, Katz JN. Decreasing medical complications for total knee arthroplasty: effect of critical pathways on outcomes. BMC Musculoskelet Disord. 2010;11:160.
4. Vorhies JS, Wang Y, Herndon JH, Maloney WJ, Huddleston JI. Decreased length of stay after TKA is not associated with increased readmission rates in a national Medicare sample. Clin Orthop Relat Res. 2012;470:166–71.
5. Bandholm T, Kehlet H. Physiotherapy exercise after fast-track total Hip and knee arthroplasty: time for reconsideration? Arch Phys Med Rehabil. 2012;93: 1292–4.
6. Parks ML. Patient-centered care for total knee arthroplasty. Orthopedics. 2013;36:203–4.
7. Weinstein SL. Nothing about You... without You. J Bone Joint Surg Am. 2005;87:1648–52.
8. Berwick DM. What "patient-centered" should mean: confessions of an extremist. Health Aff. 2009;28:w555–65.
9. Berwick DM, Nolan TW, Whittington J. The triple Aim: care, health. And Cost Health Aff. 2008;27:759–69.
10. Bourne RB, Chesworth BM, Davis AM, Mahomed NN, Charron KDJ. Patient satisfaction after total knee arthroplasty: Who is satisfied and Who is Not? Clin Orthop Relat Res. 2009;468:57–63.
11. Nam D, Nunley RM, Barrack RL. Patient dissatisfaction following total knee replacement a growing concern? Bone Joint J. 2014;96–B:96–100.
12. Vissers MM, Bussmann JB, Verhaar JAN, Busschbach JJV, Bierma-Zeinstra SMA, Reijman M. Psychological factors affecting the outcome of total Hip and knee arthroplasty: a systematic review. Semin Arthritis Rheum. 2012;41:576–88.
13. Dunbar MJ, Haddad FS. Patient satisfaction after total knee replacement: new inroads. Bone Joint J. 2014;96–B:1285–6.
14. Culliton SE, Bryant DM, Overend TJ, MacDonald SJ, Chesworth BM. The relationship between expectations and satisfaction in patients undergoing primary total knee arthroplasty. J Arthroplast. 2012;27:490–2.
15. Hamilton DF, Lane JV, Gaston P, Patton JT, MacDonald D, Simpson AHRW, et al. What determines patient satisfaction with surgery? A prospective cohort study of 4709 patients following total joint replacement. BMJ Open. 2013;3:e002525.
16. O'Neill T, Jinks C, Ong BN. Decision-making regarding total knee replacement surgery: A qualitative meta-synthesis. BMC Health Serv Res. 2007;7:1–9.
17. Conner-Spady BL, Marshall DA, Hawker GA, Bohm E, Dunbar MJ, Frank C, et al. You'll know when you're ready: a qualitative study exploring how patients decide when the time is right for joint replacement surgery. BMC Health Serv Res. 2014;14:454.
18. Carr T, Teucher UC, Casson AG. Time while waiting Patients' experiences of scheduled surgery. Qual Health Res. 2014;24:1673–85.
19. Webster F, Perruccio AV, Jenkinson R, Jaglal S, Schemitsch E, Waddell JP, et al. Where is the patient in models of patient-centred care: a grounded theory study of total joint replacement patients. BMC Health Serv Res. 2013;13:531.
20. Leov J, Barrett E, Gallagher S, Swain N. A qualitative study of pain experiences in patients requiring hip and knee arthroplasty. J Health Psychol. 2015;1359105315597054.
21. Lucas B, Cox C, Perry L, Bridges J. Pre-operative preparation of patients for total knee replacement: An action research study. Int J Orthop Trauma Nursing. 2013;17:79–90.
22. Sjöling M, Norbergh K-G, Malker H, Asplund K. What information do patients waiting for and undergoing arthroplastic surgery want? Their side of the story. J Orthop Nurs. 2006;10:5–14.
23. Jeffery AE, Wylde V, Blom AW, Horwood JP. "It's there and I'm stuck with it": Patients' experiences of chronic pain following total knee replacement surgery. Arthritis Care Res. 2011;63:286–92.
24. Lane JV, Hamilton DF, MacDonald DJ, Ellis C, Howie CR. Factors that shape the patient's hospital experience and satisfaction with lower limb arthroplasty: an exploratory thematic analysis. BMJ Open. 2016;6:e010871.
25. Westby MD, Backman CL. Patient and health professional views on rehabilitation practices and outcomes following total hip and knee arthroplasty for osteoarthritis:a focus group study. BMC Health Serv Res. 2010;10:119.
26. Jacobson AF, Myerscough RP, Delambo K, Fleming E, Huddleston AM, Bright N, et al. Patients' perspectives on total knee replacement: AJN. Am J Nurs. 2008;108:54–63.
27. Gustafsson BÅ, Ekman S-L, Ponzer S, Heikkilä K. The hip and knee replacement operation: an extensive life event. Scand J Caring Sci. 2010;24: 663–70.
28. Webster F, Perruccio AV, Jenkinson R, Jaglal S, Schemitsch E, Waddell JP, et al. Understanding why people do or do not engage in activities following total joint replacement: a longitudinal qualitative study. Osteoarthr Cartil. 2015;23:860–7.
29. Harding PA, Holland AE, Hinman RS, Delany C. Physical activity perceptions and beliefs following total hip and knee arthroplasty: a qualitative study. Physiother Theory Pract. 2015;31:107–13.
30. Beaton DE, Clark JP. Qualitative research: a review of methods with use of examples from the total knee replacement literature. J Bone Joint Surg Am. 2009;91:107–12.
31. Pope C, Mays N. Qualitative research: reaching the parts other methods cannot reach: an introduction to qualitative methods in health and health services research. BMJ. 1995;311:42–5.
32. Barker KL. How can qualitative research be utilised in the NHS when re-designing and commissioning services? British J Pain. 2015;9:70–2.
33. Leech NL, Onwuegbuzie AJ. A typology of mixed methods research designs. Qual Quant. 2007;43:265–75.
34. Lincoln YS, Guba EG. Naturalistic inquiry. Newbury Park: SAGE Publications; 1985.
35. Sandelowski M. Sample size in qualitative research. Res Nurs Health. 1995;18: 179–83.
36. Mays N, Pope C. Rigour and qualitative research. BMJ. 1995;311:109–12.

37. Farley FA, Weinstein SL. The case for patient-centered care in orthopaedics. J Am Acad Orthop Surg. 2006;14:447–51.
38. Trebble TM, Hansi N, Hydes T, Smith MA, Baker M. Process mapping the patient journey: an introduction. BMJ. 2010;341:c4078.
39. Alami S, Boutron I, Desjeux D, Hirschhorn M, Meric G, Rannou F, et al. Patients' and Practitioners' views of knee osteoarthritis and its management: a qualitative interview study. PLoS One. 2011;6:e19634.
40. Showalter A, Burger S, Salyer J. Patients' and their spouses' needs after total joint arthroplasty: a pilot study. Orthop Nurs. 2000;19:49.
41. Gustafsson BÅ, Ponzer S, Heikkilä K, Ekman S-L. The lived body and the perioperative period in replacement surgery: older people's experiences. J Adv Nurs. 2007;60:20–8.
42. Perry MAC, Hudson S, Ardis K. If I didn't have anybody, what would I have done?" Experiences of older adults and their discharge home after lower limb orthpaedic surgery. J Rehabil Med. 2011;43:916–22.
43. Haanstra TM, van den Berg T, Ostelo RW, Poolman RW, Jansma IP, Cuijpers P, et al. Systematic review: Do patient expectations influence treatment outcomes in total knee and total hip arthroplasty? Health Qual Life Outcomes. 2012;10:152.
44. Noble PC, Fuller-Lafreniere S, Meftah M, Dwyer MK. Challenges in outcome measurement: discrepancies between patient and provider definitions of success. Clin Orthop Relat Res. 2013;471:3437–45.
45. Youm J, Chenok K, Belkora J, Chan V, Bozic KJ. The emerging case for shared decision making in orthopaedics. J Bone Joint Surg Am. 2012;94:1907–12.
46. Bozic KJ, Belkora J, Chan V, Youm J, Zhou T, Dupaix J, et al. Shared decision making in patients with osteoarthritis of the Hip and knee. J Bone Joint Surg Am. 2013;95:1633–9.
47. Mann C, Gooberman-Hill R. Health care provision for osteoarthritis: Concordance between what patients would like and what health professionals think they should have. Arthritis Care Res. 2011;63:963–72.
48. Montin L, Suominen T, Leino-Kilpi H. The experiences of patients undergoing total hip replacement. J Orthop Nurs. 2002;6:23–9.
49. Cheng RTS, Klainin-Yobas P, Hegney D, Mackey S. Factors relating to perioperative experience of older persons undergoing joint replacement surgery: an integrative literature review. Disabil Rehabil. 2015;37:9–24.
50. Polit DF, Beck CT. Generalization in quantitative and qualitative research: Myths and strategies. Int J Nurs Stud. 2010;47:1451–8.
51. Kamath AF, Horneff JG, Gaffney V, Israelite CL, Nelson CL. Ethnic and gender differences in the functional disparities after primary total knee arthroplasty. Clin Orthop Relat Res. 2010;468:3355–61.
52. Lavernia CJ, Alcerro JC, Contreras JS, Rossi MD. Ethnic and racial factors influencing well-being, perceived pain, and physical function after primary total joint arthroplasty. Clin Orthop Relat Res. 2011;469:1838–45.
53. Mota REM, Tarricone R, Ciani O, Bridges JFP, Drummond M. Determinants of demand for total hip and knee arthroplasty: a systematic literature review. BMC Health Serv Res. 2012;12:225.

11

Tibial component rotation in total knee arthroplasty

Peter Z. Feczko[*], Bart G. Pijls, Michael J. van Steijn, Lodewijk W. van Rhijn, Jacobus J. Arts and Peter J. Emans

Abstract

Background: Both the range of motion (ROM) technique and the tibial tubercle landmark (TTL) technique are frequently used to align the tibial component into proper rotational position during total knee arthroplasty (TKA). The aim of the study was to assess the intra-operative differences in tibial rotation position during computer-navigated primary TKA using either the TTL or ROM techniques. The ROM technique was hypothesized to be a repeatable method and to produce different tibial rotation positions compared to the TTL technique.

Methods: A prospective, observational study was performed to evaluate the antero-posterior axis of the cut proximal tibia using both the ROM and the TTL technique during primary TKA without postoperative clinical assessment. Computer navigation was used to measure this difference in 20 consecutive knees of 20 patients who underwent a posterior stabilized total knee arthroplasty with a fixed-bearing polyethylene insert and a patella resurfacing.

Results: The ROM technique is a repeatable method with an interclass correlation coefficient (ICC2) of 0.84 ($p < 0.001$). The trial tibial baseplate was on average 4.56 degrees externally rotated compared to the tubercle landmark. This difference was statistically significant ($p = 0.028$). The amount of maximum intra-operative flexion and the pre-operative mechanical axis were positively correlated with the magnitude of difference between the two methods.

Conclusions: It is important for the orthopaedic surgeon to realise that there is a significant difference between the TTL technique and ROM technique when positioning the tibial component in a rotational position. This difference is correlated with high maximum flexion and mechanical axis deviations.

Keywords: Total knee arthroplasty, Tibial rotation, ROM technique, TTL technique, Computer navigation

Background

Rotational alignment of the components in total knee arthroplasty (TKA) is an important factor for both survival and the performance of the prostheses [1, 2]. The majority of the attention has focussed on the rotational alignment of the femoral component [3–6], which has resulted in the widespread use of the transepicondylar axis and the antero-posterior axis (Whiteside's Line) of the distal femur as the reference axes for the rotational alignment of the femoral component [3–6].

However there is more discussion about the rotational alignment of the tibial component in part because of the difficulty of clinically assessing tibial component rotation. Furthermore, a whole range of anatomical landmarks can

be used, including the medial border of the tibial tuberosity, the medial third of the tibial tuberosity, the anterior tibial crest, the posterior tibial condylar line, the second ray and the first web space of the foot. Aligning the tibial component to the tibial tubercle is one of the most popular landmark methods [7–9]. The disadvantage of all anatomical landmark techniques is that they do not account for femoro-tibial kinematics [10]. To address this problem, the ROM technique was introduced; in this technique, the rotational alignment of the tibial tray is determined through conformity to the femoral component when the knee is put through a series of full flexion-extension cycles [11]. However, the position of the tibial tray is not exclusively determined by the femoral component but is also influenced by the extensor mechanism, the patellar component, the ligament balancing and the tibial cut [12, 13]. The rationale behind the ROM technique lies

* Correspondence: p.feczko@mumc.nl
Department of Orthopaedic Surgery, Maastricht University Medical Centre, P.O. Box 58006202 AZ Maastricht, The Netherlands

in the theoretical advantage of aligning the tibial component in relation to the femoral component while respecting the soft tissue torsion forces to create optimal femoro-tibial kinematics [14]. For this method to work, the femoral component should be positioned accurately. Using computer-assisted surgery may improve the accuracy of positioning [15].

Several studies have demonstrated variability in the relationships between different landmarks and techniques for establishing rotational alignment of tibial components in total knee arthroplasty [11, 16–18]. A review reported that there is no gold standard measurement of tibial component rotation [18]. Whether the ROM technique is a repeatable method, and whether there is a significant difference in tibial component rotational position between the TTL technique and the ROM technique in computer navigated TKA with patella resurfacing remains unanswered questions in the literature. The primary purpose of this study was therefore to intra-operatively evaluate the repeatability of the ROM technique. The secondary outcome was to evaluate the difference in rotational alignment of the trial tibial component with the use of the TTL and ROM techniques during computer-navigated TKA with patella resurfacing . Additionally, the factors that influenced the positioning of the trial tibial component with both techniques were investigated. Postoperative clinical and radiological data were not collected.

Methods

A prospective, observational study of 20 consecutive primary posterior stabilized TKAs in 20 patients with fixed-bearing polyethylene inserts (Scorpio Flex PS, Stryker Corporation, Mahwah, NJ USA) was performed by a single surgeon (MvS).

Data collection began with 10 consecutive TKAs to determine whether there was a difference between the alignment techniques and if so to gather data to perform a power analysis. Using the acquired data, we determined that a total of 20 subjects were needed to achieve 90 % power assuming a minimum detectable difference of 5.0 degrees, a standard deviation of 7.7 degrees and a significance level of alpha < 0.05.

The mean pre-operative mechanical leg axis was 3.65° ± SD 7.15 of varus. The mean pre-operative mechanical leg axis of the varus knees ($N = 15$) was 7.0° ± SD 4.05, of the valgus knees ($N = 5$) was −6.4° ± SD −4.15.

Positive values indicated varus alignment, negative values indicated valgus alignment.

The mean posterior slope was 1.5° ± SD 1.02.

Ethics and consent

The Medical Ethics Committee of the Maastricht University Medical Centre has concluded that the described research does not apply to the Dutch Medical Research involving Human Subjects Act (WMO), therefore the patient was not required to provide consent regarding the use of the material.

Furthermore, every patient in the Maastricht University Medical Centre is provided with information regarding these kinds of studies. If they do not wish to contribute to these studies, this information will be included in their file. The patient involved in this study did not make an objection against the use of his/her material for research purposes.

Patient demographics

The patient demographics are summarized in Table 1.

Operative procedure

The Stryker Knee Navigation System (Stryker Navigation System II, version 3.1) was used in this study. The prosthesis (Scorpio PS Stryker Howmedica Osteonics, Allendale, NJ USA) used in these surgeries allows five degrees of rotation between the tibial insert and the femoral component. In all cases, a tourniquet was applied for the entire duration of the surgery. After a standard midline skin incision and a medial parapatellar arthrotomy, the active wireless trackers of the navigation system were fixed to the femur and tibia. The required landmarks were entered into the navigation computer, and the rotation centre of the hip was determined by a special algorithm executed in customized software. The transepicondylar axis of the distal femur and the Whiteside's line were set in each case exactly perpendicular to each other to improve the accuracy of the positioning the femoral component. The femoral component was aligned parallel to the transepicondylar axis. The AP axis of the proximal tibia was determined by placing the tip of the pointer on the centre of the line between the intercondylar eminences and aligning it to the medial 1/3 of the tibial tubercle . This AP axis was saved in the navigation program as 0 degrees of rotation. The proximal tibial and distal femoral cuts were performed and examined with the navigation system. The tibial posterior slope was set according to the patient's natural slope. The polyethylene insert (Scorpio-Flex PS fixed bearing tibial insert) had an additional four degrees of posterior down-slope. The rotation of the femoral component was oriented according to the transepicondylar line and the AP axis (Whiteside's

Table 1 Patient demographics. Positive values indicated varus alignment, negative values indicated valgus alignment

	Age (years)	Preoperative Leg axis (degrees varus)	Sex (Male/Female)	Side (Right/Left)	Preoperative ROM (degrees)	Preoperative flexion contracture (degrees)
Mean ± SD	69.8 ± 10	3.7 ± 7.2	8/12	10/10	117 ± 16	5.6 ± 4.7

Line) of the distal femur as currently advised in literature [3, 5, 17]. After soft tissue balancing and achievement of the maximal range of motion, the patella was prepared. The patellar button position may affect femoro-tibial kinematics; therefore, all of the trial components, including the patella and the PS tibial trial insert, were placed before the tibial component was subjected to the ROM technique. One navigation tracker was applied to the alignment handle of the trial tibial tray to check the position according to the given 0 degrees of rotation. Flexion and extension were measured intra-operatively after the approach was made and the trackers were placed. Positive values for extension represent hyperextension, while negative values represent flexion contracture.

The tibial component was inserted and checked for smooth movement on the tibial cut surface. The knee was then put through five full flexion-extension cycles while the surgeon held the ankle only. During the ROM cycles, no hands were touching the knee to prevent manual manipulation, and no varus/valgus stress was applied. The movement was followed on the navigation computer to confirm that no varus/valgus stress was applied. After performing the ROM cycles, the rotational position of the trial tibial component was recorded as indicated by the navigation computer. Positive values indicated that the trial component was in internal rotation according to the given TTL axis, and negative values indicated that the trial component was in external rotation. While this measurement was being acquired, the patella was lying in the patellar groove to facilitate optimal patellofemoral tracking and to prevent lateral pull on the patella tendon that could cause the tibia to rotate externally. The rotational position was noted (measurement 1). After removing and reinserting the components, the ROM technique was applied two additional times with five full flexion-extension movements and corresponding subsequent measurements from the navigation system (measurement 2 and 3).

After completing the operative procedure, the final tibial tray was cemented up to 1/3 of the medial border of the tibial tubercle.

Statistics

The statistical analyses were performed with SPSS statistical software (Version 12, SPSS Inc., Chicago, IL USA). The reproducibility of the ROM-technique was evaluated using the intra-class correlation coefficient (ICC). For each target, there was one 'rater'(MvS) who performed the three consecutive attempts at positioning the tibial component using the ROM technique. Since the exact same rater made ratings on every patient and it was assumed that both patients and observer were drawn randomly from larger populations, the ICC2 was used [19]. The ICC2 reflects the reliability of this single

rater. Means were compared with paired T-tests in cases of normal distributions [20]. A level of $p < 0.05$ was considered statistically significant. The mean of the 3 ROM measurements was used to evaluate the difference between the ROM and TTL techniques. We evaluated potential factors associated with the difference between the ROM and TTL technique including, leg axis, intra-operative flexion, intra-operative extension and posterior slope. (Table 2) The associations between each variable and the difference between the ROM and TTL were examined with univariable regression analyses. Factors that were associated with the outcome in univariable analyses (p-values < 0.20) were included in multivariable regression analyses. In multivariable regression analyses p-values < 0.05 were considered significant. Regression coefficients with their 95 % confidence intervals are reported.

Results

The tibial component can be reliable positioned in terms of rotation using the ROM technique, as demonstrated by an ICC2 = 0.84 (95 % CI (0.70–0.93); $p < 0.001$). The ICC2 = 0.84 of tibial component positioning using the ROM technique indicating nearly perfect repeatability. Because the ROM technique was nearly perfectly reliable, the means of the 3 ROM measurements were used to evaluate the difference between the two techniques. With the ROM technique, the tibial component was on average 4.56 (± SD 8.59) degrees externally rotated compared to the tubercle landmark. This difference was statistically significant $p = 0.028$.

It appeared from the multivariable regression analyses that more valgus pre-operative mechanical leg axis (–0.54 (95%CI –0.98 - -0.10); $p = 0.019$), intra-operative flexion (0.57 (95%CI 0.13 – 1.00); $p = 0.014$) and intra-operative extension (1.41 (95%CI 0.50 – 2.32); $p = 0.005$) were associated with a greater difference between tibial component positioning using the ROM and TTL techniques. (Table 3) These results indicate that increasing the pre-operative varus mechanical leg alignment by 1 degree resulted in an increase in the external rotation of the tibial component of 0.54 degrees relative to the tibial tubercle using the ROM technique.

Table 2 Outcome and available covariates assessed for inclusion in the regression model. Positive values for extension represent hyperextension, while negative values indicate flexion contracture

Variables	Mean ± SD	(range)
Difference ROM and TTL (°)	−4.6 ± 8.6	(−27.0 to 11.5)
Varus mechanical leg axis (°)	3.7 ± 7.2	(−13.0 to 15.0)
Intra-operative flexion (°)	121.9 ± 6.7	(108.0 to 134.0)
Intra-operative extension (°)	−0.1 ± 3.0	(−5.5 to 7.0)
Posterior slope (°)	1.5 ± 1.0	(0.0 to 3.5)

Table 3 Results of univariable and multivariable regression analyses

Variable	Univariable analysis		Multivariable analysis	
	coefficient (95%CI)	p-value	coefficient (95%CI)	p-value
Varus mechanical leg axis	−0.58 (−1.09 to −0.05)	0.030	−0.54 (−0.98 to −0.10)	0.019
Intra-operative flexion	0.82 (0.33 to 1.31)	0.002	0.57 (0.13 to 1.00)	0.014
Intra-operative extension	1.19 (−0.09 to 2.48)	0.070	1.41 (0.50 to 2.32)	0.005
Posterior slope	2.63 (−1.31 to 6.56)	0.180	0.04 (−3.05 to 3.13)	0.979

In the varus knees, the tibial component was on average 5.9 (± SD 8.7) degrees externally rotated; in the valgus knees, the mean external rotation was 0.4 (± SD 7.6) degrees relative to the tibial tubercle. The differences between the rotational alignments using the ROM and TTL techniques in both the varus and valgus knees were not statistically significant ($p = 0.221$).

The cut posterior slope (0.04 (95%CI −3.05 − 3.13); $p = 0.979$) was not significantly related to the difference in the rotational alignment of the tibial component according to the tibial tubercle in either the ROM or TTL techniques.

Discussion

This study revealed that the ROM technique is a repeatable method for aligning the tibial component. Using the ROM technique, the tibial component was on average 4.56 (± SD 8.59) degrees externally rotated compared to the tubercle landmark. Our result is in contradiction with Ikeuchi et al. [11] They found that using the ROM technique results in a more internally rotated position of the tibial component en found also widely variable results. However in line with our findings, Berhouet [21] and Chotanaputhi [22] found the ROM technique reproducible and the alignment of the tibial tray was externally rotated in comparison with the medial border of the tibial tubercle and the posterior tibial condyle line respectively. Ikeuchi [11] used cruciate-retaining (CR) TKA components without patellar resurfacing. The mean posterior slope of the cut tibia was 5 degrees and they compared the position of the tibial component related to the Akagi line [23]. The amount of tibial slope, the design of the prosthesis and the patella resurfacing all might have influenced the outcome. Rossi [24] stated that the ROM technique is a reproducible method to establish tibial rotation during TKA, having found that components were positioned in 0.35 external rotation to the Akagi line.

Using anatomical landmarks for the rotational alignment of the femoral and tibial components is a widely accepted method. Alignment to the medial 1/3 of the tibial tubercle (Insall's reference [25]) is based on papers of Nicoll [26], Lawrie [27], Lützner [28] and Yin [29], who found the medial 1/3 of the tibial tubercle the most accurate and reliable anatomical landmark. However,

determining the component positions separately can lead to rotational mismatch between the femoral and tibial components [30]. Using the dynamic ROM technique may allow for the tibial tray to align itself according to the femoral component position, ligament balancing and extensor mechanism alignment.

Retrieval and biomechanical studies have indicated that femoro-tibial rotational mismatches cause increased contact stress on the tibial insert and patellar component that leads to accelerated polyethylene wear [31–33]. Steinbrück et al. [34] recommended the rotational alignment of the tibial component to the medial 1/3 of the tibial tubercle to achieve the lowest retro-patellar pressure. Using the ROM technique the tibial component was externally rotated by a mean 4.56 degrees respect the tibial tubercle which might have resulted in increased retro-patellar peak pressure. Kim et al [35] found the best survival rate when tibial component was aligned between 2 degrees of internal rotation to 5 degrees of external rotation to the medial 1/3 of the tibial tubercle. External rotational errors were not associated with pain in a study of Nicoll [26].

To measure the rotational difference between the ROM and TTL techniques in degrees may not be easy during TKAs that are performed without navigation. Computer navigation is an ideal method for measuring the difference in trial tibial tray position between the TTL and ROM techniques given its reported accuracy of one degree [36]. Furthermore, the use of computer navigation can help to optimize the femoral component position, which is crucial for the performance of the ROM technique. [15, 37] Computer navigation has no advantage regarding the identification of the correct positions of the anatomical landmarks, but it does have advantages in comparing the positions of the landmarks to other landmarks (e.g., the transepicondylar axis to Whiteside's line) and positioning the implants according the identified landmarks.

Huddleston et al. [16] found that when the ROM technique is applied to varus knees, the antero-posterior axis of the tibial tray is significantly more externally rotated then when this technique is applied to valgus knees. The same result was found in our study, although this difference did not reach statistical significance likely because our study was underpowered regarding this aspect. However, the pre-operative mechanical leg axis was correlated with the difference between the ROM and TTL techniques ($p = 0.019$). With increasing pre-operative varus alignment, the ROM technique results in increasing external rotation of the tibial component.

The maximum degrees of flexion ($p = 0.014$) and extension ($p = 0.005$) during surgery were also correlated with the difference between the ROM technique and the tubercle landmark in this study, which indicates that the use of the ROM technique for a patient with great preoperative flexion would result in a more internally rotated tibial component position compared with a patient with less preoperative flexion.

Limitations of the study
The number of patients (observations) in our study is rather low. Various studies have suggested that for each variable studied in multiple regression analysis at least 10 observations are required [38–40] although a recent study showed that this number could be lower in certain circumstances [41]. The results should therefore be interpreted with some caution.

Clinical and radiological data were not collected post-operatively. Therefore, no results are available regarding potential differences in clinical outcomes between the two techniques. It is known that a tourniquet affects the intra-operative patello-femoral tracking [42, 43]. Therefore, it is likely that the tourniquet had some effect on the tibial component rotational alignment in the ROM technique. The use of a tourniquet during all of the operations and keeping it inflated while performing the ROM cycles might have affected our results.

Although tibial rotational alignment is also effected by ligament balancing, we did not measure the gaps intra-operatively.

The design of the prosthesis (CR or PS version) and the design of the tibial tray (symmetric or anatomical) may also have influence on the outcome [44].

Conclusions
The ROM technique is a repeatable intra-operative method for determining the rotational position of the tibia trial component. Because the best method to determine the intra-operative position of the tibia component is still under debate, TKA surgeons should be aware that there is a difference between the ROM and TTL methods, particularly in patients with high peri-operative ranges of motion and/or high pre-operative varus/valgus alignment.

Competing interests
The authors declare that they have no competing interests.

Author's contribution
PF wrote and submitted the article, BP participated in the design of the study and collected the data, MS participated in the design of the study and performed the operations, LvR gave final approval of the version to be submitted, JA performed the statistical analysis, PE helped in the interpretation of the data and revised the article. All authors read and approved the final manuscript.

References
1. Hofmann S, Romero J, Roth-Schiffl E, Albrecht T. Rotational malalignment of the components may cause chronic pain or early failure in total knee arthroplasty. Orthopade. 2003;32(6):469–76.
2. Incavo SJ, Wild JJ, Coughlin KM, Beynnon BD. Early Revision for Component Malrotation in Total Knee Arthroplasty. Clin Orthop Relat Res. 2007;458:131–6.
3. Eisenhuth SA, Saleh KJ, Cui Q, Clark CR, Brown TE. Patellofemoral instability after total knee arthroplasty. Clin Orthop Relat Res. 2006;446:149–60.
4. Luo CF. Reference axes for reconstruction of the knee. Knee. 2004;11(4):251–7.
5. Benjamin J. Component alignment in total knee arthroplasty. Instr Course Lect. 2006;55:405–12.
6. Poilvache PL, Insall JN, Scuderi GR, Font-Rodriguez DE. Rotational landmarks and sizing of the distal femur in total knee arthroplasty. Clin Orthop Relat Res. 1996;331:35–46.
7. Siston RA, Goodman SB, Patel JJ, Delp SL, Giori NJ. The high variability of tibial rotational alignment in total knee arthroplasty. Clin Orthop Relat Res. 2006;452:65–9.
8. Fitzpatrick C, Fitzpatrick D, Auger D, Lee J. A tibial-based coordinate system for three-dimensional data. Knee. 2007;14(2):133–7.
9. Fuiko R, Kotten B, Zettl R, Ritschl P. The accuracy of palpation from orientation points for the navigated implantation of knee prostheses. Orthopade. 2004;33(3):338–43.
10. Tao K, Cai M, Zhu Y, Lou L, Cai Z. Aligning the tibial component with medial border of the tibial tubercle—is it always right? Knee. 2014;21(1):295–8.
11. Ikeuchi M, Yamanaka N, Okanoue Y, Ueta E, Tani T. Determining the rotational alignment of the tibial component at total knee replacement: a comparison of two techniques. J Bone Joint Surg Br. 2007;89(1):45–9.
12. Moreland JR. Mechanisms of failure in total knee arthroplasty. Clin Orthop Relat Res. 1988;226:49–64.
13. Miller MC, Zhang AX, Petrella AJ, Berger RA, Rubash HE. The effect of component placement on knee kinetics after arthroplasty with an unconstrained prosthesis. J Orthop Res. 2001;19(4):614–20.
14. Eckhoff DG, Metzger RG, Vandewalle MV. Malrotation associated with implant alignment technique in total knee arthroplasty. Clin Orthop Relat Res. 1995;321:28–31.
15. Hernandez-Vaquero D, Noriega-Fernandez A, Fernandez-Carreira JM, Fernandez-Simon JM, Llorens De Los Rios J. Computer-assisted surgery improves rotational positioning of the femoral component but not the tibial component in total knee arthroplasty. Knee Surg Sports Traumatol Arthrosc. 2014;22(12):3127–34.
16. Huddleston JI, Scott RD, Wimberley DW. Determination of neutral tibial rotational alignment in rotating platform TKA. Clin Orthop Relat Res. 2005;440:101–6.
17. Middleton FR, Palmer SH. How accurate is Whiteside's line as a reference axis in total knee arthroplasty? Knee. 2007;14(3):204–7.
18. Gromov K, Korchi M, Thomsen MG, Husted H, Troelsen A. What is the optimal alignment of the tibial and femoral components in knee arthroplasty? Acta Orthop. 2014;85(5):480–719.
19. Shrout PE, Fleiss JL. Intraclass correlations: uses in assessing rater reliability. Psychol Bull. 1979;86:420–8.
20. Petrie A. Statistics in orthopaedic papers. J Bone Joint Surg Br. 2006;88(9):1121–36.
21. Berhouet J, Beaufils P, Boisrenoult P, Frasca D, Pujol N. Rotational positioning of the tibial tray in total knee arthroplasty: a CT evaluation. Orthop Traumatol Surg Res. 2011;97:699–704.
22. Chotanaphuti T, Panichcharoen W, Laoruengthana A. Comparative study of anatomical landmark technique and self-aligned tibial component rotation determined by computer-assisted TKA. J Med Assoc Thai. 2012; 95 Suppl 10:S37–41.
23. Akagi M, Oh M, Nonaka T, Tsujimoto H, Asano T, Hamanishi C. An anteroposterior axis of the tibia for total knee arthroplasty. Clin Orthop Relat Res. 2004;420:213–9.
24. Rossi R, Buzzone M, Bonasia DE, Marmotti A, Castoldi F. Evaluation of tibial rotational alignment in total knee arthroplasty: a cadaver study. Knee Surg Sports Traumatol Arthrosc. 2010;18:889–93.

25. Insall JN, Binazzi R, Soudry M, Mestriner LA. Total Knee Arthroplasty. Clin Orthop Relat Res. 1985;192:13–22.

26. Nicoll D, Rowley DI. Internal rotational error of the tibial component is a major cause of pain after total knee replacement. J Bone Joint Surg [Br]. 2010;92-B:1238–44.

27. Lawrie CM, Noble PC, Ismaily SK, Stal D, Incavo SJ. The Flexion-Extension Axis of the Knee and its Relationship to the Rotational Orientation of the Tibial Plateau. J Arthroplasty. 2011;26(6 Suppl):53–58.e1.

28. Lützner J, Krummenauer F, Günther KP, Kirschner S. Rotational alignment of the tibial component in total knee arthroplasty is better at the medial third of tibial tuberosity than at the medial border. BMC Musculoskelet Disord. 2010;11:57.

29. Yin L, Chen K, Guo L, Cheng L, Wang F, Yang L. Knee alignment in the transverse plane during weight-bearing activity and its implication for the tibial rotational alignment in total knee arthroplasty. Clin Biomech (Bristol, Avon). 2015;30(6):565–71.

30. Lee DH, Seo JG, Moon YW. Synchronisation of tibial rotational alignment with femoral component in total knee arthroplasty. Int Orthop. 2008;32(2):223–7.

31. D'Lima DD, Chen PC, Colwell Jr CW. Polyethylene contact stresses, articular congruity, and knee alignment. Clin Orthop Relat Res. 2001;392:232–8.

32. Wasielewski RC, Galante JO, Leighty RM, Natarajan RN, Rosenberg AG. Wear patterns on retrieved polyethylene tibial inserts and their relationship to technical considerations during total knee arthroplasty. Clin Orthop Relat Res. 1994;299:31–43.

33. Chowdhury EA, Porter ML. A study of the effect of tibial tray rotation on a specific mobile bearing total knee arthroplasty. J Arthroplasty. 2005;20(6):793–7.

34. Steinbrück A, Schröder C, Woiczinski M, Müller T, Müller PE, Jansson V, et al. Influence of tibial rotation in total knee arthroplasty on knee kinematics and retropatellar pressure: an in vitro study. Knee Surg Sports Traumatol Arthrosc. 2015;11.

35. Kim YH, Park JW, Kim JS, Park SD. The relationship between the survival of total knee arthroplasty and postoperative coronal, sagittal and rotational alignment of knee prosthesis. Int Orthop. 2014;38(2):379–85.

36. Pitto RP, Graydon AJ, Bradley L, Malak SF, Walker CG, Anderson IA. Accuracy of a computer-assisted navigation system for total knee replacement. J Bone Joint Surg Br. 2006;88(5):601–5.

37. Kim SH, Lee HJ, Jung HJ, Lee JS, Kim KS. Less femoral lift-off and better femoral alignment in TKA using computer –assisted surgery. Knee Surg Traumatol Arthrosc. 2013;21(12):2877–83.

38. Harrell FE, Lee KL, Mark DB. Multivariable prognostic models: issues in developing models, evaluating assumptions and adequacy, and measuring and reducing errors. Stat Med. 1996;15:361–87.

39. Concato J, Peduzzi P, Holford TR, Feinstein AR. Importance of events per independent variable in proportional hazards analysis. I. Background, goals, and general strategy. J Clin Epidemiol. 1995;48:1495–501.

40. Peduzzi P, Concato J, Feinstein AR, Holford TR. Importance of events per independent variable in proportional hazards regression analysis. II. Accuracy and precision of regression estimates. J Clin Epidemiol. 1995;48:1503–10.

41. Vittinghoff E, McCulloch CE. Relaxing the rule of ten events per variable in logistic and Cox regression. Am J Epidemiol. 2007;165:710–8.

42. Komatsu T, Ishibashi Y, Otsuka H, Nagao A, Toh S. The effect of surgical approaches and tourniquet application on patellofemoral tracking in total knee arthroplasty. J Arthroplasty. 2003;18(3):308–12.

43. Husted H, Toftgaard JT. Influence of the pneumatic tourniquet on patella tracking in total knee arthroplasty: a prospective randomized study in 100 patients. J Arthroplasty. 2005;20(6):694–7.

44. Stulberg SD, Goyal N. Which Tibial Tray Design Achieves Maximum Coverage and Ideal Rotation: Anatomic, Symmetric, or Asymmetric? An MRI-based study. J Arthroplasty. 2015;30:1839–41.

12

Use of autogenous onlay bone graft for uncontained tibial bone defects in primary total knee arthroplasty

Jung-Ro Yoon, In-Wook Seo and Young-Soo Shin* (ID)

Abstract

Background: The use of autogenous bone graft is a well-known technique for reconstruction of tibial bone defects in primary total knee arthroplasty (TKA). In cases where the size of the bone graft is inappropriate, the stability of bone graft fixation and subsequent bone graft to host bone incorporation may be compromised. We describe a simple and reliable technique of reconstruction in a proximal tibia bone defect at the time of primary TKA by using autogenous onlay bone graft (AOBG).

Methods: Records were reviewed of 19 patients (mean age, 72 years) who underwent primary TKA using AOBG without the additional allogenous bone or metal augments, between August 2013 and August 2014.

Results: Mean Knee Society score (KSS) in the 22 knees was significantly higher postoperatively than preoperatively (92 ± 4 vs. 30 ± 7, $P < 0.001$). The mean range of motion (ROM) in the 22 knees, which was $106 \pm 12°$ preoperatively, improved to $112 \pm 10°$ at last follow-up, but this this difference was not significant ($P = 0.32$). No migration of implants and presence of radiolucent lines at the bone cement-prosthesis interface were observed. Furthermore, the serial radiographs of 19 patients had a mean time of 3.2 months (range, 2.7–4.4 months) for solid union with cross trabeculation between the proximal tibial bone and graft.

Conclusions: This simple AOBG supplement technique may biologically promote graft to host bone healing by enhancing fixation stability without the additional fixatives and assist the surgeon in managing the varying nature of uncontained bone defects.

Keywords: Bone defect, Bone graft, Knee reconstruction, Knee replacement

Background

A severe tibial bone defect in primary total knee arthroplasty (TKA) is one of the biggest challenges to treat for the surgeon, which can lead to a poorly balanced tibial component. Moreover, an uncontained defect is associated with a resultant angular deformity that is usually posterior and medial in a more than 20° varus knee from primary TKA [1]. The management of bone defects on the tibial aspect can vary depending on the size and location of the loss of bone, and it is necessary to consider other patient specific factors such as age, functional requirements, and bone quality. Various surgical options are available, including a thicker tibial bone resection, filling in the defect with methylmethacrylate cement, alone or with screws, and the use of metal augments [2, 3]. However, in certain situations, such as the presence of an uncontained, moderate, single condyle defect involving an area of 50% with a depth > 5 mm, a desirable surgical outcome may be difficult to achieve and bone graft may be needed. Although allogenous bone has now gained wide acceptance as a source of bone graft for primary or revision TKA owing to enhanced surgical and fixation techniques and increased functional outcomes, it has been reported to result in complications, such as risk of disease transmission, nonunion, collapse or resorption of the graft [4]. In overcoming these disadvantages, we describe

* Correspondence: sysoo3180@naver.com
Department of Orthopedic Surgery, Veterans Health Service Medical Center, 61 Jinhwangdoro-gil, Gangdong-Gu, Seoul 134-791, Korea

a simple and reliable technique to reconstruct bone defects of the proximal tibia at the time of primary TKA by using autogenous onlay bone graft (AOBG) to ensure higher graft healing rates and lower infection rate without the use of an additional allogenous bone or metal augments. It was hypothesized that this method would achieve reliable clinoradiographic outcomes in these patients.

Methods
Inclusion criteria and enrolled patients
Between August 2013 and August 2014, 19 patients (22 knees) were performed primary TKA using AOBG. The present study included 19 patients (10 women and 9 men) with a hip-knee-ankle (HKA) of 20° or more on preoperative long-standing anteroposterior radiographs (Fig. 1). The diagnosis was degenerative osteoarthritis in all cases. Patients with valgus knees, rheumatoid knees and medial bone defects <5 mm were excluded. The average patient age was 72 years (range, 57–85 years) at the time of surgery. At follow-up evaluation, the patients were assessed clinically using Knee Society score (KSS) and range of motion (ROM). Postoperative radiographs and computed tomography (CT) scanning were analyzed for the presence of implant migration, defined as a vertical or angular displacement of the implant by 3 mm or 3°, respectively [5], and presence of radiolucent lines of ≥1 mm running parallel to the implant margins at the bone cement-prosthesis interface [6]. 2 orthopaedic surgeons measured the radiographic variables twice in all 19 patients, with a 2-week interval between measurements. This study was approved by the Ethics Committee of our institution (2016–11-001), and all patients provided written informed consent. The study was registered with the Republic of Korea Clinical Trials Registry (Identifier Number: KCT0002328).

Surgical technique
The initial tibial proximal bone cut is performed using a standard tibial cutting guide. We reconstructed tibial defects with AOBG in primary TKA using a minimum of five steps.

1) Measuring the defect size and recipient bed preparation
   The size of the tibial defect is measured using gauze shaped to fit the defect precisely after 8 to 10 mm of bone is resected from the lateral tibial condyle. Sizing is followed by predrilling and burring the recipient defect bed until bleeding occurs, otherwise unsuccessful incorporation and failure of the graft may occur (Fig. 2).
2) Bone graft preparation

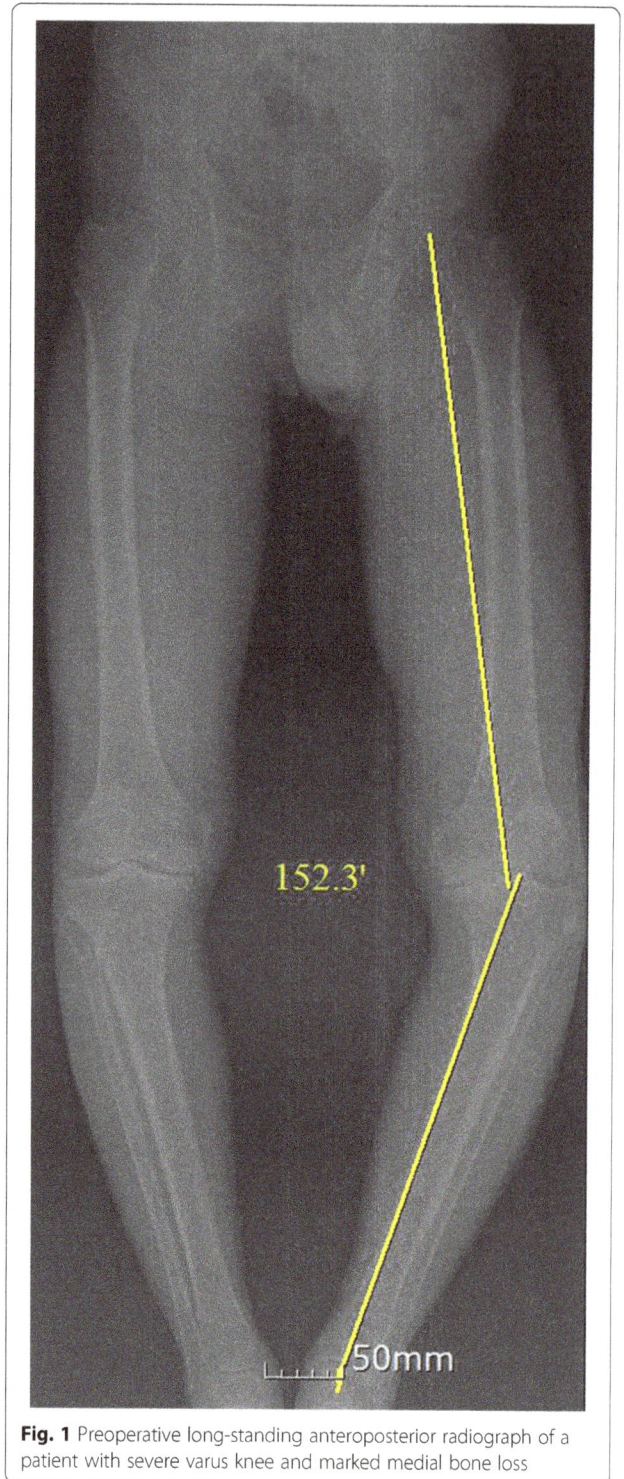

Fig. 1 Preoperative long-standing anteroposterior radiograph of a patient with severe varus knee and marked medial bone loss

Autogenous bone from the posterior condylar bone (used for smaller defects) or proximal tibial bone (used for larger defects) is fashioned carefully depending on the size of the previously measured gauze using a combination of saw cuts, bony rongeurs, and a high speed burr so there is a match

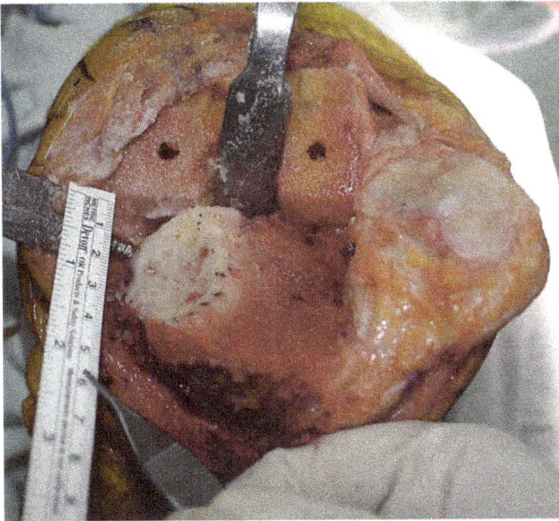

Fig. 2 An intraoperative photograph showing delineation of severe tibial bone defects

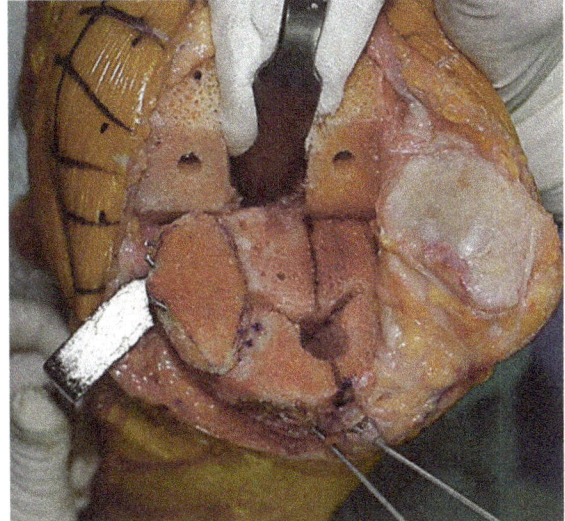

Fig. 3 Uncontained defects of the posteromedial tibial condyle can be reconstructed with an autogenous onlay bone graft (AOBG) using provisional Kirschner wires

between the graft shape and the lesion to be filled, where the cartilage is peeled off and the subchondral bones are exposed. While creating an interference fit it is important to ensure that the bone graft diameter is not smaller than the diameter of the bone defect.

3) Bone graft fixation using provisional Kirschner wires
Two 2 mm Kirschner wires are used to provisionally stabilize the AOBG to the host bone from back to front in parallel and aimed at a level below the anticipated joint line for the tibial component and in a position that does not interfere with the peg of the tibial component. In addition, the two Kirschner wires should pull forward as much as possible to make it easier to remove (Fig. 3).

4) Final fitting
Once the AOBG is coapted, the portion of the AOBG that protrudes above the anticipated joint line is removed using an oscillating saw in a rough cut manner; a protrusion to the margin is trimmed by a bony rongeur. The AOBG frequently interrupts the approach to the medullary canal of the tibia. The medullary canal is first accessed with an oscillating saw and an osteotome, by which the surgeon creates a hole to advance through areas of the AOBG. This pre-made hole is expanded to pass intramedullary reamers into the canal.

5) Cementing and Kirschner wires removal
It is of the utmost importance that cement not be allowed to permeate the gap between the graft and recipient defect bed. An excellent way to prevent this from occurring is to fill the empty space with any remaining graft fragments and apply a small portion of cement to the upper surface of the tibia along the line of the graft and the recipient defect bed (Fig. 4a, b). The Kirschner wires are withdrawn after fixation of the tibial component with cement that will harden.

Postoperative rehabilitation for our patient was the same as for patients without bone grafting in that weight-bearing and continuous passive motion is not limited. In cases with patients who undergo further release of medial structures such as the femoral origin of the MCL to obtain a rectangular mediolateral gap in some severe varus knees, a hinged brace is used for six weeks postoperatively [7].

Statistical analysis
Statistical analyses were performed using SPSS statistical software version 20 (IBM Corp., Armonk, NY, USA). The preoperative and last follow-up KSS, ROM were analyzed using a paired-samples t-test. A P-value <0.05 was considered statistically significant. The reliabilities of measurements of radiographic alignment and time to union were determined by calculating the intraclass correlation coefficient (ICC) and the standard error of measurement, with ICC values >0.75, $0.4–0.75$, and <0.4 representing good, fair, and poor reliability/accuracy, respectively. At an alpha level of 0.05 and a power of 0.8, we performed a post hoc power analysis to detect a mean difference of 5 points for KSS from before to after surgery. This study included 19 patients, with adequate power, to detect

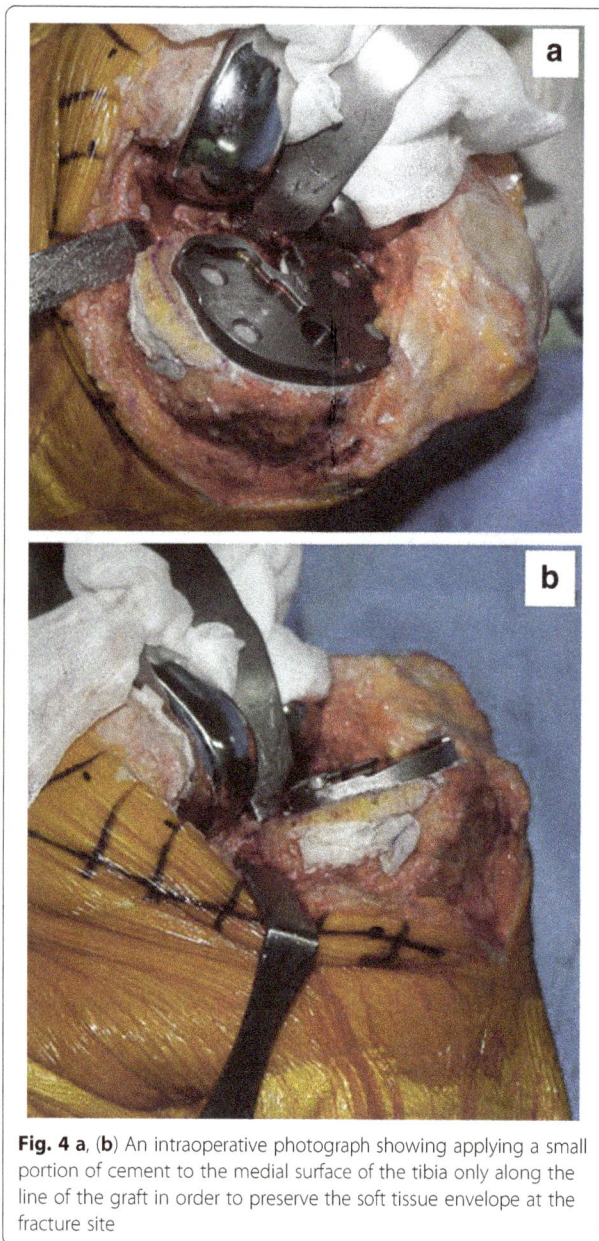

Fig. 4 a, (**b**) An intraoperative photograph showing applying a small portion of cement to the medial surface of the tibia only along the line of the graft in order to preserve the soft tissue envelope at the fracture site

significant differences in KSS (0.823) from before to after surgery.

Results

The intra- and inter-observer reliabilities of the radiographic variables including time to union (0.769–0.856) and alignment (0.755–0.848) were satisfactory. The group was comprised of 10 women and nine men with a mean age of 72 years (range, 57–85 years) at the time of surgery. The mean depth of medial tibial defects, anteroposterior width, and mediolateral width were 12.0 mm (range, 9–20 mm), 33.2 mm (range, 28–44 mm), and 15.0 mm (range, 10–25 mm). The average follow-up period was 30.2 months (range, 24–36 months). Table 1

presents detailed data for uncontained defects in all cases. Mean KSS in the 22 knees was significantly higher postoperatively than preoperatively (92 ± 4 vs. 30 ± 7, $P < 0.001$). The mean ROM in the 22 knees, which was $106 \pm 12°$ preoperatively, improved to $112 \pm 10°$ at last follow-up, but this difference was not significant ($P = 0.32$). None of patients experienced migration of implants and presence of radiolucent lines (Fig. 5a, b). Furthermore, the serial radiographs of 22 knees had a mean time of 3.2 months (range, 2.7–4.4 months) for solid union with cross trabeculation between the proximal tibial bone and graft (Fig. 6a, b). No a major complication, such as perioperative wound infection, was encountered in the present study.

Discussion

This simple technique to compensate for bone defects on the medial tibial condyle during primary TKA using the AOBG has proven to be quite effective regarding higher graft healing rates and lower infection rate.

The use of methylmethacrylate cement, independently or with screws, is a good option to fill contained defects ≤5 mm; additionally, bone grafts or metal augments may be used to offer support for tibial components for bone defects ≥5 mm [8]. Contained defects are ideal for impacted morselized bone grafts, which were found to be

Table 1 Baseline characteristics included in this study

Case No	Age (year)	Gender	Location	Source of grafting	Uncontained defect measurements (mm)			Follow-up (months)
					Depth	AP width	ML width	
1	77	F	PM	PCB	9	30	12	32
2	75	M	PM	PCB	10	32	15	28
3	82	F	PM	PCB	10	30	14	30
4	57	M	PM	PTB	14	35	16	24
5	65	M	PM	PCB	10	32	14	28
6	75	F	PM	PTB	15	38	16	32
7	72	M	PM	PCB	10	30	15	26
8	71	F	PM	PCB	10	30	12	30
9	68	M	PM	PTB	12	32	16	27
10	81	F	PM	PCB	10	30	15	28
11	74	F	PM	PTB	17	40	18	36
12	85	F	PM	PTB	14	36	15	34
13	72	M	PM	PTB	12	30	14	32
14	58	M	PM	PCB	10	32	12	30
15	74	M	PM	PTB	20	44	25	34
16	69	F	PM	PCB	10	30	14	28
17	79	F	PM	PTB	14	34	15	31
18	76	M	PM	PTB	18	40	20	29
19	77	F	PM	PCB	9	28	10	32
20	65	M	PM	PCB	10	32	14	30
21	59	F	PM	PTB	11	34	15	33
22	75	F	PM	PCB	10	32	12	30

AP anteroposterior, *ML* mediolateral, *PM* posteromedial, *F* female, *M* male, *PCB* posterior condylar bone, *PTB* proximal tibial bone

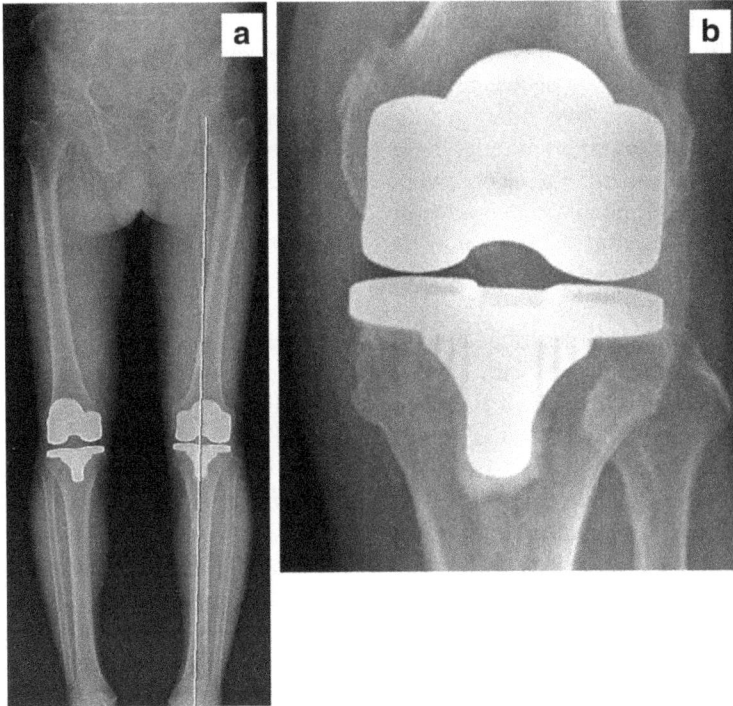

Fig. 5 a Postoperative long-standing anteroposterior and (**b**) anteroposterior radiographs at year of an 72-year-old woman with the AOBG showed no migration of implants and presence of radiolucent lines at the bone cement-prosthesis interface

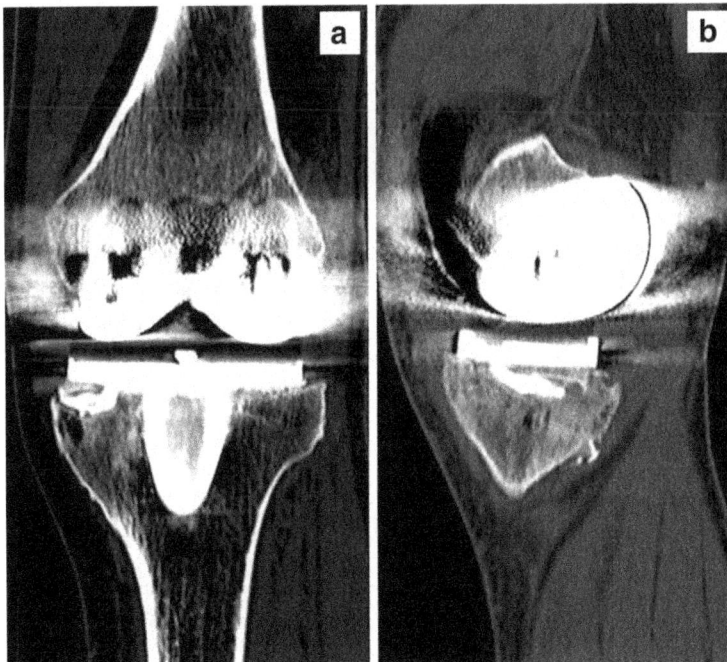

Fig. 6 a Postoperative anteroposterior and (**b**) lateral CT scans at 1 year, demonstrating autograft incorporation with cross trabeculation between the proximal tibial bone and graft

not recommended for repairing uncontained defects, because the cortical rim is considerable to ensure stability of the tibial component. In uncontained defects involving ≥50% of single tibial condyle, the use of structural allografts is recommended because they offer greater initial stability [9]. However, many shortcomings have been associated with the use of structural allografts, such as risk of disease transmission, nonunion, collapse or resorption of the graft [4, 10]. Another consideration is that they often require a longer period of limited weight bearing to allow for union of the grafts with the host bone. In addition, Whittaker et al. [11] described how to use metal augments in uncontained defects with moderate and severe bone loss ≥50% and ≥5 mm of the tibial condyle. However, there are some disadvantages, including further resection of bone to create a proper off-the-shelf augment fit and elevated cost. In an attempt to overcome these shortcomings, autogenous bone graft has been used for uncontained defects with marked bone loss of the tibial condyle; it is an advantageous method that improves graft union rates and bone stock preservation [12–14].

One study evaluating prerequisites for complete graft incorporation in 24 primary or revision knees reported that pertinent coverage of the graft by the component can prevent resorption of unstressed graft which may contribute to failure by collapse [1]. However, our study included one case of undersized tibial component on the cortical wall of the proximal tibia related to an our unintentional error during the initial learning curve. This suggests that limited coverage of the cortical wall of the proximal tibia may be related to early aseptic loosening especially with the standard tibial component. Nevertheless, we found no evidence of graft resorption or the need for revision surgery due to loosening of the tibial component. One reason for the better outcomes observed in the present study may be the use of autogenous bone obtained from posterior condylar bone or proximal tibial bone to augment bone defects on the medial tibial condyle, in cases where defect sizes are moderate with a depth of 5 to 20 mm in primary TKA, leading to a lower infection rate. However, the free-hand technique described earlier for the preparation of tibial bone defects may be somewhat technically demanding. Another factor that can explain the positive outcomes may be the soft tissue wall around the medial aspect of the proximal tibia, which can prevent the grafted bone from disintegrating after surgery. Furthermore, the AOBG can be harvested with little addition to the surgical time, and can be easily obtained without the additional fixatives, effectively creating the original shape of the medial tibial condyle in all cases by allowing the use of standard components for the primary system without tibial stem extenders. For additional fixatives, graft union rates have shown similar results across studies regardless of the presence of screws. One study classified tibial bone defects by their position and extent in 30 primary TKA cases without screw fixation treated with autogenous bone grafts. Nonunion between the graft and host bone occurred in one slant-peripheral-type case, resulting in 96.6% survivorship of autogenous bone grafts at 6.8 years [13]. In contrast, another study evaluating an autologous bone graft procedure attached the proximal portion of the tibial resection using two cannulated cancellous screws; the authors found that the screws were responsible for rigid initial fixation with a high rate of bony union at 6.6 years, which helped maintain long-term alignment [14]. Thus, we modified the surgical method to use temporary K wires instead of countersunk screws with more compression and less bone cement permeation under the graft. Additional surgical procedures, such as insertion of multiple screws may lead to fragmentation of the grafted bone, resulting in early failure of knee replacement [12].

We acknowledge the limitations of this article as it has a relatively small number of patients and short term follow-up study. However, it is not easy to find the appropriate indication of AOBG. In case of an uncontained, moderate, single condyle defect involving an area of 50% with a depth > 5 mm, surgeons may prefer use of allogenous bone or metal augments, because it does provide a simple way to reestablish the joint line without resecting the entire bone surface down to the level of the defect and offers the potential for early weight-bearing. Therefore, from a practical standpoint it is difficult to design and conduct randomized controlled trials comparing simple AOBG supplement technique and other techniques for a proximal tibia bone defect at the time of primary TKA.

Conclusions

This simple AOBG supplement technique may biologically promote graft to host bone healing by enhancing fixation stability without the additional fixatives and assist the surgeon in managing the varying nature of uncontained bone defects, thereby preventing the risk of infection in primary TKA if this surgical technique is accurately performed.

Abbreviations

AOBG: Autogenous onlay bone graft; CT: Computed tomography; KSS: Knee society score; ROM: Range of motion; TKA: Total knee arthroplasty

Acknowledgements

The authors would like to thank Ms. Jae-Ok Park for her help in preparing the manuscript.

Funding

No benefits in any form have been received or will be received from a commercial party related directly or indirectly to the subject of this article, nor have any funds been received in support of this study.

Authors' contributions

JRY conceived of the study, and participated in its design. IWS carried out the acquisition of data and statistical analysis. YSS participated in the study design and wrote the manuscript. All authors read and approved the final manuscript.

Consent for publication

Written consent to publish the clinical information for all individual participants included in the study was obtained.

Competing interests

The authors declare that they have no competing interests.

References

1. Kharbanda Y, Sharma M. Autograft reconstructions for bone defects in primary total knee replacement in severe varus knees. Indian J Orthop. 2014;48:313–8.
2. Dennis DA. Repairing minor bone defects: augmentation & autograft. Orthopedics. 1998;21:1036–8.
3. Huten D. Femorotibial bone loss during revision total knee arthroplasty. OrthopTraumatol Surg Res. 2013;99:S22–33.
4. Schmitz HC, Klauser W, Citak M, Al-Khateeb H, Gehrke T, Kendoff D. Three-year follow up utilizing tantal cones in revision total knee arthroplasty. J Arthroplast. 2013;28:1556–60.
5. Chockalingam S, Scott G. The outcome of cemented vs. cementless fixation of a femoral component in total knee replacement (TKR) with the identification of radiological signs for the prediction of failure. Knee. 2000;7:233–8.
6. Shannon BD, Klassen JF, Rand JA, Berry DJ, Trousdale RT. Revision total knee arthroplasty with cemented components and uncemented intramedullary stems. J Arthroplast. 2003;18:27–32.
7. Lee SY, Yang JH, Lee YI, et al. A novel medial soft tissue release method for varus deformity during total knee arthroplasty: femoral origin release of the medial collateral ligament. Knee Surg Relat Res. 2016;28:153–60.
8. Lonner JH, Lotke PA, Kim J, Nelson C. Impaction grafting and wire mesh for uncontained defects in revision knee arthroplasty. Clin Orthop Relat Res. 2002;404:145–51.
9. Dorr LD, Ranawat CS, Sculco TA, McKaskill B, Orisek BS. THE CLASSIC: bone graft for Tibial defects in Total knee Arthroplasty. Clin Orthop Relat Res. 2006;446:4–9.
10. Lee KJ, Bae KC, Cho CH, et al. Radiological stability after revision of infected total knee arthroplasty using modular metal augments. Knee Surg Relat Res. 2016;28:55–61.
11. Whittaker JP, Dharmarajan R, Toms AD. The management of bone loss in revision total knee replacement. J Bone Joint Surg Br. 2008;90:981–7.
12. Ahmed I, Logan M, Alipour F, et al. Autogenous bone grafting of uncontained bony defects of tibia during total knee arthroplasty a 10-year follow up. J Arthroplast. 2008;23:744–50.
13. Watanabe W, Sato K, Itoi E. Autologous bone grafting without screw fixation for tibial defects in total knee arthroplasty. J Orthop Sci. 2001;6:481–6.
14. Hosaka K, Saito S, Oyama T, et al. Union, knee alignment, and clinical outcomes of patients treated with autologous bone grafting for medial tibial defects in primary total knee arthroplasty. Orthopedics. 2017;40:e604–8.

13

Improved knee biomechanics among patients reporting a good outcome in knee-related quality of life one year after total knee arthroplasty

Josefine E. Naili[1*], Per Wretenberg[2], Viktor Lindgren[3], Maura D. Iversen[1,4,5], Margareta Hedström[6] and Eva W. Broström[1]

Abstract

Background: It is not well understood why one in five patients report poor outcomes following knee arthroplasty. This study evaluated changes in knee biomechanics, and perceived pain among patients reporting either a good or a poor outcome in knee-related quality of life after total knee arthroplasty.

Methods: Twenty-eight patients (mean age 66 (SD 7) years) were included in this prospective study. Within one month of knee arthroplasty and one year after surgery, patients underwent three-dimensional (3D) gait analysis, completed the Knee Injury and Osteoarthritis Outcome Score (KOOS), and rated perceived pain using a visual analogue scale. A "good outcome" was defined as a change greater than the minimally detectable change in the KOOS knee-related quality of life, and a "poor outcome" was defined as change below the minimally detectable change. Nineteen patients (68%) were classified as having a good outcome. Groups were analyzed separately and knee biomechanics were compared using a two-way repeated measures ANOVA. Differences in pain between groups were evaluated using Mann Whitney *U* test.

Results: Patients classified as having a good outcome improved significantly in most knee gait biomechanical outcomes including increased knee flexion-extension range, reduced peak varus angle, increased peak flexion moment, and reduced peak valgus moment. The good outcome group also displayed a significant increase in walking speed, a reduction (normalization) of stance phase duration (% of gait cycle) and increased passive knee extension. Whereas, the only change in knee biomechanics, one year after surgery, for patients classified as having a poor outcome was a significant reduction in peak varus angle. No differences in pain postoperatively were found between groups.

Conclusion: Patients reporting a good outcome in knee-related quality of life improved in knee biomechanics during gait, while patients reporting a poor outcome, despite similar reduction in pain, remained unchanged in knee biomechanics one year after total knee arthroplasty. With regards to surgeon-controlled biomechanical factors, surgery may most successfully address frontal plane knee alignment. However, achieving a good outcome in patient-reported knee-related quality of life may be related to dynamic improvements in the sagittal plane.

Keywords: Gait, Knee, Biomechanics, Joint replacement, Quality of Life, Function, Osteoarthritis

* Correspondence: josefine.naili@ki.se
The work was performed at Karolinska Institutet, Karolinska University Hospital, Stockholm, Sweden.
[1]Department of Women's and Children's Health, Karolinska Institutet, MotorikLab, Q2:07, Karolinska University Hospital, 171 76 Stockholm, Sweden
Full list of author information is available at the end of the article

Background

The majority of patients with knee osteoarthritis report decreased pain and improved function following total knee arthroplasty (TKA), yet nearly one in five report limited function, persistent disability, and reduced quality of life (QoL) [1–3]. The reasons for persistent disability in this subset of patients are not well understood [1]. Patient satisfaction after TKA is associated with patient-reported outcomes and clinician assessments [4], although surgeons tend to report greater satisfaction with surgical results than patients [5]. In a study investigating factors associated with patient satisfaction after TKA, the authors found no differences between satisfied and dissatisfied patients with regards to clinical examination findings, performance-based function, and radiography, although perceived knee pain differed between the groups, wherein satisfied patients reported lower postoperative pain levels [6].

Patient-reported outcomes are frequently used for evaluating pain and function following TKA. The Knee Injury and Osteoarthritis Outcome Score (KOOS) is one of few disease-specific instruments for patients with knee osteoarthritis that includes a subscale measuring knee-related QoL. The knee-related QoL subscale evaluates knee-specific mental and social aspects of function and requires patients to reflect upon the impact of knee symptoms on their QoL [7]. This subscale may be considered the most emotionally sensitive part of the questionnaire as it evaluates awareness and lifestyle changes related to the knee [7]. The knee-related QoL subscale is the most responsive KOOS subscale when outcomes are measured at six and 12 months after TKA [7]. Additionally, 90% of patients with TKA consider this subscale to be extremely or very important [8].

At one year follow-up, studies using three dimensional (3D) gait analysis to evaluate outcomes after TKA have shown that knee biomechanics and gait pattern do not return to normal after surgery [9–12]. Knee kinematics and kinetics during gait continue to deviate compared to healthy controls, as represented by reduced knee flexion-extension range, reduced peak flexion moments, and increased external knee adduction moments [9, 10]. The frequency and severity of anterior knee pain after TKA appear to partially be explained by a retained higher preoperative external knee flexion moment [13]. To the best of our knowledge, no prior studies have evaluated change in knee biomechanics during gait in patients grouped according to their postoperative self-reported outcome. Therefore, the primary aim of this study was to evaluate change in knee biomechanics during gait among patients reporting a good or a poor outcome in knee-related QoL, respectively. Secondly, we wanted to evaluate if the good or poor outcome groups reported differences in perceived pain postoperatively.

Methods

Participants

Between the years 2010 and 2014, 40 patients were recruited from two orthopedic departments in Stockholm County, Sweden (Ortho Center, Löwenströmska Hospital and the Department of Orthopedics at Karolinska University Hospital). Inclusion criteria were: being scheduled for TKA within one month due to primary knee osteoarthritis, the ability to walk 10 m repeatedly without assistance of a walking aid, and the ability to understand verbal and written information in Swedish. Exclusion criteria were: other severe joint pain or previous major orthopedic surgery in the lower extremities (including traumatic knee injury), rheumatoid arthritis, neurological disorder, diabetes mellitus, body mass index (BMI) > 40, and/or other medical condition affecting walking ability. All patients that met inclusion and exclusion criteria and accepted participation were included in this prospective cohort study [11]. Twenty-five age and gender matched, healthy controls without any known musculoskeletal disease or neurological disorder were recruited through acquaintances between the years 2013–2015. The control group was matched to the osteoarthritis group by age strata across five age groups (40–49, 50–59, 60–69, 70–79, 80–89 years of age). The mean age of the control group was 66 years (SD 10), and they had a mean BMI of 24.9 (SD 2.9). The present study is a secondary analysis and therefore, participants and methods are described more in detail elsewhere [11]. The study was approved by Stockholm's regional ethical review board (DNR: 2010/1014-31/1), and all study participants provided written informed consent in accordance with the Declaration of Helsinki.

Out of the 40 patients included at baseline, 28 patients (18 females), with a mean age of 66 (SD 7) years, completed the one year follow-up. Reasons for not completing the one year follow up were: not going through with the planned surgery ($n = 2$), post-operative infection causing re-operation ($n = 2$), TKA in the contralateral limb within the following year ($n = 5$), death ($n = 1$), pelvic fracture during the following year ($n = 1$), and cancer diagnosis ($n = 1$). Patients who did not complete the one year follow up ($n = 12$) did not differ statistically from the studied group with regards to distribution of age, gender, weight, height, BMI or duration of years with symptomatic knee osteoarthritis.

Setting and procedures

Baseline evaluations were performed within one month prior to surgery (mean 20 (SD 13) days) and postoperative evaluations one year after surgery (mean 12 (SD 0.9) months). Three-dimensional gait data and patient-reported outcomes were collected at the Motion Analysis Laboratory at Karolinska University Hospital, Solna,

Sweden. Each test session started with a physical examination. Passive range of motion of the lower extremity joints were recorded using a goniometer with the patient in a supine position for all measures except hip extension which was recorded with the patient in a prone position. Anthropometric measures were recorded using calibrated scales. After the initial examination, 35 retro-reflective markers were placed on anatomical landmarks (head, trunk, pelvis, lower and upper extremities), according to the conventional biomechanical model Plug-In-Gait (Vicon Motion Systems Ltd, Oxford, UK) [14].

Three-dimensional gait analysis

Three-dimensional gait data were collected using an eight camera system (Vicon Motion Systems Ltd, Oxford, UK) (sampling rate 100 Hz), and two force plates embedded in the floor (Kistler, Winterthur, Switzerland) (1000 Hz). Kinematic, kinetic, and time and distance parameters were collected simultaneously. Kinetics were expressed as internal moments (forces from muscles, ligaments and tendons acting on the specific joint). The studied kinematic variables included knee flexion-extension range during an entire gait cycle, peak knee flexion angle in swing phase, and peak varus angle during stance phase. The studied kinetic variables during stance phase included peak knee flexion moment, peak knee extension moment, and peak knee valgus moment. Patients were instructed to walk barefoot at self-selected speed along a defined 10 m walkway. Recordings were made in two directions (back and forth). Approximately five gait trials, with clean force plate strikes, were analyzed for each patient at each test session. Gait variables from these strides were averaged to obtain one value for each variable of interest, for each patient, at each test session. Raw motion capture data were filtered in a Woltring Filter [15] with a mean squared error setting of 15, and 3D gait kinematics and kinetics were computed according to the Plug-in-Gait model [14]. The gait kinematics and kinetics data were then exported to the software program MATLAB®, R2014a (The MathWorks, Inc, Natick, MA, USA) where discrete values (maxima, minima) were computed for the participants.

Perceived pain

After completing the gait trials, patients rated their perceived pain experienced during the gait trials using a visual analogue scale (VAS) where 0 represents "no pain" and 100 mm represents "severe pain" [16].

Patient-reported outcomes

The KOOS was used to evaluate patient-reported pain, symptoms, function in activities of daily living (ADL), function in sport and recreation, and knee-related QoL

[17]. KOOS generates a final score for each separate subscale, ranging from 0-100, where 0 represent "severe difficulties" and 100 "no problems at all". Adequate test-retest reliability (intra class correlation range 0.85 – 0.9) has been reported for all subscales [18]. The questionnaire is widely used, and is valid and responsive to change in patients with knee osteoarthritis receiving both conservative [19] and surgical treatment [20].

Radiological classification

According to standard practice at each hospital, preoperative standing anterior-posterior radiographs were taken. Two experienced orthopedic surgeons together performed the classification of radiographic severity of osteoarthritis (for the knee joint as a whole) according to the modified Kellgren and Lawrence's (KL) classification [21] (Table 1).

Knee replacement surgery and postoperative rehabilitation

The surgical procedures were performed by seven different senior orthopedic surgeons from two hospitals, all using a posterior cruciate ligament retaining cemented TKA (PFC-Sigma, DePuy, Johnson & Johnson, Warsaw, Poland). Surgeons were equally distributed across the two groups. After surgery, patients were allowed full weight bearing (together with use of an appropriate walking aid), and unrestricted range of motion. The postoperative rehabilitation was performed according to the standard practice at each hospital (in-patient physiotherapy <1 week). Thereafter, patients received rehabilitation in a primary care setting of their choice, which lasted for a median duration of 3 months (range 1-6 months) in the good outcome group and 5 months (range 1-6 months) in the poor outcome group.

Classification of outcome

The minimally detectable change (MDC) of KOOS knee-related QoL is reported to be 21.1 points one year after TKA [8, 22], and this was used as a cut-off to classify individuals postoperative outcome as either a "good outcome" (change ≥ MDC), or a "poor outcome" (change < MDC). The MDC is a statistical estimate that provides a threshold for interpretation of a measurement [23]. When a change score exceeds this threshold, there is reasonable certainty that it represents a true change, and not a measurement error [23]. The MDC is not an absolute value, and should be considered a guideline [23]. In this sample, 19 (68%) out of 28 patients reported change greater than the MDC in KOOS knee-related QoL at the one year follow-up, and were classified as having a good outcome (Fig. 1). Nine patients reported change smaller than 21.1 points in knee-related QoL and were classified as having a poor outcome. The good

Table 1 Baseline characteristics, within one month prior to knee arthroplasty. Patients are grouped according to postoperative change in knee-related Quality of Life

	Good outcome group, n = 19	Poor outcome group, n = 9	Difference between groups, p-value
Female, n	12	6	0.856
Age, years, mean (SD)	67.3 (7.7)	62.4 (5.4)	0.1
Height (cm), median (range)	170 (156-184)	163 (159-181)	0.438
Weight (kg), mean (SD)	82.8 (11.8)	83.5 (14.3)	0.892
BMI (m2/kg), mean (SD)	29 (4.6)	30 (5.1)	0.614
Symptom duration, years, median (range)	10 (1.5-26)	8 (1-20)	0.263
Kellgren and Lawrence score (1-4b)			
1-2	-	-	
3a, n	0	1	0.321
3b, n	1	3	0.084
4a, n	7	1	0.214
4b, n	11	4	0.689
Knee Injury and Osteoarthritis Outcome Score, 0-100			
Pain, mean (SD)	48 (14)	40 (17)	0.218
Symptoms, median (range)	32 (18-89)	32 (18-75)	0.699
Activities of Daily Living, mean (SD)	62 (11)	46 (19)	*0.007*
Sport and Recreation, median (range)	15 (0-60)	15 (0-80)	0.809
Knee-related Quality of Life, mean (SD)	30 (13)	24 (9)	0.251

Poor outcome was defined as change below the minimally detectable change (21.1) in knee-related Quality of Life of KOOS
Italicized p-value indicating a significant difference (p<0.05)

and poor outcome groups were analyzed separately and compared (Table 1).

Statistical analysis

A significance level was set at p <0.05 and data analyses were performed using IBM SPSS Statistics version 22 (Chicago, IL, USA). Depending on data distribution, means with standard deviation and medians with range, were used to describe the explored variables. Normal distribution of data was assessed using Shapiro-Wilk's test and Q-Q plots. Sample size calculations were made a priori for the primary analysis with another aim [11].

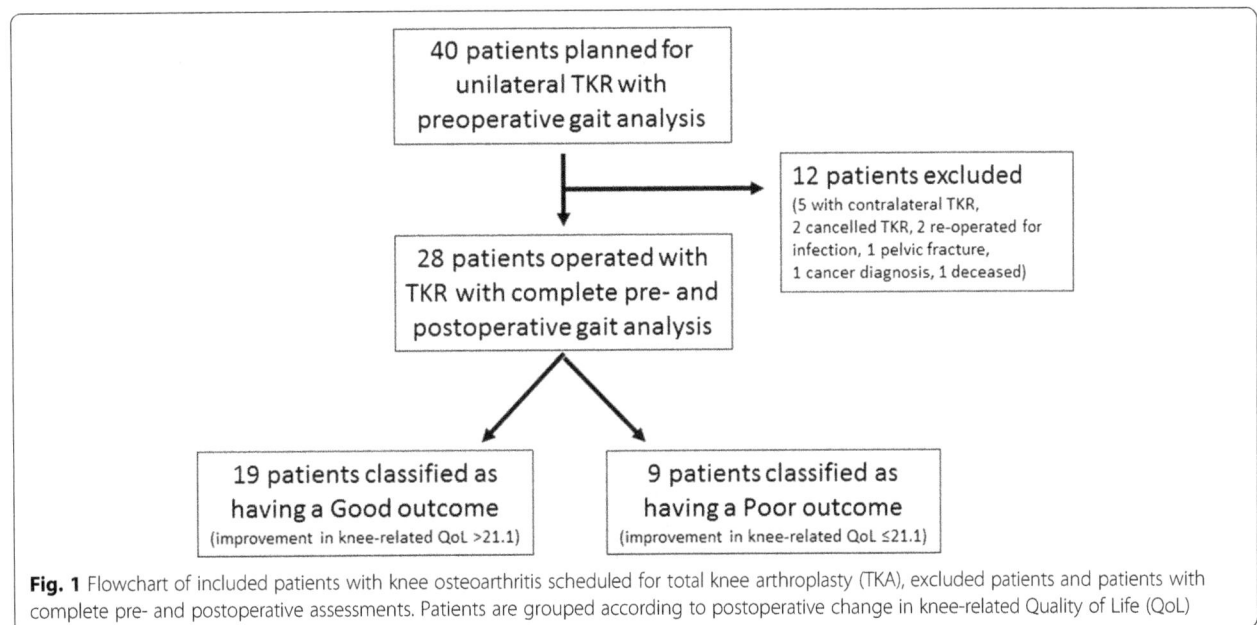

Fig. 1 Flowchart of included patients with knee osteoarthritis scheduled for total knee arthroplasty (TKA), excluded patients and patients with complete pre- and postoperative assessments. Patients are grouped according to postoperative change in knee-related Quality of Life (QoL)

In this secondary analysis, post hoc power analyses were performed with regards to change in knee gait biomechanics. The sample size of the good outcome group ($n = 19$) had sufficient power (range 93-99%) to detect significant differences in knee flexion-extension range, peak varus angle and peak valgus moment within the group [24]. Power for the corresponding variables within the poor outcome group ($n = 9$) was low (range 23-55%) [24]. Knee gait biomechanics, passive range of knee motion, and time and distance parameters were analyzed using a two-way repeated measures ANOVA with the within groups factor Time (prior to TKA and one year post TKA) and the between groups factor Group (the good outcome group and the poor outcome group) and the interaction Group*Time. The Group*Time interaction refers to the statistical test of whether the response profile for one group is the same as for the other group. In case of a significant interaction, simple effects were tested, i.e. effects of one factor holding the levels of the other factor fixed. To adjust for preoperative differences between groups an ANCOVA was performed. Receiver operating characteristic (ROC) curves

were calculated to evaluate whether change in knee gait biomechanics could be used to correctly classify patients into either the good or poor outcome group. The area under the ROC curve (AUC) and 95% confidence intervals (CI) were calculated. An AUC of at least 0.70 was considered to be appropriate [25]. Differences in baseline data and change in VAS pain raw scores between the good and the poor outcome group were evaluated using independent samples t-tests and Mann Whitney U test, depending on data distribution. Fisher's exact test was used to determine whether the proportion of patients differed between the groups with regards to the KL classification of radiographic severity of osteoarthritis.

Results

Preoperative differences between groups

The good outcome group presented with significantly less knee flexion-extension range (5°) during gait preoperatively (Fig. 2), compared to the poor outcome group ($p = 0.004$) (Table 2). The proportion of patients with less radiographic changes (a KL score of 3b) were larger in the poor outcome

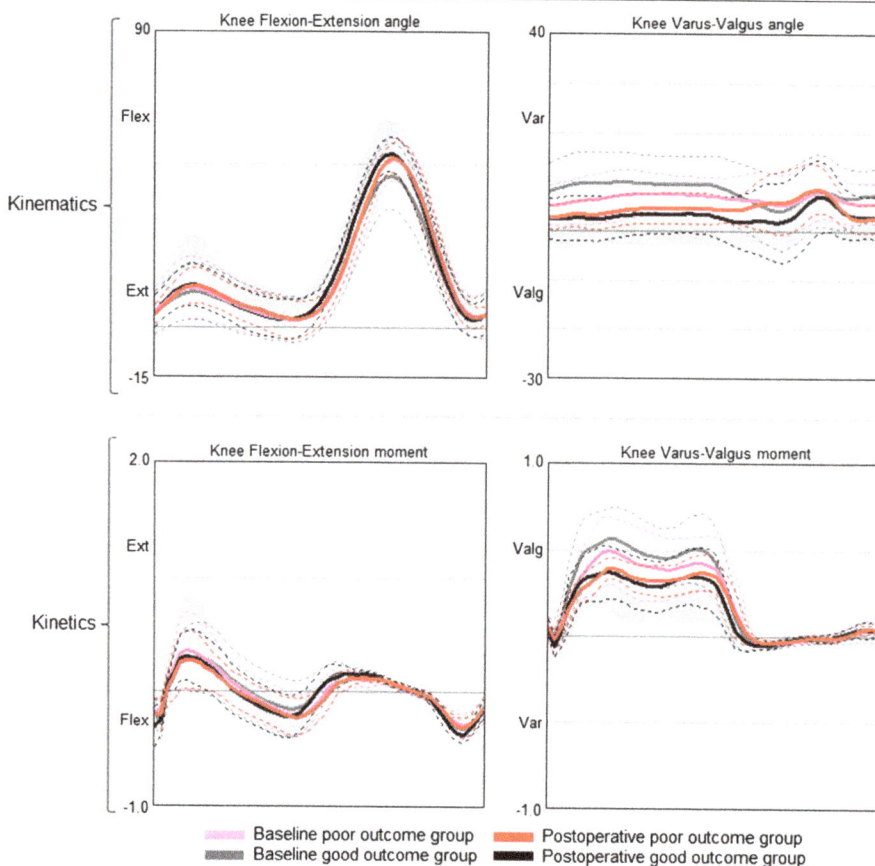

Fig. 2 Knee kinematics (degrees) and kinetics (Nm/kg) at baseline and at one year follow-up. Patients are grouped according to postoperative change in knee-related Quality of Life; the good outcome group ($n = 19$), the poor outcome group ($n = 9$). The solid lines represents the mean for each group, respectively. The dashed lines represent ± 1 standard deviation for each group, respectively. The shaded area represents the mean ± 1 standard deviation of an age matched healthy control group ($n = 25$)

Table 2 Passive range of knee motion, knee gait biomechanics, and time and distance parameters at baseline and one year after total knee arthroplasty. Patients are grouped according postoperative change in knee-related quality of life

	Control group n = 25	Good outcome group, n = 19		Poor outcome group, n = 9		Effect of interactions	Within group differences	Between group differences	Postop Δ adj. for baseline
	Reference	Baseline	Postoperative	Baseline	Postoperative		p	p	p
Passive range of knee motion, degrees									
Flexion, mean (SD)	136 * ‖ (5)	119 (15)	115 (10)	124 (16)	112 (14)	0.182	a) 0.306 **b) 0.025**	c) 0.375 d) 0.516	-
Extension, mean (SD)	2 (4)	−5 (7)	0 (3.5)	0 (7)	0 (6)	0.152	**a) 0.007** b) 0.814	c) 0.187 d) 0.880	-
Knee kinematics during gait, degrees									
Peak flexion, mean (SD)	54 * ‖ (4)	48 (10)	53 (6)	53 (6)	52 (4)	0.081	**a) 0.004** b) 0.973	c) 0.175 d) 0.782	-
Flex-Ext range, mean (SD)	57 ‖ (5)	45 (6)	53 (5)	52 (5)	50 (6)	**0.003**	**a) 0.000** b) 0.471	**c) 0.009** d) 0.275	e) 0.143
Peak varus angle during stance, mean (SD)	3.2 * (3.3)	10.5 (6.1)	5.7 (4.8)	8.5 (4.3)	5.6 (2.4)	0.246	**a) 0.000** **b) 0.042**	c) 0.375 d) 0.953	-
Knee kinetics during gait, Nm/kg									
Peak flexion moment, mean (SD)	−0.54 ‖ (0.17)	−0.41 (0.11)	−0.49 (0.15)	−0.41 (0.10)	−0.38 (0.11)	**0.044**	**a) 0.009** b) 0.540	c) 0.966 d) 0.054	-
Peak extension moment, mean (SD)	0.50 * ‖ (0.10)	0.43 (0.19)	0.37 (0.15)	0.39 (0.29)	0.33 (0.21)	0.976	a) 0.171 b) 0.324	c) 0.672 d) 0.555	-
Peak valgus moment, mean (SD)	0.60 * ‖ (0.10)	0.60 (0.18)	0.44 (0.16)	0.54 (0.18)	0.46 (0.06)	0.154	**a) 0.000** b) 0.069	c) 0.428 d) 0.797	-
Time and distance parameters									
Walking speed, m/s, mean (SD)	1.3 ‖ (0.2)	1.1 (0.2)	1.2 (0.2)	1.1 (0.2)	1.1 (0.2)	0.288	**a) 0.022** b) 0.721	c) 0.593 d) 0.086	-
Stance phase, % of gait cycle, mean (SD)	60.3 ‖ (1.0)	62.5 (2.6)	61.3 (1.8)	62 (1.8)	61.7 (1.6)	0.184	**a) 0.005** b) 0.642	c) 0.603 d) 0.484	-

a) *p*-value indicating differences between preoperative and postoperative assessment within the **good outcome group**
b) *p*-value indicating differences between preoperative and postoperative assessment within the **poor outcome group**
c) *p*-value indicating differences between the good and the poor outcome group **preoperatively**
d) *p*-value indicating differences between the good and the poor outcome group **postoperatively**
e) *p*-value indicating **postoperative** differences between groups **adjusted for preoperative values**
* indicating a significant difference ($p < 0.05$) between control group and the **good outcome group postoperatively**
‖ indicating a significant difference ($p < 0.05$) between control group and the **poor outcome group postoperatively**

group, although not statistically different ($p = 0.08$) (Table 1). Preoperatively, the poor outcome group reported significantly lower scores in the KOOS ADL subscale (Table 1). In both the good and the poor outcome groups several patients had gone through previous knee arthroscopy. These arthroscopic surgeries were done for diagnostic purposes for some, and in some cases it was due to degenerative meniscal tears (the tears were not repaired, only resected). The number of participants with a previous history of knee arthroscopy were equally distributed in the two groups (11 out of 19 in the good outcome group (57%), and 5 out of 9 in the poor outcome group (56%).

Change in knee biomechanics within the good outcome group

The good outcome group displayed significant improvements in the majority of knee gait biomechanics variables

(Fig. 2). During gait, peak knee flexion angle increased by 5°, knee flexion-extension range increased by 8°, peak varus angle was reduced by 4.8°, peak flexion moment increased by 0.08 Nm/kg, and peak valgus moment was reduced by 0.16 Nm/kg (Table 2). The good outcome group also displayed a significant increase in walking speed, a reduction (normalization) of stance phase duration (% of gait cycle), and increased passive range of knee extension by 5° (Table 2).

Change in knee biomechanics within the poor outcome group

The poor outcome group displayed a significant reduction in peak varus angle during stance phase by 2.9° ($p = 0.042$) (Table 2). Aside from that, no other knee gait biomechanics outcomes, or passive knee joint range of motion showed any significant change one year after surgery

(Table 2). Baseline data and postoperative results, for each individual classified as having a poor outcome, are presented separately (Table 3).

Postoperative differences between groups

At the postoperative evaluation, there were no differences between the good and the poor outcome groups, other than a tendency for the good outcome group to demonstrate larger increases in peak flexion moment during stance phase ($p = 0.054$) (Table 2).

Differences in change in pain between the groups

No differences were found between the groups with regards to change in perceived pain during gait trials assessed with VAS, or in perceived pain during gait trials at the postoperative assessment (Table 4).

Predictive value of change in knee gait biomechanics on knee-related QoL post TKA

Receiver operating characteristic (ROC) curves showed that smaller change in flexion-extension range, and change in peak flexion moment had a good ability to predict a poor outcome post TKA (Fig. 3). The AUC was 0.83 for change in flexion-extension range (CI 0.67 – 0.98), and 0.77 for change in peak flexion moment (CI 0.59 – 0.94). The ability to predict a poor outcome in knee related QoL for the other evaluated knee gait biomechanics outcomes were low (Fig. 3).

Postoperative differences between TKA patients and control group

At the one year follow-up, both the good and the poor outcome groups presented with significantly lower passive range of knee flexion, lower peak flexion angle during gait, lower peak extension moment, and lower peak valgus moment compared to controls (Table 2). The good outcome group was comparable to the control group with regards to walking speed and stance phase duration, while the poor outcome group walked with a reduced walking speed and with a longer stance phase duration as compared to controls (Table 2). The poor outcome group had a significantly lower flexion-extension range, and lower peak flexion moment compared to the control group (Table 2).

Discussion

This study evaluated change in knee biomechanics during gait among TKA patients classified as having a good or a poor outcome based on postoperative change in knee-related QoL. We found that patients reporting a good outcome in knee-related QoL one year following TKA displayed significant improvements in most knee biomechanical outcomes during gait. Whereas, the only change found at one year after surgery for patients classified as having a poor outcome was a significant reduction in peak varus angle. Even though the sample of patients classified as having a poor outcome was small, data indicate that these patients, who had less severe progression of OA, remained unchanged in knee biomechanics after surgery.

Preoperatively, the good outcome group presented with significantly smaller knee flexion-extension range during gait compared to the poor outcome group. Thus, the good outcome group had a larger potential to improve in knee flexion-extension range after surgery, which they did. The good outcome group displayed significant improvements in most knee biomechanics outcomes during gait, however, these improvements were not necessarily clinically relevant. The increase in flexion-extension range of 8° in the good outcome group seems to be clinically relevant, as

Table 3 Passive range of knee motion and knee biomechanics during gait at baseline and at one year following total knee arthroplasty among patients reporting a poor outcome in knee-related quality of life

	Passive range of motion				Knee biomechanics during gait									
	Knee flexion		Knee extension		Flexion-extension range		Peak varus angle during stance		Peak flexion moment		Peak extension moment		Peak valgus moment	
	Degrees				Degrees				Nm/kg					
ID	Baseline	Postop	Baseline	Postop	Baseline	Postop	Baseline	Postop	Baseline	Postop	Baseline	Postop	Baseline	Postop
1	120	110	−15	0	49.2	51.7	1.5	2.2	−0.42	−0.47	0.23	0.50	0.32	0.48
2	140	125	5	5	56.2	54.5	12.2	8.9	−0.46	−0.41	0.31	0.24	0.51	0.48
3	115	105	10	0	48.5	53.8	4.7	2.2	−0.51	−0.54	0.22	0.23	0.40	0.40
4	120	100	0	−5	50.9	55.9	7.9	7.1	−0.44	−0.39	1.11	0.79	0.57	0.52
5	140	130	5	5	55.4	54.9	16.0	6.3	−0.43	−0.36	0.21	0.42	0.84	0.45
6	90	115	−5	−5	55.0	50.0	7.4	6.4	−0.37	−0.33	0.17	0.21	0.26	0.35
7	130	105	0	5	50.9	39.8	6.2	7.7	−0.39	−0.43	0.49	0.13	0.60	0.42
8	130	90	−5	−10	58.7	49.1	10.8	3.7	−0.48	−0.32	0.32	0.17	0.65	0.56
9	135	130	0	5	42.1	41.5	9.9	5.8	−0.16	−0.15	0.44	0.30	0.68	0.47

Table 4 Perceived pain during gait trials among patients with knee osteoarthritis preoperatively, one year after total knee arthroplasty, and differences in change between groups. Patients are grouped according postoperative change in knee-related quality of life

	Good outcome group, $n = 19$	Poor outcome group, $n = 9$	Difference between groups, p-value
Perceived pain during gait trials, 0-100			
Preoperative VAS, median (range)	35 (4-79)	45 (4-74)	0.09
Postoperative VAS, median (range)	0 (0-18)	1 (0-50)	0.188
Change in VAS, median (range)	−30 (-4 - -79)	−42 (5 - -72)	0.455

VAS visual analog scale

the ROC curve analysis showed that a smaller change in flexion-extension range was indicative of a poor outcome in knee-related QoL. In the good outcome group, we also found increased passive range of knee extension and increased knee flexion moment, which we interpret as improved ability to load the knee joint during the latter part of the stance phase. We interpret this increased knee flexion moment as a reflection of patients' improved confidence in knee joint function, reduced pain, and possibly improved muscle strength as pain has subsided and patients are able to be more physically active. These factors are likely captured in their improved knee-related QoL scores [8]. Pasquier et al. found that improvement in passive knee flexion after TKA was greater for knees with low preoperative flexion, in opposition to knees with preoperative flexion at 110° or larger [26]. In the present

study, both groups presented with passive knee flexion larger than 110° preoperatively, and after surgery both groups displayed a slight reduction in passive knee flexion, although not statistically changed. Based on our data, it does not appear to be any clear relationship between passive range of motion and dynamic flexion-extension range during gait.

In the poor outcome group, peak varus angle during stance phase was the only biomechanical variable that improved significantly following surgery. The postoperative degree of varus angle during stance phase, in both the good and poor outcome group, is in agreement with findings of others [27]. Orishimo et al. reported the varus angle to decrease at six months after surgery, but to increase again at the one year follow-up [27]. This, even though static radiographs displayed patients were

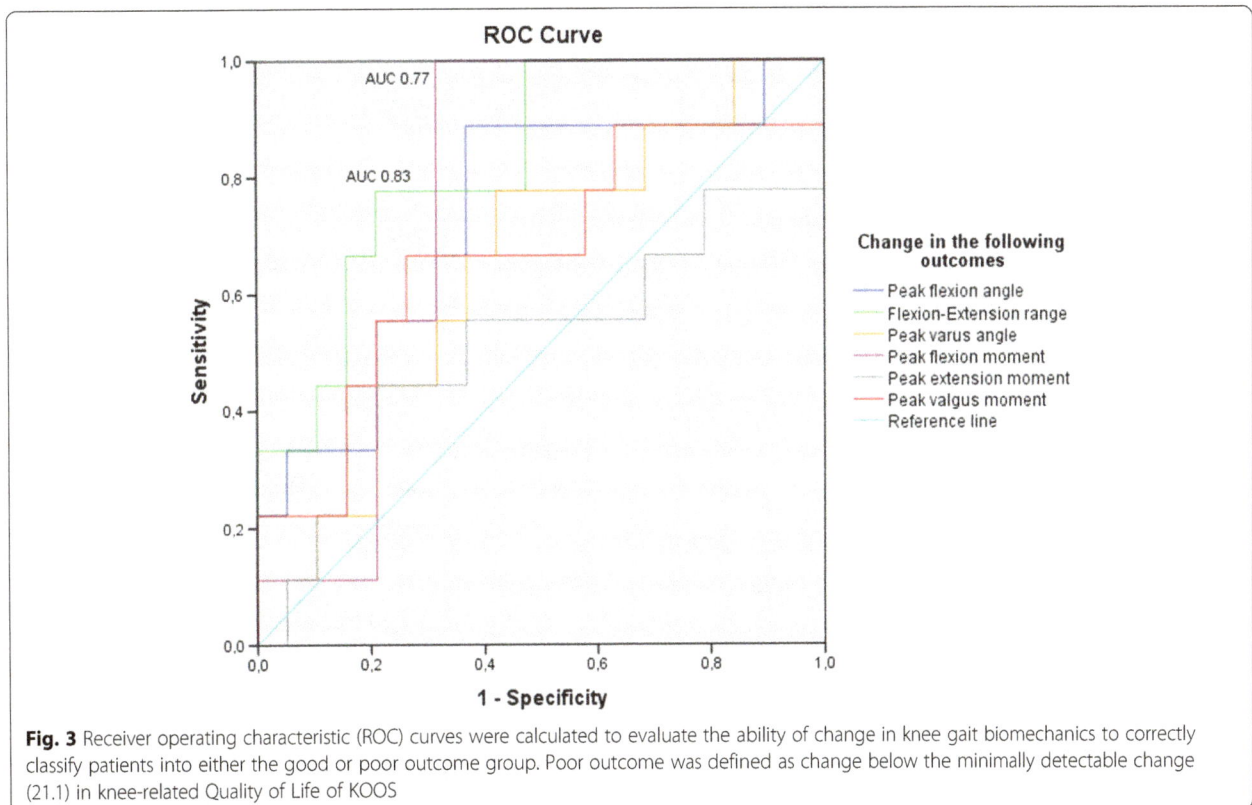

Fig. 3 Receiver operating characteristic (ROC) curves were calculated to evaluate the ability of change in knee gait biomechanics to correctly classify patients into either the good or poor outcome group. Poor outcome was defined as change below the minimally detectable change (21.1) in knee-related Quality of Life of KOOS

aligned in a more normalized (neutral) position [27]. Prodromos et al. evaluated the predictive value of static knee alignment on dynamic loading of the knee during gait among patients treated with a high tibial osteotomy and reported it to be low [28]. Further, the authors also found recurrent varus alignment among tibial osteotomy patients presenting with a high external knee adduction moment preoperatively [28]. Similar findings have been reported by Rodriguez et al. who found that dynamic loading patterns of the knee could not be determined by static alignment alone [29]. The results from the ROC curve analysis indicate that smaller change in knee flexion-extension range, and in peak flexion moment are a good predictors of a being classified as having poor outcome after TKA surgery. With regards to surgeon-controlled factors, frontal plane alignment may be the biomechanical factor surgery most successfully can address. However, achieving a good outcome in patient-reported knee-related QoL may not be related to improvements in knee alignment in the frontal plane, but rather to dynamic improvements in flexion-extension range.

Conflicting results have been reported for the influence of preoperative factors and their association with a poor outcome after TKA [30, 31]. Baker et al. reported preoperative variables to have a marginal influence on postoperative satisfaction [30], while results from Judge et al. showed that worse preoperative mental health was a predictor of poor patient-reported outcome [31]. Smith et al. reported the frequency and severity of knee pain post TKA to be partially explained by preoperative joint loading patterns during gait [13]. Scott and colleagues reported that patient expectations, poor mental health, and other musculoskeletal pain had an impact on satisfaction, although the largest determinant of satisfaction after TKA was the level of pain reduction [3]. Using a VAS to monitor perceived pain during gait trials, we found no differences in perceived pain between the good and the poor outcome group. These data suggest pain may not be the primary reason for lower knee-related QoL in the poor outcome group, and that VAS is not sensitive enough to differentiate between groups. Knoop et al. identified five different "clinical" phenotypes in patients with knee osteoarthritis [32], where clinical outcomes differed among these phenotypes. The authors suggest interventions may need to be adapted to these clinical phenotypes [32]. Due to the small samples in the present study, it is not meaningful to classify patients according to these phenotypes, although if we were to speculate, we would expect there to be some individuals in the poor outcome group that fit the description of the phenotype called "minimal joint disease". It is possible that these individuals may not have had severe joint damage but had pain. Thus, beyond pain relief they did

not view the surgery as impacting their knee-related QoL. Future studies should explore whether biomechanical response to knee arthroplasty is different across different clinical phenotypes. It would also be of importance to assess muscle strength pre- and postoperatively, as well as closely monitoring compliance to postoperative rehabilitation.

The number of patients classified as having a poor outcome was higher than expected, compared to previous studies reporting proportions of around 20% of patients with poor outcomes [1–3]. Using the MDC of knee-related QoL as a cut-off for a good or poor outcome, we found a larger percentage of patients with a poor outcome (32%) within our sample. This result may be related to the use of the knee-related QoL subscale which may be a more sensitive measure at one year after surgery, as this is the subscale reported that best demonstrates the improvement occurring between 6 and 12 months [8]. As pain reduction occurs earlier in the postoperative phase, the knee-related QoL subscale is able to capture improvements that takes longer time, such as awareness, ability to trust in the knee, and knee-related lifestyle changes [8]. The percentage of dissatisfied patients is reported to be even higher when evaluating the ability to perform activities of daily living as compared to pain outcomes [2], and this may also be reflected in the subscale knee-related QoL. The higher proportion of patients classified as having a poor outcome could possibly be a consequence of chance in this small sample size. If the MDC cut-off level is a too sensitive measure this would actually minimize the differences, as some patients could have been considered having a good outcome if another measure was used. Hence, some patients classified as having a good outcome might actually be included in the poor outcome group, which we believe makes our results more conservative. It is important to point out, that the MDC is a statistical estimate, and should not be confused with a threshold of what is a *minimal important difference* (MID) [33]. According to King, the MID of a patient-reported outcome will likely depend on the baseline values from which the patients starts, and may differ between groups and settings [33].

Limitations of this study includes that it is a secondary analysis of a prospective cohort study, thus, a priori power calculations were conducted with another aim. Post hoc power calculations deemed sufficient for comparisons within the good outcome group, while power was low in the poor outcome group. The sample size of the poor outcome group may predispose the results towards type II error in reporting no significant change, therefore conclusions are limited. Additionally, we did not monitor aspects of the postoperative rehabilitation, other than record the duration, nor did we have data on muscle strength which we also consider to be limitations

Improved knee biomechanics among patients reporting a good outcome in knee-related quality of life...

107

of the present study. The strengths of this study include the use of objective measures of knee biomechanics during gait combined with the use of reliable, valid and responsive patient-reported instruments for assessing outcome after TKA. The total sample size is consistent with, and even larger than similar studies using 3D gait analysis [27, 34]. Furthermore, data were collected prospectively with an acceptable rate of follow-up. Seven different senior orthopedic surgeons performed the surgeries making the results generalizable to patients with osteoarthritis treated with TKA in the orthopedic community.

Conclusion

In this prospective cohort study, we evaluated changes in knee biomechanics among patients classified as having either a good or a poor outcome in knee-related QoL one year after TKA. We found that patients classified as having a good outcome in knee-related QoL improved in knee biomechanics during gait, while patients classified as having a poor outcome, despite similar reduction in pain, remained unchanged in knee biomechanics one year after TKA. With regards to surgeon-controlled factors, frontal plane alignment may be the biomechanical factor surgery most successfully can address. However, achieving a good outcome in patient-reported knee-related QoL may not be related to improvements in knee alignment in the frontal plane, but rather to dynamic improvements in knee flexion-extension.

Abbreviations

3D: Three-dimensional; ADL: Activities of daily living; BMI: Body mass index; KL: Kellgren and lawrence; KOOS: Knee injury and osteoarthritis outcome score; MDC: Minimally detectable change; MID: Minimal important difference; QoL: Quality of life; TKA: Total knee arthroplasty; VAS: Visual analogue scale

Acknowledgment

The authors acknowledge physiotherapist Anna-Clara Esbjörnsson and data technician Mikael Reimeringer at the Motion Analysis Laboratory at Karolinska University Hospital for helping with the data collection.

Funding

This study was supported by grants from Karolinska Institutet, Stiftelsen Promobilia, and the Swedish Rheumatism Foundation. Study sponsors had no involvement in study design, collection, analysis and interpretation of data; in the writing of the manuscript; or in the decision to submit the manuscript for publication.

Authors' contributions

JEN, PW, EWB: Conception and design. JEN, MH: Acquisition of data. JEN: Data analysis. JEN, PW: drafting the article. JEN, PW, VL, MI, MH and EWB have made substantial contributions in the interpretation of data, revising the article critically and all approved of the final version for submission.

Competing interests

Each author certifies that he or she has no commercial associations that might pose a conflict of interest in connection with the submitted article. The author declare that he/she has no competing interests.

Consent for publication

Not applicable.

Author details

[1]Department of Women's and Children's Health, Karolinska Institutet, MotorikLab, Q2:07, Karolinska University Hospital, 171 76 Stockholm, Sweden. [2]Department of Orthopedics, School of Medical Sciences, Örebro University and Örebro University Hospital, Örebro, Sweden. [3]Department of Molecular Medicine and Surgery, Karolinska Institutet, L1:00, Karolinska University Hospital, 171 76 Stockholm, Sweden. [4]Department of Physical Therapy, Movement & Rehabilitation Sciences, Bouve College of Health Sciences, Northeastern University, 360 Huntington Avenue, Boston, MA 02115, USA. Division of Rheumatology, Immunology, and Allergy, Brigham and Women's Hospital, Harvard Medical School, Boston, MA, USA. [6]Department of Clinical Science, Intervention and Technology, Karolinska Institutet, Karolinska University Hospital, K54, 141 86 Stockholm, Sweden.

References

1. Wylde V, Dieppe P, Hewlett S, Learmonth ID. Total knee replacement: is it really an effective procedure for all? Knee. 2007;14(6):417–23.
2. Bourne RB, Chesworth BM, Davis AM, Mahomed NN, Charron KDJ. Patient satisfaction after total knee arthroplasty Who is satisfied and Who is Not? Clin Orthop Rel Res. 2010;468(1):57–63.
3. Scott CE, Howie CR, MacDonald D, Biant LC. Predicting dissatisfaction following total knee replacement: a prospective study of 1217 patients. J Bone Joint Surg Brit. 2010;92(9):1253–8.
4. Becker R, Doring C, Denecke A, Brosz M. Expectation, satisfaction and clinical outcome of patients after total knee arthroplasty. Knee Surg Sports Traumatol Arthrosc. 2011;19(9):1433–41.
5. Bullens PH, van Loon CJ, de Waal Malefijt MC, Laan RF, Veth RP. Patient satisfaction after total knee arthroplasty: a comparison between subjective and objective outcome assessments. J Arthroplasty. 2001;16(6):740–7.
6. Ali A, Sundberg M, Robertsson O, Dahlberg LE, Thorstensson CA, Redlund-Johnell I, Kristiansson I, Lindstrand A. Dissatisfied patients after total knee arthroplasty: a registry study involving 114 patients with 8-13 years of followup. Acta Orthop. 2014;85(3):229–33.
7. Roos EM, Lohmander LS. The knee injury and osteoarthritis outcome score (KOOS): from joint injury to osteoarthritis. Health Qual Life Outcomes. 2003;1:64.
8. Roos EM, Toksvig-Larsen S. Knee injury and osteoarthritis outcome score (KOOS) - validation and comparison to the WOMAC in total knee replacement. Health Qual Life Outcomes. 2003;1:17.
9. Milner CE. Is gait normal after total knee arthroplasty? systematic review of the literature. J Orthop Sci. 2009;14(1):114–20.
10. McClelland JA, Webster KE, Feller JA. Gait analysis of patients following total knee replacement: a systematic review. Knee. 2007;14(4):253–63.
11. Naili JE, Iversen MD, Esbjornsson AC, Hedstrom M, Schwartz MH, Hager CK, Brostrom EW. Deficits in functional performance and gait one year after total knee arthroplasty despite improved self-reported function. Knee Surg Sports Traumatol Arthrosc. 2016. doi:10.1007/s00167-016-4234-7.
12. Yoshida Y, Mizner RL, Ramsey DK, Snyder-Mackler L. Examining outcomes from total knee arthroplasty and the relationship between quadriceps strength and knee function over time. Clin Biomech (Bristol, Avon). 2008;23(3):320–8.
13. Smith AJ, Lloyd DG, Wood DJ. Pre-surgery knee joint loading patterns during walking predict the presence and severity of anterior knee pain after total knee arthroplasty. J Orthop Res. 2004;22(2):260–6.
14. Davis R, Ounpuu S, Tybursk D, Gage J. A gait analysis data collection and reduction technique. Hum Mov Sci. 1991;10(5):575.

15. Woltring HJ. A Fortran package for generalized, cross-validatory spline smoothing and differentiation. Adv Eng Softw. 1986;8(2):104–13. 1978.

16. Kahl C, Cleland J. Visual analogue scale, numeric pain rating scale and the McGill pain questionnaire: an overview of psychometric properties. Phys Ther Rev. 2005;10(2):123–8.

17. Roos E, Roos H, Lohmander L, Ekdahl C, Beynnon B. Knee injury and osteoarthritis outcome score (KOOS)–development of a self-administered outcome measure. J Orthop Sports Phys Ther. 1998;28(2):88–96.

18. Collins NJ, Prinsen CA, Christensen R, Bartels EM, Terwee CB, Roos EM. Knee Injury and Osteoarthritis Outcome Score (KOOS): systematic review and meta-analysis of measurement properties. Osteoarthr Cartil. 2016.

19. Ageberg E, Nilsdotter A, Kosek E, Roos EM. Effects of neuromuscular training (NEMEX-TJR) on patient-reported outcomes and physical function in severe primary hip or knee osteoarthritis: a controlled before-and-after study. BMC Musculoskelet Disord. 2013;14:232.

20. Steinhoff AK, Bugbee WD. Knee Injury and Osteoarthritis Outcome Score has higher responsiveness and lower ceiling effect than Knee Society Function Score after total knee arthroplasty. Knee Surg Sports Traumatol Arthrosc. 2014. doi:10.1007/s00167-014-3433-3.

21. Dieppe P, Judge A, Williams S, Ikwueke I, Guenther KP, Floeren M, Huber J, Ingvarsson T, Learmonth I, Lohmander LS, et al. Variations in the pre-operative status of patients coming to primary hip replacement for osteoarthritis in European orthopaedic centres. BMC Musculoskelet Disord. 2009;10:19.

22. Collins NJ, Misra D, Felson DT, Crossley KM, Roos EM. Measures of knee function: international knee documentation committee (IKDC) subjective knee evaluation form, knee injury and osteoarthritis outcome score (KOOS), knee injury and osteoarthritis outcome score physical function short form (KOOS-PS), knee outcome survey activities of daily living scale (KOS-ADL), lysholm knee scoring scale, oxford knee score (OKS), western ontario and McMaster universities osteoarthritis index (WOMAC), activity rating scale (ARS), and tegner activity score (TAS). Arthritis Care Res. 2011;63(Suppl 11):S208–228.

23. Beaton DE, Bombardier C, Katz JN, Wright JG, Wells G, Boers M, Strand V, Shea B. Looking for important change/differences in studies of responsiveness. OMERACT MCID working group. Outcome measures in rheumatology. Minimal clinically important difference. J Rheumatol. 2001;28(2):400–5.

24. Faul F, Erdfelder E, Lang A-G, Buchner A. G*power 3: a flexible statistical power analysis program for the social, behavioral, and biomedical sciences. Behav Res Methods. 2007;39:175–91.

25. de Vet HCW, Terwee CB, Mokkink LB, Knol DL. Measurement in medicine: a practical guide. Cambridge: Cambridge University Press; 2011.

26. Pasquier G, Tillie B, Parratte S, Catonne Y, Chouteau J, Deschamps G, Argenson JN, Bercovy M, Salleron J. Influence of preoperative factors on the gain in flexion after total knee arthroplasty. Orthop Traumatol Surg Res. 2015;101(6):681–5.

27. Orishimo KF, Kremenic IJ, Deshmukh AJ, Nicholas SJ, Rodriguez JA. Does total knee arthroplasty change frontal plane knee biomechanics during gait? Clin Orthop Relat Res. 2012;470(4):1171–6.

28. Prodromos CC, Andriacchi TP, Galante JO. A relationship between gait and clinical changes following high tibial osteotomy. J Bone Joint Surg Am. 1985;67(8):1188–94.

29. Rodriguez JA, Bas MA, Orishimo KF, Robinson J, Nicholas SJ. Differential Effect of Total Knee Arthroplasty on Valgus and Varus Knee Biomechanics During Gait. J Arthroplast. 2016. doi:10.1016/j.arth.2016.06.061

30. Baker PN, Rushton S, Jameson SS, Reed M, Gregg P, Deehan DJ. Patient satisfaction with total knee replacement cannot be predicted from pre-operative variables alone: a cohort study from the national joint registry for england and wales. Bone Joint J. 2013;95-B(10):1359–65.

31. Judge A, Arden NK, Cooper C, Kassim Javaid M, Carr AJ, Field RE, Dieppe PA. Predictors of outcomes of total knee replacement surgery. Rheumatology (Oxford). 2012;51(10):1804–13.

32. Knoop J, van der Leeden M, Thorstensson CA, Roorda LD, Lems WF, Knol DL, Steultjens MP, Dekker J. Identification of phenotypes with different clinical outcomes in knee osteoarthritis: data from the Osteoarthritis Initiative. Arthritis Care Res. 2011;63(11):1535–42.

33. King MT. A point of minimal important difference (MID): a critique of terminology and methods. Expert Rev Pharmacoecon Outcomes Res. 2011;11(2):171–84.

34. van den Boom LG, Halbertsma JP, van Raaij JJ, Brouwer RW, Bulstra SK, van den Akker-Scheek I. No difference in gait between posterior cruciate retention and the posterior stabilized design after total knee arthroplasty. Knee Surg Sports Traumatol Arthrosc. 2014;22(12):3135–41.

14

Association between activity limitations and pain in patients scheduled for total knee arthroplasty

Ilana M. Usiskin, Heidi Y. Yang, Bhushan R. Deshpande, Jamie E. Collins, Griffin L. Michl, Savannah R. Smith, Kristina M. Klara, Faith Selzer, Jeffrey N. Katz and Elena Losina[*]

Abstract

Background: Historically, persons scheduled for total knee arthroplasty (TKA) have reported severe pain with low demand activities such as walking, but recent data suggests that TKA recipients may have less preoperative pain. Little is known about people who elect TKA with low levels of preoperative pain. To better understand current TKA utilization, we evaluated the association between preoperative pain and difficulty performing high demand activities, such as kneeling and squatting, among TKA recipients.

Methods: We used baseline data from a randomized control trial designed to improve physical activity following TKA. Prior to TKA, participants were categorized according to Western Ontario and McMaster Universities Osteoarthritis Index (WOMAC) Pain scores: Low (0–25), Medium (26–40), and High (41–100). Within each group, limitations in both low demand and high demand activities were assessed.

Results: The sample consisted of 202 persons with a mean age of 65 (SD 8) years; 21 %, 34 %, and 45 % were categorized in the Low, Medium, and High Pain groups, respectively. Of the Low Pain group, 60 % reported at least one of the following functional limitations: limited flexion, limp, limited walking distance, and limitations in work or housework. While only 12 % of the Low Pain group reported at least moderate pain with walking on a flat surface, nearly all endorsed at least moderate difficulty with squatting and kneeling.

Conclusions: A substantial number of persons scheduled for TKA report Low WOMAC Pain (≤25) prior to surgery. Persons with Low WOMAC Pain scheduled for TKA frequently report substantial difficulty with high demand activities such as kneeling and squatting. Studies of TKA appropriateness and effectiveness for patients with low WOMAC Pain should include measures of these activities.

Keywords: Total knee arthroplasty, Osteoarthritis, Pain, Functional limitations

Abbreviations: BMI, Body Mass Index; BWH, Brigham and Women's Hospital; KOOS, Knee injury and Osteoarthritis Outcome Score; MHI-5, Mental Health Inventory; OA, Osteoarthritis; OAI, Osteoarthritis Initiative; SD, Standard deviation; SPARKS, Study of Physical Activity Rewards After Knee Surgery; TKA, Total knee arthroplasty; WOMAC, Western Ontario and McMaster Universities Osteoarthritis Index

* Correspondence: elosina@partners.org
Orthopaedic and Arthritis Center for Outcomes Research, Department of
Orthopaedic Surgery, Brigham and Women's Hospital, 75 Francis Street,
BC-4016, Boston, MA 02115, USA

Background

Total knee arthroplasty (TKA) is a common and effective surgery for end-stage knee osteoarthritis (OA), with over 600,000 TKAs performed each year in the US [1, 2]. Historically, only persons with severe pain, extensive structural changes, and limited range of motion have been considered candidates for TKA [3–5]. However, more recently, younger individuals reporting less severe pain on low demand activities such as walking are opting for TKA, and the number of younger persons electing to undergo the procedure is predicted to increase [6–10]. These trends raise questions about the characteristics of persons with low pain on basic activities who undergo TKA.

The Western Ontario and McMaster Universities Osteoarthritis Index (WOMAC) has been widely used to evaluate candidates for TKA and to measure the effectiveness of the surgery [11–14]. The WOMAC Pain scale asks about pain while lying down, sitting, standing, walking on a flat surface, and climbing stairs. While the activities captured by the WOMAC Pain scale range in difficulty, we refer to these items as "low demand" activities compared to more difficult mobility-related activities such as running and jumping, which we refer to as "high demand" activities. We also consider squatting, kneeling, and twisting to be high demand activities, as these methods of changing body position can be challenging for persons with knee conditions. These five high demand activities are measured by the Knee injury and Osteoarthritis Outcomes Score (KOOS) Sports and Recreational Activity scale.

Numerous studies have pointed to high WOMAC Pain prior to TKA as a risk factor for a poor outcome, as well as for lower satisfaction with the surgery [15, 16]. However, persons with low WOMAC Pain prior to surgery remain an understudied group in terms of their outcomes and expectations for surgery. Preoperative expectations have been shown to be associated with surgical satisfaction, although there are some conflicting reports about this connection, and no literature yet exists on how these expectations differ in patients with low WOMAC Pain prior to surgery [17–20]. In the absence of substantial pain with low demand activities, it is important to understand the characteristics of patients with low WOMAC Pain and what may be driving them to seek TKA.

Persons scheduled for TKA with low WOMAC Pain may have activity limitations in domains beyond those measured by the WOMAC Pain scale. While patients may not typically choose to undergo TKA in order to return to rigorous activities such as skiing or running, TKA recipients often report that movements such as kneeling and pivoting are important to their quality of life, and they may seek TKA in order to participate more

fully or re-engage in recreational activities such as gardening [21–23].

Moreover, existing suggestions for TKA appropriateness criteria are limited and heavily weigh symptoms related to the execution of low demand activities [3, 24–26]. These reports consider patients without severe pain with walking or other low demand activities to be inappropriate candidates for TKA, regardless of age or radiographic severity [3, 25]. It is therefore unclear how to determine the appropriateness of TKA in persons with low WOMAC Pain, and such determinations require a better understanding of these patients' characteristics prior to surgery. We hypothesized that TKA recipients reporting low levels of pain with low demand activities will be limited in high demand activities such as squatting and kneeling.

Methods

Study design

We analyzed preoperative baseline data from the Study of Physical Activity Rewards after Knee Surgery (SPARKS), a randomized controlled clinical trial (RCT) aimed at establishing the efficacy of a behavioral economics-based intervention for improving physical activity following TKA. The sample size for this proof of concept RCT was based on increases in physical activity post-TKA due to a behavioral intervention and was estimated at 200. Patients with knee OA scheduled to undergo a unilateral TKA at Brigham and Women's Hospital (BWH) in Boston were enrolled from January 2014 to January 2016. Participants completed baseline questionnaires and wore Fitbit Zip accelerometers (Fitbit Inc, San Francisco, CA) for one week prior to TKA. The trial was approved by the Partners Healthcare Institutional Review Board and is registered on https://ClinicalTrials.gov (identifier NCT01970631).

Enrollment

Persons scheduled to undergo a primary, unilateral TKA at BWH were eligible for the study if they were over 40 years old, had an underlying diagnosis of OA, were not planning to undergo another surgery within six months, did not have inflammatory arthritis, dementia, epilepsy, Parkinson's disease, or neuropathy, and did not live in a nursing home. Subjects needed to be willing and able to use a Fitbit Zip accelerometer and to complete questionnaires online. Eligible subjects who agreed to participate met with a research assistant for a baseline visit, during which written informed consent was obtained and the patient was provided a Fitbit and instructions for its use.

Assessments and outcome measures

The baseline questionnaire, which participants completed within 8 weeks of surgery, included demographic and clinical characteristics, quality of life, pain and functional status, and limitations in demanding recreational activities. Demographic information included age, sex, body mass index (BMI), race, education level, and employment status. We relied on the expert opinion of our orthopedic colleagues to identify the functional limitations that patients often cite as key reasons to undergo TKA. These included: inability to fully bend or extend knee, limp, limited walking distance, and pain interference with work or housework. Mental health was evaluated with the Mental Health Inventory (MHI-5), a 5-item questionnaire measuring anxiety and depressive feelings scaled from 0 to 100, with lower scores indicative of worse mental health [27, 28]. Health-related quality of life was calculated using the EuroQol EQ-5D-3L instrument, which is a self-rating of general health across five domains: mobility, self-care, usual activities, pain/discomfort, and anxiety/depression. Responses to each of the five domains were converted to a summary score on a 0 to 1 scale, with 1 representing the best quality of life, using published crosswalk index values [29]. Range of motion was self-reported using the validated method of Gioe and colleagues, in which study participants were presented with pictures of knees positioned at varying levels of flexion and extension [30, 31].

Pain and functional status was measured using the WOMAC Pain and Function scales [11]. Limitations in demanding recreational activities were measured using the Sport and Recreational Activity subscale of the Knee injury and Osteoarthritis Outcome Score (KOOS), which measures the difficulty that respondents experience with certain high demand activities (twisting, squatting, kneeling, jumping, and running) [22, 32]. Study participants were asked to rate the difficulty they experienced performing each of these five activities on a 5-level Likert scale ranging from no difficulty to extreme difficulty. A composite KOOS Sport and Recreational Activity subscore was calculated for participants who answered at least 3 of the 5 items [22]. Responses to the WOMAC Pain and Function scales and the KOOS Sport and Recreational Activity scale were scaled to range from 0 to 100, with 100 corresponding to the worst health status.

At the baseline visit, participants were asked to wear a Fitbit Zip accelerometer for seven consecutive days. An average number of daily steps was calculated using only the days with at least 8 h of wear time.

Analytic approach

Subjects were stratified by preoperative WOMAC Pain level: Low (0–25), Medium (26–40), and High (41–100). The WOMAC Pain group cutoffs were made based on distributional assumptions and to increase the transparency of interpretation of pain group status. The cutoffs also avoid overstating a 'dose-response' relationship. Defining pain groups based on WOMAC pain <25, 26–40,

and >40 had meaningful clinical interpretation. Almost all the patients (41 out of 43) with WOMAC Pain <=25 endorsed mostly none, mild or moderate pain on each item with at most one item above moderate pain. Most of the patients (40 out of 68) with WOMAC pain 26–40 endorsed moderate to extreme pain on at least two items, with at most three items with moderate to extreme pain. Those in the High pain group generally had to endorse moderate, severe or extreme pain, with 57 out of the 91 patients in this group endorsing moderate to extreme on all items. We evaluated the association between preoperative WOMAC Pain group and demographic features, clinical characteristics, and daily step count. We also evaluated the responses to each of the five individual items on both the WOMAC Pain and the KOOS Sport and Recreational Activity subscales. Demographic and clinical features were summarized as means and standard deviations (SD) for continuous variables and as proportions for categorical variables.

In order to assess functional limitations not captured by the WOMAC Pain subscale, we evaluated four clinically-meaningful characteristics: range of motion, limp, walking distance, and limitations in work or housework. We dichotomized each of these four variables to identify patients with clinically-relevant functional limitations: flexion ≤100°, at least moderate limp, limited to walking fewer than five blocks, or at least moderate limitations in work or housework. At least moderate limp and at least moderate limitations in work or housework included responses of moderate, severe, or extreme on a five-item Likert scale. We calculated the number of patients in each WOMAC Pain group who had 0, 1, or 2 or more of these four functional limitations.

Tests for trend across pain groups were conducted for demographic and clinical characteristics using the Jonckheere–Terpstra test for continuous variables and the Cochran–Mantel–Haenszel test for categorical variables. P-values reported in this manuscript refer to overall linear trends across the three WOMAC Pain groups. Statistical significance was indicated at a two-sided p-value less than 0.05. Statistical analysis was performed using SAS v9.4 (Cary, NC, USA).

Results

Sample characteristics

Two hundred fifty-one patients agreed to participate in the SPARKS study. Our study sample comprises the 202 participants who completed the baseline questionnaire, wore the Fitbit for the appropriate number of days, underwent surgery, and were ultimately randomized. Participants were 57 % female, had a mean age of 65 years (SD 8), and had a mean BMI of 31 (SD 6) (Table 1). Patients who were eligible for the study but did not agree to participate or could not be contacted

Table 1 Demographic characteristics of the sample of subjects scheduled for TKA by WOMAC pain group

	WOMAC Pain Group				p-value (trend)
	Low (0–25) n = 43 (21 %)	Medium (26–40) n = 68 (34 %)	High (41–100) n = 91 (45 %)	Overall n = 202	
Age: mean (SD)	68 (7)	66 (8)	64 (7)	65 (8)	0.001
Female: no. (%)	16 (37 %)	38 (56 %)	61 (67 %)	115 (57 %)	0.001
BMI: mean (SD)	29 (5)	31 (6)	32 (6)	31 (6)	0.04
Race					0.06
White	41 (95 %)	63 (93 %)	78 (86 %)	182 (90 %)	
Non-White	2 (5 %)	5 (7 %)	13 (14 %)	20 (10 %)	
Education: no. (%)					0.04
Graduated from college	34 (79 %)	48 (71 %)	56 (62 %)	138 (68 %)	
Did not graduate from college	9 (21 %)	20 (29 %)	35 (38 %)	64 (32 %)	
Employment Status: no. (%)					0.34
Employed full- or part-time	24 (57 %)	40 (60 %)	44 (50 %)	108 (55 %)	
Not working	18 (43 %)	27 (40 %)	44 (50 %)	89 (45 %)	

had a mean age of 68 years (SD 9) and were 64 % female.

The pain groups were as follows: 21 % Low Pain, 34 % Medium Pain, and 45 % High Pain. The mean age of the study subjects was 68 years (SD 7), 66 years (SD 8), and 64 years (SD 7) (p = 0.001) in the Low, Medium, and High Pain groups, respectively (Table 1). The Low Pain group was 63 % male, and the Medium and High Pain groups were 44 % and 33 % male, respectively (p = 0.001). The Low Pain group had a mean BMI of 29, and the Medium and High Pain groups had mean BMIs of 31 and 32, respectively (p = 0.04). Most participants were White: 95 % of the Low Pain group, 93 % of the Medium Pain group, and 86 % of the High Pain group (p = 0.06). Employment status was not associated with baseline WOMAC Pain group, with 57 % of Low Pain, 60 % of Medium Pain, and 50 % of High Pain participants reporting full or part time employment (p = 0.34). Baseline WOMAC Pain was associated with education, with 79 % of subjects in the Low Pain group, 71 % of the Medium Pain group, and 62 % of the High Pain group reporting having earned a bachelor's degree (p = 0.04).

Clinical characteristics

The overall mean WOMAC Pain score was 41 (SD 19), and the overall mean WOMAC Function score was 41 (SD 18) (Table 2). The mean WOMAC Function score for the Low Pain group was 23 (SD 11), 35 (SD 10) for the Medium Pain group, and 54 (SD 14) for the High Pain group (p <0.001). Health-related quality of life, as measured by the EQ-5D-3L, was 0.81 (SD 0.08) for the Low Pain group, 0.77 (SD 0.08) for the Medium

Pain group, and 0.64 (SD 0.18) for the High Pain group (p <0.001).

Functional limitations

We assessed four functional limitations: poor range of motion (flexion ≤100°), at least moderate limp, limited to walking less than five blocks, or at least moderate limitations in work or housework. Of those in the Low Pain group, 12 % reported flexion ≤100°, 35 % reported having at least a moderate limp, 19 % reported walking limited to five blocks, and 35 % reported at least moderate limitations in work or housework. Sixty-one percent of the Low Pain group experienced at least one functional limitation, and 23 % percent of participants in this group experienced at least two functional limitations. Of the Medium Pain group, 79 % experienced at least one and 50 % experienced at least two functional limitations. Ninety-eight percent of the High Pain group reported at least one functional limitation, with 78 % reporting two or more functional limitations (Fig. 1).

Thirty-five percent of the Low Pain group indicated that their pain at least moderately interfered with their regular work or housework, as did 63 % of the Medium Pain group and 87 % of the High Pain group (p <0.001). Pain was associated with knee extension, or the ability to completely straighten one's knee (Low Pain: 56 %, Medium Pain: 46 %, High Pain: 32 %; p = 0.006). Worse pain corresponded to less knee flexion, with 88 % of the Low Pain group able to bend their knee more than 100°, while only 84 % of the Medium Pain group and 75 % of the High Pain group could bend their knee more than 100° (p = 0.046).

Table 2 Clinical characteristics of the sample of subjects scheduled for TKA by WOMAC pain group

	WOMAC Pain Group				p-value (trend)
	Low (0–25) n = 43 (21 %)	Medium (26–40) n = 68 (34 %)	High (41–100) n = 91 (45 %)	Overall n = 202	
WOMAC Pain: mean (SD)	16 (7)	35 (4)	58 (14)	41 (12)	<0.001
WOMAC Function: mean (SD)	23 (11)	35 (10)	54 (14)	41 (18)	<0.001
HRQoL (EQ-5D-3 L Index): mean (SD)	0.81 (0.08)	0.77 (0.08)	0.64 (0.18)	0.72 (0.15)	<0.001
KOOS Sport and Activity: mean (SD)	63 (20)	68 (24)	84 (19)	74 (23)	<0.001
Knee extension: no. (%)					0.006
More than 5⁰ from straight	19 (44 %)	36 (54 %)	62 (68 %)	117 (58 %)	
Completely straight	24 (56 %)	31 (46 %)	29 (32 %)	84 (42 %)	
Knee flexion: no. (%)					0.046
100⁰ or less	5 (12 %)	11 (16 %)	23 (25 %)	39 (19 %)	
More than 100⁰	38 (88 %)	57 (84 %)	68 (75 %)	163 (81 %)	
Limp: no. (%)					0.001
Moderate to severe	15 (35 %)	29 (43 %)	57 (63 %)	101 (50 %)	
None to slight	28 (65 %)	39 (57 %)	34 (37 %)	101 (50 %)	
Walking distance: no. (%)					<0.001
Less than 5 blocks	8 (19 %)	26 (38 %)	54 (59 %)	88 (44 %)	
5 to 20 blocks	20 (48 %)	31 (46 %)	30 (33 %)	81 (40 %)	
Unlimited	14 (33 %)	11 (16 %)	7 (8 %)	32 (16 %)	
How much did pain interfere with work or housework?: no. (%)					<0.001
Moderately to extremely	15 (35 %)	43 (63 %)	79 (87 %)	137 (68 %)	
Not at all to a little bit	28 (65 %)	25 (37 %)	12 (13 %)	65 (32 %)	
Use of a supportive device: no. (%)					0.10
Yes	9 (21 %)	15 (22 %)	30 (33 %)	54 (27 %)	
No	34 (79 %)	53 (78 %)	61 (67 %)	148 (73 %)	

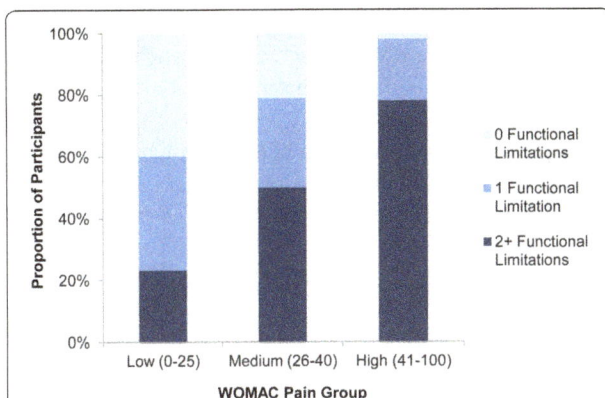

Fig. 1 The proportion of participants in each WOMAC Pain group reporting 0, 1, and 2 or more functional limitations. The four basic functional limitations analyzed include poor range of motion (self-reported flexion greater than or equal to 100⁰), limitations in work or housework (moderate or greater limitations), limp (moderate or greater), or being unable to walk more than 5 blocks. The number of these functional limitations reported (0, 1, or 2 or more) was associated with WOMAC Pain group (p < 0.001)

Activity limitations

The mean KOOS Sport and Recreational Activity score was 63 (SD 20) for the Low Pain group, 68 (SD 24) for the Medium Pain group, and 84 (SD 19) for the High Pain group (p <0.001). A considerable proportion of the subjects in the Low Pain group experienced severe or extreme difficulty performing the high demand activities measured by the KOOS Sport and Recreational Activity scale: 58 % with kneeling, 40 % with twisting, 44 % with squatting, 54 % with running, and 56 % with jumping (Fig. 2). Two-thirds of the Low Pain group, 81 % of the Medium Pain group, and 98 % of the High Pain group reported severe difficulty with at least one of the five activities measured by the KOOS Sport and Recreational Activity scale.

When we broadened the definition of difficulty with tasks to include moderate (as well as severe and extreme) difficulty, the proportion of the Low Pain group experiencing difficulty with the KOOS Sport and Recreational Activity items increased to 81 % with kneeling,

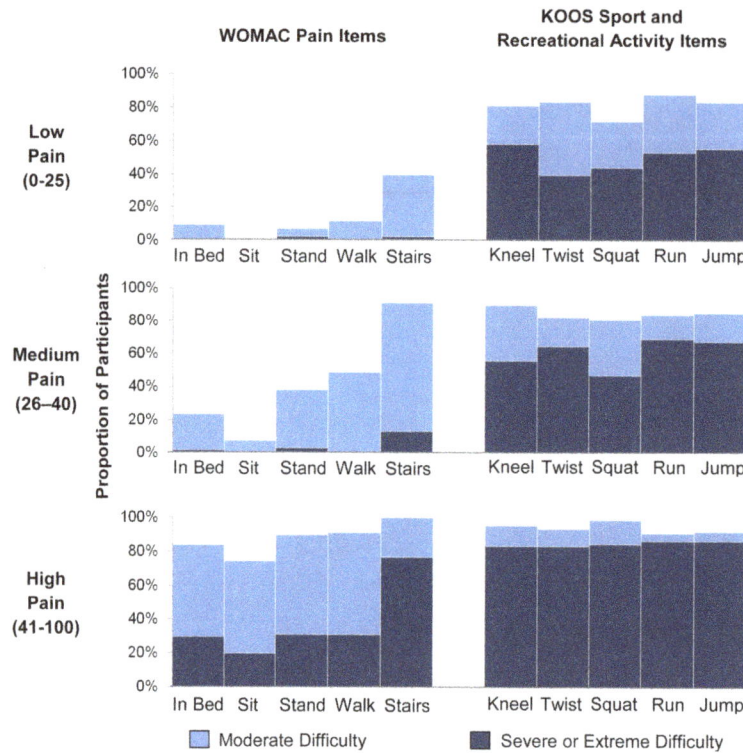

Fig. 2 The proportion of participants scheduled to undergo TKA reporting difficulty performing basic tasks (measured by the WOMAC Pain scale) and more demanding activities (measured by the KOOS Sport and Recreational Activity subscale), stratified by level of WOMAC Pain. The dark blue portions of the bars represent patients who expressed severe or extreme difficulty performing each of the WOMAC Pain or KOOS Sport and Recreational Activity items. The light blue portions of the bars show patients who reported moderate difficulty with these same items. The total height of the bars represents the proportion of patients in each WOMAC Pain group who expressed moderate or greater difficulty performing each of the tasks

84 % with twisting, 72 % with squatting, 88 % with running, and 84 % with jumping (Fig. 2). Every individual in the Low Pain group reported at least moderate difficulty performing at least one of these five high demand activities.

Discussion

This paper reports the functional and activity limitations among persons scheduled for TKA, stratified by pre-operative pain level. About one-fifth of subjects in the cohort reported Low WOMAC Pain scores (0–25) prior to surgery. However, these subjects frequently reported functional limitations such as limping or poor range of motion, as well as limitations with the high demand activities measured by the KOOS Sport and Recreational Activity scale, such as twisting, squatting, and kneeling.

Persons scheduled for TKA have been found to express goals of performing more than just low demand activities following surgery, such as returning to sports or gardening [23, 33]. A report by Noble and colleagues found that persons scheduled for TKA tend to place high importance on biomechanically-demanding activities such as kneeling and squatting, and that satisfaction

with surgery is associated with their ability to return to the activities that they deem most important [18]. Our results corroborate these and other similar findings that TKA recipients may consider improvement in the ability to engage in more demanding activities such as kneeling or gardening as being important to their decisions to undergo TKA [22, 23, 33].

Despite evidence that many TKA recipients place high importance on demanding activities, data that support TKA recipients being able to engage in high demand activities such as kneeling, squatting, and twisting after surgery are limited [19, 22, 34]. Roos and colleagues evaluated the ability of subjects to perform the activities on the KOOS Sport and Recreational Activity subscale both pre-operatively and six months post-TKA and found that TKA provided only modest increases in the number of subjects who reported being able to squat, run, jump, and twist, and decreases in the number who reported being able to kneel [22]. Additionally, Weiss and colleagues found that patients often regard kneeling and gardening as some of the most important but also some of the most difficult activities to perform following TKA [23]. The increasing numbers of patients with low

WOMAC Pain electing TKA highlights a need for more research that uses post-TKA data to evaluate the benefits of surgery specifically for patients with low WOMAC Pain. If patients are motivated to undergo TKA not by limitations in low demand activities but by the desire to return to more demanding activities, more attention should be paid to outcomes for patients with low preoperative pain that are related to performing these high demand activities. Moreover, persons with low WOMAC Pain who opt to undergo TKA may benefit from additional discussions with their surgeon regarding expectations of returning to such activities. Thorough discussions about managing expectations before indicating TKA may help to alleviate concerns about patients with low pain prior to surgery expecting improvements in high demand activities.

Additionally, future research on appropriateness criteria for TKA should account for patients who report low WOMAC Pain but who may seek surgery as a way to return to the activities that they deem important for their quality of life. Previous work on developing appropriateness criteria for TKA has included factors such as age, preoperative pain and function, and radiographic findings. Escobar and colleagues created criteria for TKA based on the RAND/UCLA Appropriateness Method, where a panel of experts rated cases as inappropriate, inconclusive, or appropriate [3]. The resulting criteria deemed patients with mild or moderate symptoms inappropriate or uncertain candidates for TKA regardless of age or radiographic severity, where moderate symptoms were defined as pain when walking on level surfaces and having some limitation in daily activities. Using Escobar's criteria, Riddle and colleagues deemed over half of 175 TKA recipients in the Osteoarthritis Initiative (OAI) to be inappropriate or inconclusive TKA candidates [3, 5]. Hawker and colleagues used a cutoff of 39 points on the combined WOMAC Pain and Function scales (out of 100 points, 100 worst) to identify patients who had OA symptoms severe enough for TKA [25]. An evaluation conducted by Ghomrawi and colleagues found poor agreement between the criteria used by Escobar and Hawker, demonstrating a critical need for consistent and relevant appropriateness standards for TKA [24].

Fifty-five percent of SPARKS participants had WOMAC Pain below 40 points, and would likely not be considered appropriate TKA candidates based on several proposed appropriateness criteria [3, 25]. These data are consistent with the assessment by Riddle and colleagues that deemed only 44 % of 175 patients in the OAI to be appropriate TKA recipients based on Escobar's criteria [3, 5]. The substantial number of TKAs in our patient sample and in the OAI that would likely be considered inappropriate based on Escobar's criteria highlights the mismatch between these criteria developed almost fifteen years ago and current practice [3].

Additionally, the substantial number of patients with low WOMAC Pain scheduled for TKA suggests that the WOMAC Pain scale is an insufficient measure of TKA appropriateness, as has been previously described [35–37]. Researchers have attempted to use other measures such as the KOOS Pain and Function subscales to aid in the assessment of TKA appropriateness, but the KOOS Sport and Recreational Activity subscale has not been explored in this capacity [35]. The use of computerized adaptive testing may be a potential option for overcoming the limitations of the WOMAC for measuring a wide range of activity and function limitations for persons considering TKA. For example, PROMIS computerized adaptive testing has been used to measure self-reported physical function in patients with arthritis and in orthopedic trauma patients [38, 39].

In the development of appropriateness criteria for TKA, it is important to recognize that pain may not be the primary focus for patients. There may be other factors besides pain on the WOMAC Pain items, such as BMI, that contribute to limitations in the high demand activities measured by the KOOS Sport and Recreational Activity subscale. In the development of appropriateness criteria for TKA, it is important to recognize that pain may not be the primary focus for patients. More work is needed to develop appropriateness criteria that account for the interplay between pain and other variables such as demographic characteristics and activity limitations. The relevance of our hypothesis that TKA recipients who report low levels of pain with low demand activities will be limited in high demand activities lies in fact that WOMAC Pain relies largely (3 out 5 items) on sedentary activities and therefore could miss the disability of the increasingly active population of TKA candidates.

We found that participants with Low Pain prior to surgery did not differ from those with Medium or High Pain with regard to the average number of steps they walked every day (Table 2). This finding is similar to that of White and colleagues, who reported that knee pain severity did not impact walking behaviors in a cohort with or at risk for knee OA [40]. Lo and colleagues also recently showed that WOMAC Pain scores did not predict physical activity levels among OAI participants with or without knee OA [41]. It is somewhat paradoxical that participants who report low WOMAC Pain and therefore experience less pain when standing or walking on flat surfaces do not walk more than those with more pain. This conveys discordance between potential capacity and performance that is often observed in knee OA cohorts, where participants who can walk without pain nonetheless choose not to [40, 41]. It is also possible that participants with low WOMAC Pain do not walk more than those with more pain because they have modified their activity to be in less pain. Our findings were not affected by missing data, since completing the baseline assessment was a key inclusion criterion for the study.

The results of this study should be viewed within the context of several limitations. The study population was recruited as a part of randomized controlled clinical trial, which introduces inherent selection bias, and the participants were recruited from a single study center. Additionally, because the study sample was obtained from a randomized controlled trial of a behavioral intervention for physical activity following TKA, subjects with low pain may have been more willing to participate. This selection bias may have enriched the proportion of subjects in our sample with low WOMAC Pain, allowing us to examine their characteristics more carefully. Individuals with severe mobility limitations were excluded from the study, and thus our sample may be more active than other TKA cohorts. This study did not include radiographs, and thus we were unable to determine the radiographic severity of subjects' knee OA, which could have influenced decisions to pursue TKA. Knee range of motion was obtained using self-report; however, participant-reported knee range of motion has been shown to match measured range of motion in a similar population with knee OA [31]. This analysis also uses single items from multi-item scales (the KOOS and the WOMAC), which have unknown validity and may compromise the reliability of the results. Our questionnaire did not give participants the option to indicate that they did not perform the high demand activities measured by the KOOS, which may have led some participants to report "extreme" difficulty with activities that they do not perform. Functional limitation items were selected based on expert opinion and were not extensively validated. In addition, we did not collect data related to motivation for TKA. Future studies should directly measure patient motivations for undergoing TKA and how satisfied they are with surgery in order to better understand why patients with low pain on low demand activities undergo TKA.

Conclusions

About one out of five subjects from the SPARKS study sample had WOMAC Pain ≤25 prior to TKA. Those with Low Pain frequently reported severe or extreme difficulty performing high demand activities, such as kneeling or squatting. We suggest that future work on determining appropriateness criteria for TKA should consider limitations beyond the low demand activities measured by the WOMAC Pain scale. Additionally, it is important that patients and surgeons discuss preoperative expectations to ensure that patients have reasonable expectations for returning to demanding activities following surgery. More research is needed to understand what motivates patients with low WOMAC Pain to seek TKA and how to measure surgical effectiveness in such patients.

Funding

This study was funded by NIH/NIAMS grants R21 AR063913 (EL), K24 AR057827 (EL), and P60 AR047782 (JNK). The sponsor had no role in study design, in the collection, analysis, and interpretation of the data, in the writing of the manuscript, or in the decision to submit the manuscript for publication.

Authors' contributions

JEC, GLM, SRS, KMK, JNK, and EL contributed to the design of the study, IMU, HYY, BRD, JEC, GLM, SRS, and KMK conducted the data acquisition, IMU, HYY, JEC, FS, and EL worked on the data analysis, and all authors were involved in the interpretation of the data. All authors were involved in drafting and critically revising the manuscript, and each author has approved the final manuscript for publication.

Authors' information

From the Orthopaedic and Arthritis Center for Outcomes Research (OrACORe) and the Policy and Innovation eValuation in Orthopedic Treatments (PIVOT) Center, Department of Orthopedic Surgery [IMU, HYY, BRD, JEC, GLM, SRS, KMK, FS, JNK, EL], Brigham and Women's Hospital; the Section of Clinical Sciences, Division of Rheumatology, Immunology and Allergy [JNK, EL], Brigham and Women's Hospital; Harvard Medical School [BRD, JEC, FS, JNK, EL]; Department of Biostatistics [EL], Boston University School of Public Health; and the Departments of Epidemiology and Environmental Health [JNK], Harvard T. H. Chan School of Public Health—all Boston, MA.

Competing interests

JNK and EL are Deputy Editors for Methodology and Biostatistics for the *Journal of Bone and Joint Surgery.*

Consent for publication

Not applicable.

References

1. Wright RJ, Sledge CB, Poss R, Ewald FC, Walsh ME, Lingard EA. Patient-reported outcome and survivorship after Kinemax total knee arthroplasty. J Bone Joint Surg Am. 2004;86-A(11):2464–70.
2. Cram P, Lu X, Kates SL, Singh JA, Li Y, Wolf BR. Total knee arthroplasty volume, utilization, and outcomes among Medicare beneficiaries, 1991–2010. JAMA. 2012;308(12):1227–36.
3. Escobar A, Quintana JM, Arostegui I, Azkarate J, Guenaga JI, Arenaza JC, Garai I. Development of explicit criteria for total knee replacement. Int J Technol Assess Health Care. 2003;19(1):57–70.
4. Quintana JM, Arostegui I, Escobar A, Azkarate J, Goenaga JI, Lafuente I. Prevalence of knee and hip osteoarthritis and the appropriateness of joint replacement in an older population. Arch Intern Med. 2008;168(14):1576–84.
5. Riddle DL, Jiranek WA, Hayes CW. Use of a validated algorithm to judge the appropriateness of total knee arthroplasty in the United States: a multicenter longitudinal cohort study. Arthritis Rheumatol. 2014;66(8):2134–43.
6. Jain NB, Higgins LD, Ozumba D, Guller U, Cronin M, Pietrobon R, Katz JN. Trends in epidemiology of knee arthroplasty in the United States, 1990–2000. Arthritis Rheum. 2005;52(12):3928–33.
7. Mehrotra C, Remington PL, Naimi TS, Washington W, Miller R. Trends in total knee replacement surgeries and implications for public health, 1990–2000. Public Health Rep. 2005;120(3):278–82.
8. Losina E, Katz JN. Total knee arthroplasty on the rise in younger patients: are we sure that past performance will guarantee future success? Arthritis Rheum. 2012;64(2):339–41.

9. Losina E, Thornhill TS, Rome BN, Wright J, Katz JN. The dramatic increase in total knee replacement utilization rates in the United States cannot be fully explained by growth in population size and the obesity epidemic. J Bone Joint Surg Am. 2012;94(3):201–7.

10. Kurtz SM, Lau E, Ong K, Zhao K, Kelly M, Bozic KJ. Future young patient demand for primary and revision joint replacement: national projections from 2010 to 2030. Clin Orthop Relat Res. 2009;467(10):2606–12.

11. Bellamy N, Buchanan WW, Goldsmith CH, Campbell J, Stitt LW. Validation study of WOMAC: a health status instrument for measuring clinically important patient relevant outcomes to antirheumatic drug therapy in patients with osteoarthritis of the hip or knee. J Rheumatol. 1988;15(12):1833–40.

12. Nilsdotter AK, Toksvig-Larsen S, Roos EM. A 5 year prospective study of patient-relevant outcomes after total knee replacement. Osteoarthritis and cartilage / OARS, Osteoarthritis Research Society. 2009;17(5):601–6.

13. Escobar A, Gonzalez M, Quintana JM, Vrotsou K, Bilbao A, Herrera-Espineira C, Garcia-Perez L, Aizpuru F, Sarasqueta C. Patient acceptable symptom state and OMERACT-OARSI set of responder criteria in joint replacement. Identification of cut-off values. Osteoarthritis Cartilage. 2012;20(2):87–92.

14. Maxwell JL, Felson DT, Niu J, Wise B, Nevitt MC, Singh JA, Frey-Law L, Neogi T. Does clinically important change in function after knee replacement guarantee good absolute function? The multicenter osteoarthritis study. J Rheumatol. 2014;41(1):60–4.

15. Judge A, Arden NK, Cooper C, Kassim Javaid M, Carr AJ, Field RE, Dieppe PA. Predictors of outcomes of total knee replacement surgery. Rheumatology (Oxford). 2012;51(10):1804–13.

16. Lizaur-Utrilla A, Gonzalez-Parreno S, Miralles-Munoz FA, Lopez-Prats FA, Gil-Guillen V. Patient-related predictors of treatment failure after primary total knee arthroplasty for osteoarthritis. J Arthroplasty. 2014;29(11):2095–9.

17. Dyck BA, Zywiel MG, Mahomed A, Gandhi R, Perruccio AV, Mahomed NN. Associations between patient expectations of joint arthroplasty surgery and pre- and post-operative clinical status. Expert Rev Med Devices. 2014;11(4):403–15.

18. Noble PC, Conditt MA, Cook KF, Mathis KB. The john insall award: patient expectations affect satisfaction with total knee arthroplasty. Clin Orthop Relat Res. 2006;452:35–43.

19. Noble PC, Gordon MJ, Weiss JM, Reddix RN, Conditt MA, Mathis KB. Does total knee replacement restore normal knee function? Clin Orthop Relat Res. 2005;431:157–65.

20. Waljee J, McGlinn EP, Sears ED, Chung KC. Patient expectations and patient-reported outcomes in surgery: a systematic review. Surgery. 2014;155(5):799–808.

21. Nakahara H, Okazaki K, Mizu-Uchi H, Hamai S, Tashiro Y, Matsuda S, Iwamoto Y. Correlations between patient satisfaction and ability to perform daily activities after total knee arthroplasty: why aren't patients satisfied? J Orthop Sci. 2015;20(1):87–92.

22. Roos EM, Toksvig-Larsen S. Knee injury and Osteoarthritis Outcome Score (KOOS) - validation and comparison to the WOMAC in total knee replacement. Health Qual Life Outcomes. 2003;1:17.

23. Weiss JM, Noble PC, Conditt MA, Kohl HW, Roberts S, Cook KF, Gordon MJ, Mathis KB. What functional activities are important to patients with knee replacements? Clin Orthop Relat Res. 2002;404:172–88.

24. Ghomrawi HM, Alexiades M, Pavlov H, Nam D, Endo Y, Mandl LA, Mushlin AI. Evaluation of two appropriateness criteria for total knee replacement. Arthritis Care Res. 2014;66(11):1749–53.

25. Hawker GA, Wright JG, Coyte PC, Williams JI, Harvey B, Glazier R, Wilkins A, Badley EM. Determining the need for hip and knee arthroplasty: the role of clinical severity and patients' preferences. Med Care. 2001;39(3):206–16.

26. Gossec L, Paternotte S, Maillefert JF, Combescure C, Conaghan PG, Davis AM, Gunther KP, Hawker G, Hochberg M, Katz JN, et al. The role of pain and functional impairment in the decision to recommend total joint replacement in hip and knee osteoarthritis: an international cross-sectional study of 1909 patients. Report of the OARSI-OMERACT Task Force on total joint replacement. Osteoarthritis Cartilage. 1909;19(2):147–54.

27. Rumpf HJ, Meyer C, Hapke U, John U. Screening for mental health: validity of the MHI-5 using DSM-IV Axis I psychiatric disorders as gold standard. Psychiatry Res. 2001;105(3):243–53.

28. Berwick DM, Murphy JM, Goldman PA, Ware Jr JE, Barsky AJ, Weinstein MC. Performance of a five-item mental health screening test. Med Care. 1991;29(2):169–76.

29. Shaw JW, Johnson JA, Coons SJ. US valuation of the EQ-5D health states: development and testing of the D1 valuation model. Med Care. 2005;43(3):203–20.

30. Gioe TJ, Pomeroy D, Suthers K, Singh JA. Can patients help with long-term total knee arthroplasty surveillance? Comparison of the American Knee Society Score self-report and surgeon assessment. Rheumatology (Oxford). 2009;48(2):160–4.

31. Collins JE, Rome BN, Daigle ME, Lerner V, Katz JN, Losina E. A comparison of patient-reported and measured range of motion in a cohort of total knee arthroplasty patients. J Arthroplasty. 2014;29(7):1378–82. e1371.

32. Gossec L, Hawker G, Davis AM, Maillefert JF, Lohmander LS, Altman R, Cibere J, Conaghan PG, Hochberg MC, Jordan JM, et al. OMERACT/OARSI initiative to define states of severity and indication for joint replacement in hip and knee osteoarthritis. J Rheumatol. 2007;34(6):1432–5.

33. Rastogi R, Davis AM, Chesworth BM. A cross-sectional look at patient concerns in the first six weeks following primary total knee arthroplasty. Health Qual Life Outcomes. 2007;5:48.

34. Huch K, Muller KA, Sturmer T, Brenner H, Puhl W, Gunther KP. Sports activities 5 years after total knee or hip arthroplasty: the Ulm Osteoarthritis Study. Ann Rheum Dis. 2005;64(12):1715–20.

35. Riddle DL, Perera RA, Jiranek WA, Dumenci L. Using surgical appropriateness criteria to examine outcomes of total knee arthroplasty in a United States sample. Arthritis Care Res. 2015;67(3):349–57.

36. Katz JN. Editorial: appropriateness of total knee arthroplasty. Arthritis Rheumatol. 2014;66(8):1979–81.

37. Collins NJ, Roos EM. Patient-reported outcomes for total hip and knee arthroplasty: commonly used instruments and attributes of a "good" measure. Clin Geriatr Med. 2012;28(3):367–94.

38. Fries JF, Cella D, Rose M, Krishnan E, Bruce B. Progress in assessing physical function in arthritis: PROMIS short forms and computerized adaptive testing. J Rheumatol. 2009;36(9):2061–6.

39. Hung M, Stuart AR, Higgins TF, Saltzman CL, Kubiak EN. Computerized adaptive testing using the PROMIS physical function item bank reduces test burden with less ceiling effects compared with the short musculoskeletal function assessment in orthopaedic trauma patients. J Orthop Trauma. 2014;28(8):439–43.

40. White DK, Tudor-Locke C, Felson DT, Gross KD, Niu J, Nevitt M, Lewis CE, Torner J, Neogi T. Do radiographic disease and pain account for why people with or at high risk of knee osteoarthritis do not meet physical activity guidelines? Arthritis Rheum. 2013;65(1):139–47.

41. Lo GH, McAlindon TE, Hawker GA, Driban JB, Price LL, Song J, Eaton CB, Hochberg MC, Jackson RD, Kwoh CK, et al. Symptom assessment in knee osteoarthritis needs to account for physical activity level. Arthritis Rheumatol. 2015;67(11):2897–904.

15

Kneeling and standing up from a chair as performance-based tests to evaluate knee function in the high-flexion range: a randomized controlled trial comparing a conventional and a high-flexion TKA design

Paul J. P. van der Ven[1], Sebastiaan van de Groes[1], Jorrit Zelle[1], Sander Koëter[2], Gerjon Hannink[1] ⓘ and Nico Verdonschot[1,3]*

Abstract

Background: We compared the functional outcome between conventional and high-flexion total knee arthroplasty (TKA) using kneeling and sit-to-stand tests at 1 year post-operative. In addition, the patient's daily functioning, pain and satisfaction were quantified using questionnaires.

Methods: We randomly assigned 56 patients to receive either a conventional or a high-flexion TKA. Primary outcomes were maximum flexion angle and maximum thigh-calf contact measured during kneeling at 1 year post operatively. Secondary outcomes were the angular knee velocity and ground reaction force ratio measured during sit-to-stand performance tests, and questionnaires.

Results: At one year post-operative, maximum knee flexion during kneeling was higher for the high-flexion TKA group (median 128.02° (range 108–146)) compared to the conventional TKA group (119.13° (range 72–135)) ($p = 0.03$). Maximum thigh-calf contact force was higher for the high flexion TKA group (median 17.82 N (range 2.98–114.64)) compared to the conventional TKA group (median 9.37 N (range 0.33–46.58))($p = 0.04$). The sit-to-stand tests showed a significantly higher angular knee velocity in the conventional TKA group (12.12 rad/s (95%CI 0.34–23.91); $p = 0.04$). There were no significant differences between groups in ground reaction force ratios and patient-reported outcome scores.

Conclusion: Although no differences were found in patient-reported outcome scores, differences in performance-based tests were clearly apparent. Standing up from a chair at 90° of knee flexion appeared to be easier for the conventional group. The kneeling test revealed significantly higher weight-bearing knee flexion for the high-flex group. Hence, if kneeling is an important activity for a patient a high-flex design may be recommendable.

Keywords: Total knee arthroplasty, High-flexion, Performance-based tests, Functional outcome, Kneeling, Sit-to-stand

* Correspondence: nico.verdonschot@radboudumc.nl
[1]611 Orthopaedic Research Laboratory, Department of Orthopaedics, Radboud University Medical Center, PO Box 9101, 6500HB Nijmegen, The Netherlands
[3]Laboratory for Biomechanical Engineering, University of Twente, Enschede, The Netherlands
Full list of author information is available at the end of the article

Background

Several types of implant designs have been manufactured in order to optimize the results after total knee arthroplasty (TKA). Range of motion (ROM) is an important outcome parameter of postoperative knee function [1–3]. High-flexion designs are aimed at accommodating larger postoperative ROM necessary for activities of daily living (ADL), such as kneeling, standing up from a low chair, sitting cross-legged, transferring in and out of bath, gardening and stair climbing [4–9].

Design features of a high-flexion TKA are typically a reduced radius and an increased thickness of the posterior femoral condyle resulting in extended condyles. In addition, specific posterior-stabilized high flexion designs have an adapted post-cam mechanism providing increased femoral rollback [9–11]. However, it remains uncertain whether these design changes actually lead to functional benefits for TKA patients.

The results of TKA are mostly assessed using physical examination, X-rays and the evaluation of patient-based questionnaires. Although patient-based questionnaires provide feasible and appropriate methods to address the concerns of patients, they are subjective and assessment is often subject to floor or ceiling effects, which limits the adequate assessment of higher functioning patients [4, 5, 11, 12]. Moreover, most questionnaires were originally not designed for use in high-flexion TKA patients (e.g. no points were scored for extra ROM beyond 125°) [4, 5].

Performance-based testing, specifically targeted at high-flexion activities, has been suggested to help to compensate for the limitations in existing scores [4, 13]. One major advantage of performance-based testing is that pain and pain-related items do not have such a large effect on functional outcome as on patient-based questionnaires [1, 14–17].

Performance-based tests, such as sit-to-stand tests [16], and kneeling [18] have been proposed to evaluate knee function after TKA in the low-flexion (≤90°) and high-flexion range (>120°), respectively. However, during kneeling, thigh-calf contact has been reported to limit flexion and can therefore obscure the potential benefit reached with high-flex TKA designs [18, 19]. In that same study, thigh–calf contact pressures were shown to exponentially increase with increasing knee flexion angles, and to reach maximum values (up to >30%BW) in maximal flexion. Therefore, in order to assess TKA systems at high flexion, flexion angles as well as thigh-calf pressures need to be recorded.

In our clinic we traditionally use a PCL-retaining, fixed bearing device. However, high-flexion TKA systems may provide advantages for patients who perform high-demand activities (such as kneeling and sit-to-stand) on a daily basis. In order to determine whether a high-flexion TKA system would provide clinically relevant benefits for our patients we set up a randomized controlled trial to compare the functional outcome of our patients treated with either a PCL-retaining or a high-flexion TKA device.

Our primary objective was to compare the functional outcome between conventional and high-flexion TKA using kneeling as a performance-based test at one year post-operative. In addition, we compared the functional outcome between conventional and high-flexion TKA using a sit-to-stand test and we quantified patient's daily functioning, pain and satisfaction using questionnaires at one year post-operative.

Methods

We performed a prospective double-blind randomized controlled trial at the department of Orthopedics of the Canisius Wilhelmina Hospital, Nijmegen, the Netherlands. The study protocol was approved by the regional ethical committee (CMO 2008/021; ABR NL21274.091.08) and was carried out in line with the Helsinki Declaration. The study was retrospectively registered in ClinicalTrials.gov under identifier NCT00899041 (date of registration: May 11, 2009).

Patients with primary osteoarthritis or arthritis secondary to rheumatoid arthritis scheduled to undergo primary TKA were considered for inclusion and were enrolled prospectively. Exclusion criteria were: other causes of arthritis, inability to complete the exercises due to contralateral arthritis, contralateral TKA or other co-morbidities, and the inability to complete the questionnaires. Endpoints were defined as death, aseptic loosening, infection, amputation, reoperation or withdrawal on request.

In our protocol we explicitly specified any foreseeable post-randomisation exclusions; 1) death of the patient, 2) aseptic loosening of the prosthesis, 3) infection of the prosthesis, 4) amputation of the leg in which the prosthesis was placed, and 5) withdrawal on own request, as in these circumstances the outcomes of interest could not be measured.

Between November 2008 and November 2012, 75 consecutive patients undergoing unilateral TKA were assessed for eligibility (Fig. 1). Nineteen patients were excluded before randomization; eight patients declined to participate and 11 patients were excluded: mentally incompetent (1 patient), presence of contralateral TKA (2 patients), bilateral osteoarthritis (8 patients).

After written informed consent had been obtained, the patients were randomly allocated to receive either a PFC Sigma FB CR (fixed-bearing, cruciate-retaining; DePuy, Leeds, UK) or a PFC Sigma RP-F PS (rotating platform, posterior stabilized, high-flexion; DePuy, Leeds, UK). Computer-generated randomization with stratification for

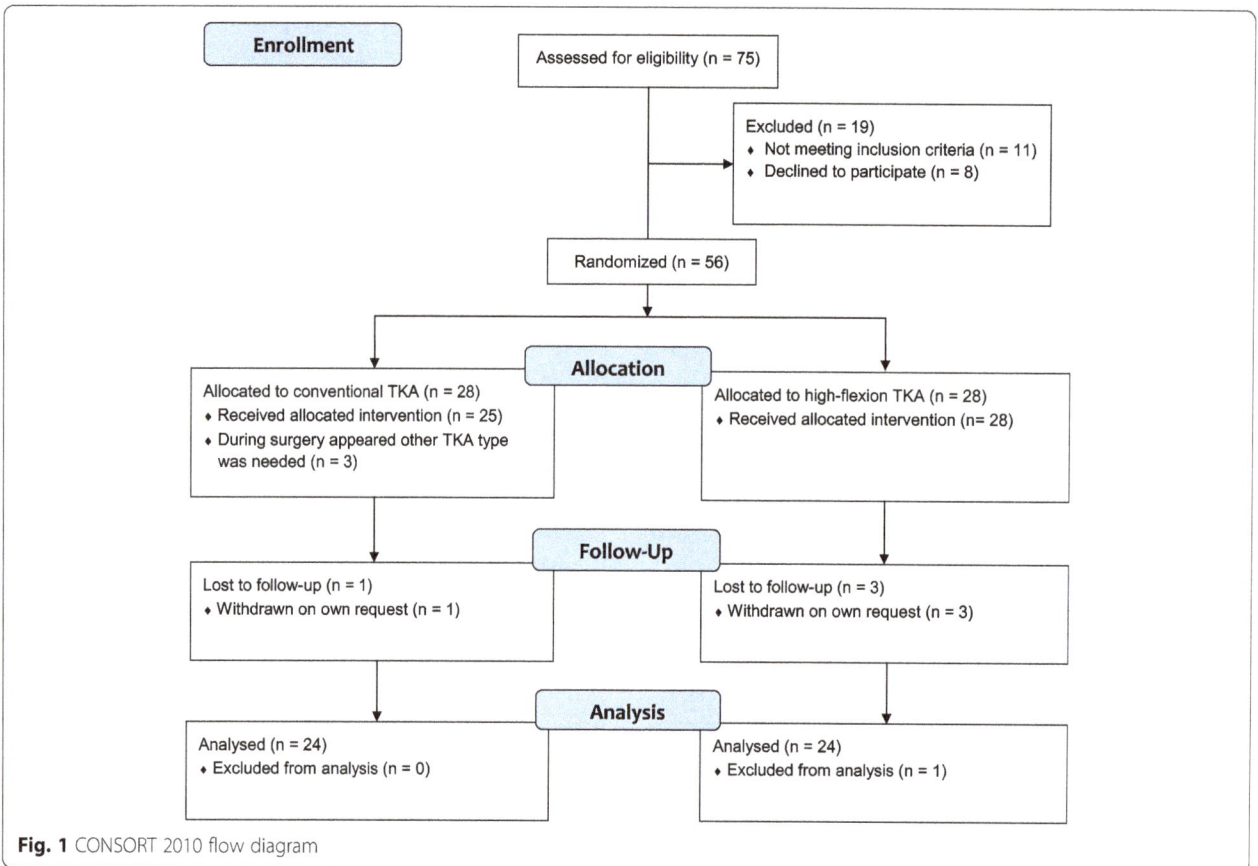

Fig. 1 CONSORT 2010 flow diagram

BMI below or above 30 kg/m^2 was performed by an independent statistician. All patients and investigators were blinded for type of implant. The day before surgery the surgeon received a sealed study number envelope with the allocated TKA.

Identical surgical techniques were used in the groups according to the manuals of the designers. Three experienced knee surgeons were involved in this study. Rehabilitation was done according to the joint-care-protocol used in our hospital, including out of bed mobilization on the first postoperative day.

Primary outcomes

The primary outcome measures were maximum flexion angle and maximum thigh-calf contact force measured during kneeling at one year post operatively. Maximal knee flexion angles during kneeling were measured using wireless accelerometers and gyroscopes (π-node, Philips, Eindhoven, the Netherlands). The accelerometers were positioned on the lateral side of both ankles, on both upper legs (10 cm above the patella) and on the sternum.

The maximal thigh-calf contact force (N) for the affected knee and unaffected knee were measured with a Conformat-pressure mapping sensor (Tekscan, Boston, USA). The pressure map was positioned in the popliteal fossa of both legs. The protocols for both measurements

have been described in detail previously [18]. The mean of three consecutive maximum flexion angle and maximal thigh-calf contact force measurements was used in statistical analysis.

Secondary outcomes

Sit-to-stand tests (STS) were used to assess the knee function in the flexion range up to 90° at one year post operatively. During STS we measured the angular knee velocity and ground reaction force ratio of both legs on the floor. The STS is a validated functional tool to assess knee patients which is selective and relatively independent of pain. The protocol has been described in detail previously [16, 20]. Angular velocity of the knee was measured using accelerometers, the ground reaction force (GRF) of each leg by two pressure plates [21]. TKA patients have been shown to produce a lower extension velocity while getting up from a chair as compared to healthy age-matched controls [15]. The ratio of ground reaction force (GRF$_{ratio}$), which demonstrates the asymmetrical functional usage of the two legs, was expressed as the GRF of the TKA side (F$_{TKA}$) divided by the GFR of the non TKA side (F$_{no\ TKA}$): GRF$_{ratio}$ = F$_{TKA}$/F$_{no\ TKA}$.

The patients' daily functioning, pain and satisfaction were assessed using the following questionnaires: Knee Society Score (KSS), Western Ontario and McMaster Universities

(WOMAC) and 0–100 Visual Analogue Scale (VAS) for pain and satisfaction (0 = no pain/extremely dissatisfied and 100 = very painful/very satisfied).

Statistical analyses

Sample size estimation showed that 21 patients per group would be required to detect a clinically relevant difference of 10° of flexion with a standard deviation of 10° in knee flexion angle [10], with an alpha of 0.05 and a power of 90%. A dropout-margin of 7 patients for each group was used, which resulted in 28 patients per group. Descriptive statistics were used to summarize the data. Shapiro-Wilk tests and normality plots were used to assess normality. Differences between conventional and high-flex TKA designs were tested using Student t-tests and Mann-Whitney-U-tests for non-parametric and normal distributed data, respectively. With non-parametric tests, a measure of effect size, r, was calculated by dividing Z by the square root of N ($r = Z/\sqrt{N}$; small $r \geq 0.1$, medium $r \geq 0.3$, and large $r \geq 0.5$) [22]. Analyses were performed using SPSS 21.0 (IBM, Chicago, USA). For all data sets, differences were considered statistically significant at p-values <0.05.

Results

After randomization of 56 patients, three patients in the conventional TKA group were excluded: two because of insufficiency of the posterior cruciate ligament and one because an additional patella component was needed to improve patella tracking. During follow-up, one patient in the conventional TKA group was withdrawn on his/her own request without providing any reason. One patient in the high-flexion TKA group was withdrawn on his/her own request because of back problems. Two other patients in the high-flexion TKA group were withdrawn on their own request without providing any reason (Fig. 1). Patient demographics and baseline values are presented in Table 1.

Complications

In the conventional TKA group, one patient had a deep venous thrombosis treated with anti-coagulants 48 days post-operative, one patient had an inadequate knee flexion post-operatively and was treated with manipulation under anesthesia, and one patient had a patellar clunk and was treated using arthroscopic debridement. At 1 year post-operative, one patient in the high-flexion TKA group presented with signs of an infected TKA. Since an infected TKA was explicitly specified as reason for post-randomisation exclusion, and this patient was unable to perform kneeling and STS movements (and therefore no measurements could be obtained) this patient was excluded from the statistical assessment. However, later it appeared that all cultured biopsies were negative.

Table 1 Patient demographics data and baseline clinical status

	Conventional TKA ($n = 24$)	High-flexion TKA ($n = 24$)
Sex (F:M)[c]	11:13	12:12
Age (yrs)[a]	64 ± 7	66 ± 8
BMI (kg/m^2)[a]	31 ± 4	32 ± 5
Thigh-calf contact force (N)[b]	15.88 (0–196.83)	9.70 (3.34–178.23)
Maximum flexion angle (°)[b]	127.7 (97–146)	126.6 (97–156)
Angular velocity (rad/s)[a]	80.56 ± 19.74	78.60 ± 18.26
GRF$_{ratio}$ (1)[a]	0.86 ± 0.29	0.84 ± 0.26
KSS[b]	103 (55–132)	104 (78–151)
WOMAC[b]	55.5 (25–94)	49.5 (8–69)
VAS$_{pain}^{b}$	43.5 (0–90)	40 (0–99)

[a]Values are mean ± SD; [b]Values are median (range); [c]Values represent numbers

Primary outcomes

Kneeling: Maximum knee flexion angle & maximum thigh-calf contact

At 1 year post-operative, maximum knee flexion during kneeling was higher for the high-flexion TKA group (median 128.02° (range 108–146°)) compared to the conventional TKA group (median 119.13° (range 72–135°)) ($U = 174$, $r = 0.32$, $p = 0.03$). Maximum thigh-calf contact force was higher for the high flexion TKA group (median 17.8 N (range 3.0–114.6 N)) than for the conventional TKA group (median 9.4 N (range 0.3–46.6 N)) ($U = 177$, $r = 0.31$, $p = 0.04$).

Secondary outcomes

Sit-to-stand: Angular knee velocity & ground reaction force ratio

At 1 year post-operative, the angular velocity measured during sit-to-stand tests was higher for the conventional TKA group (93.23 rad/s (SD 21.94)) compared to the high-flexion TKA group (81.10 rad/s (SD 17.46)) (difference 12.12 rad/s (95%CI 0.34–23.91 rad/s); $p = 0.04$). No significant differences in GRF$_{ratio}$ measurements between conventional (0.94 (SD 0.14)) and high-flexion TKA groups (0.87 (SD 0.21)) were found (difference 0.07 (95%CI -0.04 – 0.17); $p = 0.21$).

Questionnaires

At one year post-operative, no significant differences between conventional and high-flexion TKA groups in KSS, WOMAC, VAS$_{pain}$, and VAS$_{satisfaction}$ scores were found (Table 2).

Discussion

In this study we compared the functional outcome between conventional and high-flexion TKA using performance-based tests at one year follow-up. It was found that during

Table 2 Results of primary and secondary outcomes

	Conventional TKA	High-flexion TKA	p-value
	(n = 24)	(n = 24)	
Thigh-calf contact force (N)[b]	9.37 (0.33–46.58)	17.82 (2.98–114.64)	0.04[d]
Maximum flexion angle (°)[b]	119.13 (72–135)	128.02 (108–146)	0.03[d]
Angular velocity (rad/s)[a]	93.23 ± 21.94	81.10 ± 17.46	0.04[c]
GRF_{ratio} (1)[a]	0.94 ± 0.14	0.87 ± 0.21	0.21[c]
KSS[b]	179 (90–199)	193 (109–201)	0.10[d]
WOMAC[b]	12.5 (2–62)	7 (0–54)	0.10[d]
VAS_{pain}^b	4 (0–54)	5 (0–31)	0.96[d]
$VAS_{satisfaction}^b$	89.5 (4–100)	98.5 (8–100)	0.06[d]

[a]Values are mean ± SD; [b]Values are median (range); [c]Student's t-test; [d]Mann–Whitney U test

kneeling both the maximum flexion angle and thigh-calf contact force were significantly higher in the high-flexion TKA group. Sit-to-stand analyses showed no differences in asymmetry between the healthy and affected leg between conventional and high-flexion TKA group, while the patients in the conventional TKA group had a significantly higher angular velocity as compared to the high-flexion TKA group. Questionnaire scores (KSS, WOMAC and VAS scores) were similar in both groups.

Most previous clinical studies failed to show a difference between conventional TKA and high-flex TKA when using traditional outcome scores [4, 12, 13, 23, 24]. In addition, a recent study showed that current outcome measurement tools are not suited for the high flexion range [25].

In this study we found significant differences between conventional TKA and high flex TKA when using weight-bearing functional tests, but not when using traditional outcome scores proposed to evaluate knee function in the normal flexion range. The maximum knee flexion and thigh-calf contact forces during active kneeling were significantly higher in the high-flexion TKA group than in the conventional TKA group. The higher maximum thigh-calf contact in the high-flexion TKA group might be the result of the higher active flexion angle that was reached in that group. Since thigh-calf contact has been reported to limit flexion during kneeling, the flexion potential after high-flexion TKA might have been obscured by thigh-calf contact. In addition, although the surgeons used an identical surgical technique for both designs, it cannot be excluded that there were small differences in terms of treatment of the bone on the posterior region [9]. With the high-flex design more bone has to be removed at the posterior condyles, so it would be logical to also remove more posterior osteo-phytes and excessive bone that could possibly hamper high flexion. However, judging from the post-operative radiographs this could not be confirmed.

Remarkably, patients with a conventional TKA design produced a higher extension velocity during the sit-to-

stand test. A higher angular velocity has been shown to be associated with a better functional performance [15]. Although a higher active flexion angle was obtained in the high-flexion TKA group, it apparently did not lead to a better performance of the extensor mechanism. Conflicting results between different post-operative outcome measures in the evaluation of high-flexion versus conventional TKA designs have also been reported by others [4, 12, 13, 23, 24, 26].

According to several authors performance-based measurements are necessary for an adequate evaluation of high-flexion TKA [4, 12, 13, 23, 24]. Nutton et al. [23] used performance-based measurements to evaluate functional outcome following TKA with NexGen standard and high flexion components. No significant differences in outcomes between patients receiving the conventional and high flexion designs were found. They divided performance-based measurements into 'lower flexion' and 'higher flexion' activities. The lower flexion activities were walking on a flat surface, ascending and descending a slope and a flight of stairs, and sitting and rising from a high chair. The higher flexion activities were sitting and rising from a low chair, getting in and out of a bath and bending the knee to the maximum range of flexion when standing, using a stool as a step. Finally, patients were asked to crouch and rise from a crouching position (squatting), using handrails for support. Patients were not asked to kneel, as most felt anxious about performing this activity. In addition, Palmer et al. [27] reported that some TKA patients were unwilling to kneel or squat because of advice from medical staff or third parties or because of fear of harming the prosthesis, although they state that no published data exists concerning this risk. The kneeling test used in the present study might therefore be a good method to distinguish between different TKA designs as the patient is in control of the movement.

The higher active flexion in the high-flexion TKA group is probably the result of the different design features and subsequent surgical aspects of the prosthesis. First positioning of the post-cam mechanism more posterior allows the knee to flex more due to a better rollback of the femoral component. Secondly, due to the thicker posterior condyles, high-flexion TKA surgery results in a better visualization of the posterior aspect of the knee allowing better decompression of posterior osteophytes and capsular tissue [4, 9]. Osteophyte removal could lead to a higher ROM in the high-flex range. Finally, adequate tensioning of the posterior cruciate ligament in the cruciate retaining prosthesis is challenging and the outcome is less predictable than in a posterior stabilized prosthesis and may have therefore jeopardized the ROM required for a kneeling exercise.

We did not find significant differences between conventional and high-flexion TKA when using the KSS, WOMAC and VAS scores. This is in line with previous observations reported by other authors [4, 7, 12, 23]. The self-reported questionnaires have a clear ceiling effect [4, 14, 17], and this makes them less useful for higher functioning TKA patients.

Conclusion
This study showed that although no differences were found in patient-reported outcome scores, differences in performance-based tests were clearly apparent. Standing up from a chair at 90° of knee flexion appeared to be easier for the conventional group. The kneeling test revealed significantly higher weight-bearing knee flexion for the high-flex group. Hence, if kneeling is an important activity for a patient a high-flex design may be recommendable.

Abbreviations
ADL: Activities of daily living; BW: Body weight; FB CR: Fixed-bearing, cruciate-retaining; GRF: Ground reaction force; KSS: Knee Society Score; PCL: Posterior cruciate ligament; ROM: Range of motion; RP-F PS: Rotating platform, posterior stabilized; VAS: Visual Analogue Scale; WOMAC: Western Ontario and McMaster Universities

Acknowledgements
We would like to show our gratitude to the patients who made this study possible.

Funding
This study was funded by DePuy, Leeds, UK. The company had no role in the design of the study, collection, analysis, or interpretation of data or in writing the manuscript.

Authors' contributions
NV, SK, JZ designed the trial. All authors interpreted data. PvdV and GH made the statistical analyses, PvdV and SvdG wrote the first version of the manuscript. All authors (PvdV, SvdG, JZ, SK, GH, NV) critically revised different versions of the manuscript. NV is the corresponding author. All authors read and approved the final manuscript.

Consent for publication
Consent for publication was obtained from all study participants.

Competing interests
The authors declare that they have no competing interests.

Author details
[1]611 Orthopaedic Research Laboratory, Department of Orthopaedics, Radboud University Medical Center, PO Box 9101, 6500HB Nijmegen, The Netherlands. [2]Department of Orthopaedics, Canisius-Wilhelmina Hospital, Nijmegen, The Netherlands. [3]Laboratory for Biomechanical Engineering, University of Twente, Enschede, The Netherlands.

References
1. Devers BN, Conditt MA, Jamieson ML, Driscoll MD, Noble PC, Parsley BS. Does greater knee flexion increase patient function and satisfaction after total knee arthroplasty? J Arthroplast. 2011;26:178–86.
2. Padua R, Ceccarelli E, Bondi R, Campi A, Padua L. Range of motion correlates with patient perception of TKA outcome. Clin Orthop Relat Res. 2007;460:174–7.
3. Rowe PJ, Myles CM, Nutton R. The effect of total knee arthroplasty on joint movement during functional activities and joint range of motion with particular regard to higher flexion users. J Orthop Surg (Hong Kong). 2005;13:131–8.
4. Murphy M, Journeaux S, Russell T. High-flexion total knee arthroplasty: a systematic review. Int Orthop. 2009;33:887–93.
5. Noble PC, Gordon MJ, Weiss JM, Reddix RN, Conditt MA, Mathis KB. Does total knee replacement restore normal knee function? Clin Orthop Relat Res. 2005:157–65.
6. Hemmerich A, Brown H, Smith S, Marthandam SS, Wyss UP. Hip, knee, and ankle kinematics of high range of motion activities of daily living. J Orthop Res. 2006;24:770–81.
7. Tarabichi S, Tarabichi Y, Hawari M. Achieving deep flexion after primary total knee arthroplasty. J Arthroplast. 2010;25:219–24.
8. Rowe PJ, Myles CM, Walker C, Nutton R. Knee joint kinematics in gait and other functional activities measured using flexible electrogoniometry: how much knee motion is sufficient for normal daily life? Gait Posture. 2000;12:143–55.
9. Ranawat AS, Gupta SK, Ranawat CS. The P.F.C. sigma RP-F total knee arthroplasty: designed for improved performance. Orthopedics. 2006;29:S28–9.
10. Gupta SK, Ranawat AS, Shah V, Zikria BA, Zikria JF, Ranawat CS. The P.F.C. sigma RP-F TKA designed for improved performance: a matched-pair study. Orthopedics. 2006;29:S49–52.
11. Jones RE. High-flexion rotating-platform knees: rationale, design, and patient selection. Orthopedics. 2006;29:S76–9.
12. Nutton RW, Wade FA, Coutts FJ, van der Linden ML. Does a mobile-bearing, high-flexion design increase knee flexion after total knee replacement? J Bone Joint Surg Br. 2012;94:1051–7.
13. Wang Z, Wei M, Zhang Q, Zhang Z, Cui Y. Comparison of high-flexion and conventional implants in Total knee arthroplasty: a meta-analysis. Med Sci Monit. 2015;21:1679–86.
14. Marx RG, Jones EC, Atwan NC, Closkey RF, Salvati EA, Sculco TP. Measuring improvement following total hip and knee arthroplasty using patient-based measures of outcome. J Bone Joint Surg Am. 2005;87:1999–2005.
15. Boonstra MC, De Waal Malefijt MC, Verdonschot N. How to quantify knee function after total knee arthroplasty? Knee. 2008;15:390–5.
16. Boonstra MC, Schwering PJ, De Waal Malefijt MC, Verdonschot N. Sit-to-stand movement as a performance-based measure for patients with total knee arthroplasty. Phys Ther. 2010;90:149–56.
17. Terwee CB, van der Slikke RM, van Lummel RC, Benink RJ, Meijers WG, de Vet HC. Self-reported physical functioning was more influenced by pain than performance-based physical functioning in knee-osteoarthritis patients. J Clin Epidemiol. 2006;59:724–31.
18. Zelle J, Barink M, Loeffen R, De Waal MM, Verdonschot N. Thigh-calf contact force measurements in deep knee flexion. Clin Biomech (Bristol, Avon). 2007;22:821–6.
19. Zelle J, Barink M, De Waal MM, Verdonschot N. Thigh-calf contact: does it affect the loading of the knee in the high-flexion range? J Biomech. 2009;42:587–93.

20. Boonstra MC, Jenniskens AT, Barink M, van Uden CJ, Kooloos JG, Verdonschot N, et al. Functional evaluation of the TKA patient using the coordination and variability of rising. J Electromyogr Kinesiol. 2007;17:49–56.

21. Boonstra MC, van der Slikke RM, Keijsers NL, van Lummel RC, de Waal Malefijt MC, Verdonschot N. The accuracy of measuring the kinematics of rising from a chair with accelerometers and gyroscopes. J Biomech. 2006;39:354–8.

22. Fritz CO, Morris PE, Richler JJ. Effect size estimates: current use, calculations, and interpretation. J Exp Psychol Gen. 2012;141:2–18.

23. Nutton RW, van der Linden ML, Rowe PJ, Gaston P, Wade FA. A prospective randomised double-blind study of functional outcome and range of flexion following total knee replacement with the NexGen standard and high flexion components. J Bone Joint Surg Br. 2008;90:37–42.

24. Hamilton WG, Sritulanondha S, Engh CA Jr. Prospective randomized comparison of high-flex and standard rotating platform total knee arthroplasty. J Arthroplast. 2011;26:28–34.

25. Ha CW, Park YB, Song YS, Lee WY, Park YG. Are the current outcome measurement tools appropriate for the evaluation of the knee status in deep flexion range? J Arthroplast. 2016;31:87–91.

26. Long WJ, Scuderi GR. High-flexion total knee arthroplasty. J Arthroplast. 2008;23:6–10.

27. Palmer SH, Servant CT, Maguire J, Parish EN, Cross MJ. Ability to kneel after total knee replacement. J Bone Joint Surg Br. 2002;84:220–2.

16

A comparative, retrospective study of peri-articular and intra-articular injection of tranexamic acid for the management of postoperative blood loss after total knee arthroplasty

Zhenyang Mao[1,2], Bing Yue[1,2]*, You Wang[1,2], Mengning Yan[1,2] and Kerong Dai[1,2]

Abstract

Background: Intra-articular injection of tranexamic acid (TXA) is known to be effective in controlling blood loss after total knee arthroplasty (TKA). However, this method has some disadvantages, such as TXA leakage due to soft tissue release. Peri-articular injection provides an alternative to intra-articular administration of TXA. This study aimed to evaluate the effects of peri-articular injection of TXA in reducing blood loss after TKA and compare them to those of intra-articular TXA injection.

Methods: This was a retrospective analysis of 127 patients who underwent primary, unilateral TKA for knee osteoarthritis in our hospital between January 2014 and December 2014. Cases were classified into 3 comparison groups: 49 patients in the peri-articular TXA group, 36 in the intra-articular group, and 42 in the control group (TXA not administered). Demographic variables, hemoglobin (Hb) measured before and after surgery, operation time, total amount of drained volume, time of removing drains, units of blood transfused peri- and postoperatively, estimated volume of blood loss, and preoperative comorbidities were retrieved from the patients' medical charts. Statistical analyses were performed using SPSS 19.0 software.

Results: There were no significant differences of demographic variables and operation time among three groups ($P > 0.05$). Compared to the control group, both TXA groups had a significantly reduced volume of blood loss, postoperative knee joint drainage, hemoglobin concentration, time of removing drains, and need for blood transfusion ($P < 0.05$). The effects of TXA were comparable for the two methods of injection ($P > 0.05$). There were no deep venous thrombosis or thromboembolic complications in any group.

Conclusions: Peri-articular injection of TXA is as effective as an intra-articular injection in reducing postoperative blood loss during TKA. Both methods had a statistically significant benefit in reducing the change in Hb concentration, volume of joint drainage, and estimated volume of blood loss when compared to the control group. Peri-articular injection of TXA can significantly reduce the blood transfusion rate compared to the control group.

Keywords: Total knee arthroplasty, Tranexamic acid, Peri-articular injection, Intra-articular injection, Blood loss

* Correspondence: advbmp2@163.com
[1]Shanghai Key Laboratory of Orthopaedic Implants, Shanghai Ninth People's Hospital, Shanghai Jiaotong University School of Medicine, Shanghai, People's Republic of China
[2]Department of Orthopaedic Surgery, Shanghai Ninth People's Hospital, Shanghai Jiaotong University School of Medicine, 639 Zhizaoju Road, Shanghai 200011, People's Republic of China

Background

Major postoperative blood loss is one of the most common problems associated with total knee arthroplasty (TKA). Postoperative blood loss can range between 1000 mL and 2000 mL [1, 2], with 10–38 % of patients requiring transfusion of 1–2 units of blood [1–4]. Blood transfusions implicitly lead to the risk for infection, graft-versus-host disease, hemolysis, and transfusion-related acute lung injury [5]. In addition, blood products are expensive and in short supply. Therefore, controlling blood loss associated with TKA is an important clinical issue.

Several methods have been introduced to reduce TKA-associated blood loss. The administration of tranexamic acid (TXA), an antifibrinolytic agent, is currently a "hot topic" of research. Several studies have reported that intravenous (IV) administration of TXA significantly reduces postoperative blood loss and the need for transfusion [4, 6]. However, several medical conditions, most notably a history of deep venous thrombosis (DVT), cerebrovascular and cardiac disease, and renal failure, are commonly identified as comorbidities in patients undergoing TKA; they affect the use of IV-TXA. In addition, only a small percentage of the TXA solution administered by IV reaches the target location and tissue [7]. To address these clinical limitations, TXA has increasingly been administered via intra-articular injection (IAI) after TKA [7–12].

The safety and efficacy of IAI of TXA has been demonstrated in several studies [7–12]. However, the reported effectiveness of this method has been questioned. In particular, the volume of intra-articular TXA solution, usually reported to be 5–25 mL in previous studies [7, 13, 14], may be insufficient to immerse the anterior tissues of the knee joint when the patient is placed in a supine position during surgery. In addition, extensive soft tissue release, which is required in some cases to balance forces on the knee, may cause the injected TXA solution to leak from the joint.

A peri-articular injection (PAI), in which the TXA solution is injected into the soft tissue around the joint cavity before closure, is an alternative to an IAI of TXA. PAI also has the distinct advantage of allowing the surgeon to target areas that are vulnerable to postoperative bleeding, such as sites of soft tissue release and incisal edges in the synovial membrane. Therefore, our aim was to conduct a retrospective analysis of patients who underwent TKA at our hospital and were administered either IAI-TXA or PAI-TXA to evaluate the effectiveness of these two modes of TXA administration in controlling postoperative blood loss compared to patients who did not receive TXA.

Methods

TXA has been used in TKA surgeries in our hospital since May 2014. Between May 2014 and September 2014, we used an IAI of TXA in TKA as previously reported [4, 15]. However, we observed leakage of the TXA solution in some cases, especially in those who needed severe soft tissue release, and we switched to PAI of TXA in the followed TKA cases. Between January 2014 and December 2014, we retrospectively reviewed medical charts to identify patients between the ages of 50 and 80 years and in whom TKA was performed as a treatment for degenerative arthritis. Preoperative comorbidities that were thought to influence either bleeding tendency or thromboembolic tendency were recorded, as well as use of anticoagulant drugs such as warfarin and clopidogrel. All anticoagulant drugs were stopped prior to surgery, and coagulation system data were repeated and found to be normal on admission. After the retrospective review of TKA cases, 127 subjects were identified (23 male and 104 female). Of these 127 cases, 49 (8 male and 41 female) received PAI-TXA, forming the PAI-TXA group; 36 (5 male and 31 female) received IAI-TXA, forming the IAI-TXA group; and 42 patients (10 male and 32 female) were not administered TXA, forming the control group.

All surgeries were performed under general anesthesia by the same surgeon, who was a specialist in TKA procedures. A pneumatic tourniquet was prepared as a precautionary measure in case of emergent situations, such as injury to an artery, but not inflated during the surgery in those cases. A midline skin incision was made, followed by a medial para-patellar capsular approach, to expose the surgical site of the knee joint. Intra-operative hemostasis was applied in standard fashion. After bone resection of the distal femur and proximal tibia, the soft tissue balancing was performed, and the appropriate type and size of knee prosthesis components were cemented, polyethylene liners were inserted, and the patella was resurfaced. An intra-articular drain was placed in situ, followed by wound closure. For peri-articular administration of TXA, the TXA solution was injected into the soft tissues around the joint cavity, 5 to 10 mL at each point, such as posterior joint capsulae synovial membrane and ligaments, especially the sites of soft tissue release and incisal edges in the synovial membrane, before the proximal and distal components of the prosthesis were implanted. For the intra-articular administration of TXA, the TXA solution was injected into the knee joint cavity after wound closure, with the drain clamped for 15 min to allow for absorption of the TXA, and then released.

The doses of TXA were comparable to concentrations reported in previous studies of IV-TXA in TKA, showing positive effects with doses of 15 to 20 mg/kg [4, 15] and concentrations of 10–100 mg/mL for topical TXA solutions [7, 9, 14, 16]. Therefore, doses of 2 g of TXA in 80 mL normal saline were used for PAI and IAI. The contraindications of use of TXA were patients with an allergy to TXA, an actual infection, any type of cancer, atrial fibrillation and angina, stroke, rheumatoid arthritis, and revision TKA.

Postoperatively, drains were removed when the 24-h volume of drainage was less than 50 mL. Hemoglobin (Hb) was measured preoperatively and at 12 h, 24 h, and 48 h postoperatively. The change in Hb was the difference between the lowest level preoperatively and postoperatively. All patients were administered a standard course of daily oral anticoagulant (Rivaroxaban; Xarelto, Bayer Schering Pharma AG, Germany) for two weeks, starting on the first postoperative day. Patients were examined daily for clinical symptoms of DVT during the hospital stay and for 6 weeks postoperatively. Doppler ultrasonography examination was applied when there was a clinical suspicion of DVT. Once Doppler confirmed DVT, therapeutic low molecular weight heparin was administered. In addition, all patients received rehabilitation exercises that included a passive knee flexibility exercise and quadriceps femoris contraction exercise before drain removal, and the patients were allowed to walk with a walker after removal of the drain. The patients were usually discharged 14 days after surgery, unless there were wound complications. Patients had regular follow up every month for the first six months and yearly thereafter.

Demographic and clinical variables were retrieved from the patients' medical charts and included: age, sex, height, weight, body mass index, Hb measured before and after surgery to quantify change in Hb concentration preoperative platelet blood test, preoperative coagulation system data (international normalized ratio, prothrombin time, activated partial thromboplastin time), operation time,

total amount of drained volume, time of removing drains, units of blood transfused peri- and postoperatively, and preoperative comorbidities. The volume of blood loss was estimated using a previously reported method [4]. The criterion for blood transfusion was an Hb level < 8 g/dL or a postoperative Hb level between 8 and 10 g/dL with clinical signs of hemodynamic instability; this criterion was consistent with the Guidelines of the American Society of Anesthesiologists [17]. We evaluated the range of motion (ROM) to determine patients' functional outcomes at follow-up. The ROM was measured with a universal goniometer that is commonly used in clinical practice [18, 19].

Statistical analyses were performed using SPSS 19.0 software. Continuous variables were expressed as a mean ± standard deviation. Between-group differences for demographic and clinical variables were evaluated using one-way analysis of variance, and a least squared difference post-hoc test was used for variables with homogeneity of variance or Dunnett's test was used for variables with heterogeneity of variance. Between-group differences in the distribution of men and women in each group and the number of transfusions were analyzed with cross-tabulation. A value of $P < 0.05$ was considered to be statistically significant.

Results

The demographic variables for our study group are listed in Table 1, with no significant between-group differences among the three experimental groups. The postoperative volume of knee joint drainage is reported in Fig. 1. The volume was significantly lower for patients in the PAI-TXA and IAI-TXA groups compared to the control group

Table 1 The demographic data of the subjects in this study

	PAI TXA group ($n = 49$)	IAI TXA group ($n = 36$)	Control group ($n = 42$)	P value
Age (years)	68.5 ± 7.4	69.7 ± 7.2	69.6 ± 5.7	0.66
Gender (M/F)	8/41	5/31	10/32	0.48
Height (m)	1.6 ± 0.1	1.6 ± 0.1	1.6 ± 0.1	0.49
Weight (kg)	67.6 ± 11.7	65.1 ± 10.4	67.9 ± 9.3	0.44
BMI (kg/cm^2)	25.9 ± 3.7	25.6 ± 3.9	26.6 ± 3.8	0.47
Preoperative Hb (g/L)	124.3 ± 10.5	123.8 ± 10.7	125.9 ± 12.9	0.69
INR	0.98 ± 0.2	0.95 ± 0.1	0.94 ± 0.0	0.38
PT (s)	11.5 ± 2.5	11.1 ± 0.7	11.1 ± 0.6	0.33
APTT (s)	27.0 ± 4.3	27.0 ± 3.3	27.0 ± 2.9	0.99
PLT (×10^9/L)	213.7 ± 77.8	212.1 ± 63.5	212.8 ± 61.1	0.99
Operation time (min)	94.5 ± 16.4	92.1 ± 13.3	88.5 ± 10.3	0.12
Anticoagulant use, % yes	8.2	11.1	9.5	0.90
Thromboembolic tendency, % yes	14.3	11.1	14.3	0.89
Coagulopathies, % yes	2	0	0	0.20

Values are expressed as the mean ± standard deviation

PAI TXA peri-articular injection of tranexamic acid, *IAI TXA* intra-articular injection of tranexamic acid, *BMI* body mass index, *Hb* hemoglobin, *INR* international normalized ratio, *PT* prothrombin, *APTT* activated partial thromboplastin time, *PLT* platelet

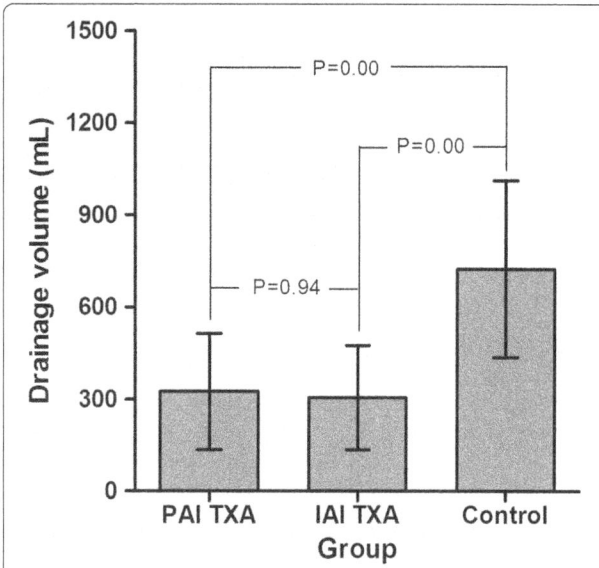

Fig. 1 The postoperative drainage volume of the three groups. Legend: The volume was significantly lower for patients in the PAI-TXA and IAI-TXA groups compared to the control group ($P < 0.05$) and was comparable for the two TXA groups ($P = 0.94$)

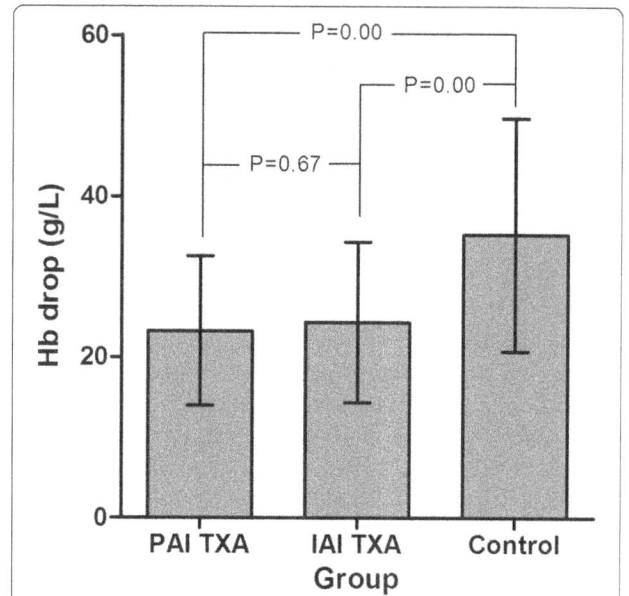

Fig. 2 The mean change in Hb concentration before and after surgery of the three groups. Legend: The mean change in Hb concentration was significantly lower for both TXA groups compared to the control group ($P < 0.05$), and had no significant difference between the PAI-TXA and IAI-TXA groups ($P = 0.67$)

($P < 0.05$), with a mean volume of 324.9 ± 189.4 mL for the PAI-TXA group, 305.0 ± 169.1 mL for the IAI-TXA group, and 724.1 ± 288.4 mL for the control group. The volume of drainage was comparable for the two TXA groups ($P = 0.94$). The times of removing drains were 36.6 ± 12.0 h for the PAI-TXA group, 42.6 ± 13.0 h for the IAI-TXA group, and 63.8 ± 13.6 h for the control group. The times of removal were comparable for the two TXA groups ($P = 0.13$), but were both significantly shorter than that of the control group ($P < 0.05$).

The mean change in Hb concentration was significantly lower for both TXA groups compared to the control group ($P < 0.05$), with a mean reduction of the Hb concentration of 23.2 ± 9.3 g/L in the PAI-TXA group, 24.3 ± 10.0 g/L in the IAI-TXA group, and 33.3 ± 14.4 g/L in the control group. The amount of change in Hb concentration was comparable for the PAI-TXA and IAI-TXA groups ($P = 0.67$) (Fig. 2).

The estimated volume of blood loss was significantly lower for patients in the PAI-TXA group (872.8 ± 333.3 mL) and IAI-TXA group (914.2 ± 469.4 mL) compared to patients in the control group (1487.1 ± 975.7 mL) ($P < 0.05$). Again, there was no significant difference between the two TXA groups ($P = 0.96$) (Fig. 3).

The number of patients requiring blood transfusions is reported in Table 2. The rate of blood transfusion was comparable for both TXA groups ($P = 0.71$), with 8 patients receiving a transfusion in the PAI-TXA group and 7 patients receiving a transfusion in the IAI-TXA group. In comparison, 16 patients required a blood transfusion in the control group, a transfusion rate that

was significantly higher than in the PAI-TXA group, but not significantly different compared to the IAI-TXA group ($P = 0.07$) (Table 2).

We divided the patients who did and did not use anti-coagulants into three groups to investigate whether the

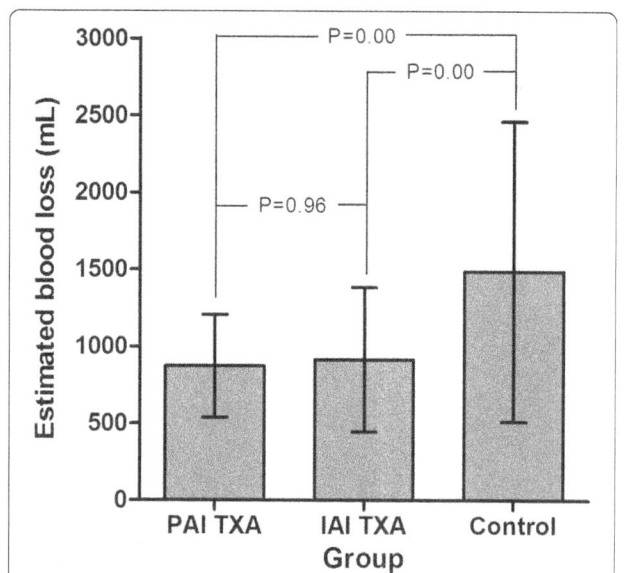

Fig. 3 The estimated volume of blood loss of the three groups. Legend: The estimated volume of blood loss was significantly lower for patients in the PAI-TXA and IAI-TXA group compared to those in the control group ($P < 0.05$). There was no significant difference between the two TXA groups ($P = 0.96$)

Table 2 The number of patients requiring blood transfusions in the three groups

Groups	Number of Patients with Transfusions (%)	P Value (Compared to PAI TXA Group)	P Value (Compared to IAI TXA Group)	P Value (Compared to Control Group)
PAI TXA Group (n = 49)	8 (16.32)	N/A	0.71	0.02
IAI TXA Group (n = 36)	7 (19.44)	0.71	N/A	0.07
Control Group (n = 42)	16 (38.10)	0.02	0.07	N/A

PAI TXA peri-articular injection of tranexamic acid, *IAI TXA* intra-articular injection of tranexamic acid

anticoagulation usage would impact the volume of knee joint drainage, drop in Hb, and estimated blood loss after TKA (Table 3). We found that there was no significant difference between the patients who did and did not use anticoagulation therapy in the PAI, IAI, and control groups (P > 0.05). The results were comparable between patients who did not use anticoagulation therapy in the PAI and IAI groups (P > 0.05). However, there was a significant difference between these patients and those who did not use anticoagulants in the control group. There was no significant difference among the three subgroups when anticoagulation was used (P > 0.05) (Table 3).

There was no DVT or thromboembolic complication in any group. No surgical site or wound complications occurred. All patients had satisfactory ROM results after surgery. At the first three-month follow-up visit, no significant difference was found among the three groups (P > 0.05) (Table 4). At this follow-up visit, patients' ROM reached 120°.

Discussion

The main findings of the current study were that PAI of TXA is as effective as IAI of TXA in reducing postoperative blood loss during TKA. Both methods had a statistically significant benefit in reducing the change in Hb concentration, volume of joint drainage, and estimated volume of blood loss when compared to a control group.

TXA is a well-known antifibrinolytic agent used to decrease blood loss in various surgical and other medical circumstances, such as in the management of craniocerebral trauma, postpartum hemorrhage, hemophilia hemorrhaging, and menorrhea [20–23]. Recently, IV and topical intra-operative administration of TXA have been reported to reduce postoperative blood loss and the consequent need for blood transfusion after TKA [6, 10, 24]. Several meta-analysis have provided evidence that IV administration of TXA does not increase the risk for DVT [25, 26]; however, Raveendran et al.[27] considered that the effects of TXA on thromboembolic events and mortality remain uncertain. Therefore, topical administration of TXA has been considered a safe alternative to IV administration, limiting the systemic absorption of TXA while providing the benefit of directly increasing drug activity at the application site. Wong et al.[8] found that the plasma levels detected in patients using topical TXA were significantly less than in patients receiving an equivalent IV-administered dose.

Topical TXA has become the routine form of care since Seo et al.[16] reported their findings of the effectiveness of

Table 3 Subgroup analysis of patients on anticoagulants

Anticoagulation use or not	PAI-N (n = 45)	PAI-U (n = 4)	P value	IAI-N (n = 32)	IAI-U (n = 4)	P value	Control-N (n = 38)	Control-U (n = 4)	P value	P*	P**
Drainage volume (mL)	324.7 ± 182.1	327.5 ± 296.0	0.98	299.1 ± 172.7	352.5 ± 148.9	0.56	732.4 ± 289.6	645.0 ± 305.1	0.57	0.00,	0.21,
										0.90,	0.90,
										0.00,	0.18,
										0.00	0.15
Hb drop (g/L)	23.2 ± 8.8	23.5 ± 15.5	0.96	23.9 ± 10.0	28.0 ± 9.8	0.44	32.4 ± 14.0	42.0 ± 18.16	0.21	0.00,	0.24,
										0.80,	0.68,
										0.00,	0.11,
										0.00	0.22
Estimated blood loss (mL)	860.6 ± 343.2	1009.7 ± 150.8	0.40	861.4 ± 457.27	1336.1 ± 337.5	0.06	1486.1 ± 1002.3	1496.5 ± 787.4	0.98	0.00,	0.43,
										0.99	0.40,
										0.00,	0.60,
										0.00	0.97

Values are expressed as a mean ± standard deviation
PAI peri-articular injection, *IAI* intra-articular injection, *U* anticoagulation used, *N* anticoagulation not used
*P**: Differences (Three groups, PAI-N vs. IAI-N, PAI-N vs. Control-N, IAI-N vs. Control-N) among subgroups of PAI-N, IAI-N, and Control-N
*P***: Differences (three groups, PAI-U vs. IAI-U, PAI-U vs. Control-U, IAI-U vs. Control-U) among subgroups of PAI-U, IAI-U, and Control-U

Table 4 Follow-up ROM of the patients in the three groups

	One month	Two months	Three months
PAI TXA Group (n = 49)	97.8 ± 5.8	110.6 ± 5.2	124.0 ± 4.3
IAI TXA Group (n = 36)	96.5 ± 5.1	109.6 ± 4.4	125.4 ± 4.1
Control Group (n = 42)	96.9 ± 5.2	108.5 ± 7.4	125.0 ± 4.0
P value	0.53	0.22	0.29

Values are expressed as a mean ± standard deviation
ROM range of motion, PAI TXA peri-articular injection of tranexamic acid,
IAI TXA intra-articular injection of tranexamic acid

intra-articular administration of TXA in reducing the volume of blood loss and transfusion rate, compared to IV administration. After surgical hemostasis is achieved, a topical application of TXA can reduce topical fibrinolysis and consequently stabilize clot formation and promote microvascular hemostasis, thereby decreasing bleeding [28, 29].

In the majority of studies evaluating the clinical benefits of topical use of TXA, the application method has been an IAI [9–12]. However, the following limitations of IAI of TXA have been noted. In some studies, the volume of intra-articular TXA solution applied ranged only from 5 mL to 25 mL [7, 13, 14]. This low volume of solution may not be sufficient to immerse all soft tissues of the knee joint effectively, particularly when the patient is placed in the supine position for surgery. This would compromise the effectiveness of TXA in controlling bleeding at the sites near the anterior aspect of the knee joint. In addition, in some cases of advanced knee osteoarthritis, extensive soft tissue release is required to achieve soft tissue balance. Such extensive soft release would allow leakage of intra-articular TXA into surrounding tissues. A PAI of TXA, in contrast, would improve permeation of TXA into the deeper soft tissues of the knee joint and avoid TXA leakage. Furthermore, a peri-articular method of administration allows selective application of TXA to potential sites of bleeding, such as released soft tissues and the incisal margin areas in synovial membrane. Finally, a PAI simplifies postoperative management of the patient by eliminating the need to clamp the drain, as required with intra-articular administration.

Postoperative anemia increases the risk for postoperative complications, including wound complications, poor functional recovery, and a longer hospital stay due to the potential need for blood transfusion [3]. In our study, PAI of TXA was effective in lowering the volume of postoperative blood loss and blood transfusion in patients undergoing primary unilateral TKA. PAI-TXA also reduced the volume of postoperative joint drainage, leading to an earlier removal of the drain. The volume of postoperative drainage of 324.9 ± 189.4 mL in patients in the PAI-TXA group, within 48 h, was similar to volumes of 297 ± 196 mL reported by Alshryda et al. (intra-articular) [9] and 401 ± 82.4 mL reported by Roy et al.

(intra-articular) [14]. In addition, the effectiveness of PAI-TXA in reducing the volume of postoperative blood loss and preserving Hb concentrations in our study is consistent and comparable with the findings of previous studies reported by Georgiadis et al. (intra-articular) [6], Wong et al. (intra-articular) [8], and Aguilera et al. (intravenous) [30].

The method for topical administration of TXA, however, has remained a controversial issue in clinical practice. Maniar et al.[15] evaluated five different methods of TXA administration, reporting that an IAI, compared to no intervention, reduced the volume of blood loss but had no discernible effects on postoperative joint drainage volume. Sarzaeem et al.[31] compared IV administration of TXA to two topical methods, IAI and peri-articular irrigation (not injection), to a control group. Among the TXA groups, IAI of TXA led to less blood loss compared to IV administration, and IV administration led to less blood loss than irrigation of the knee joint with TXA. In our study, we found that both PAI and IAI of TXA significantly reduced the blood loss and wound drainage after TKA compared to the control group.

TXA is a synthetic analog of the amino acid lysine, and it serves as an antifibrinolytic. Although few adverse effects have been reported in the orthopedic field, concerns about thromboembolism persist. Many studies show that IV or IAI of TXA during TKA was not associated with a significant incidence of DVT [7, 8, 14, 16]. In the current study, no DVT or thromboembolic complication was found, confirming the results of those studies.

Anticoagulant drugs may influence bleeding. In our study, we divided each group into two subgroups, the anticoagulation not used subgroup and the anticoagulation used subgroup, in order to investigate the impact of anticoagulation use on the volume of knee joint drainage, drop in Hb, and estimated blood loss. There was no significant difference among the three anticoagulation used subgroups (P > 0.05), which were inconsistent with the results among the three groups; this may be attributed to the small sample size of these three subgroups, which only had 4 patients each. Further well-designed studies may be needed to understand if anticoagulant drug use would influence the therapeutic effect of TXA.

The limitations of our study need to be acknowledged. Foremost, as a retrospective study with a relatively small sample size, the level of evidence is low. In addition, we did not measure systemic blood levels of TXA and, therefore, the level of TXA leaked from the soft tissue and joint space of the knee into the systemic circulation could not be determined. Furthermore, avoiding TXA leakage is thought to be a theoretical advantage of the PAI method. In our experience, no TXA leakage occurred using this method. Due to our small sample size, further well-designed randomized controlled trials will be required to investigate if avoiding TXA leakage is an actual advantage of the PAI method compared to the IAI method,

Conclusions

The peri-articular injection of TXA is as effective as the intra-articular injection in reducing postoperative blood loss in TKA, while possessing several potential advantages.

Abbreviations

DVT: Deep venous thrombosis; Hb: Hemoglobin; IAI-TXA: Intra-articular injection of TXA; PAI-TXA: Peri-articular injection of TXA; ROM: Range of motion; TKA: Total knee arthroplasty; TXA: Tranexamic acid

Acknowledgement

None.

Funding

Authors have received funding from the National Natural Science Foundation of China (No. 81472119, 81672196). Shanghai Municipal Education Commission Gaofeng Clinical Medicine Grant Support (No. 20161423).

Authors' contributions

All authors contributed equally to this work. ZM analyzed and interpreted the clinical data. BY, YW, MY and KD performed the surgery. ZM and BY were major contributors in writing the manuscript. All authors read and approved the final manuscript.

Competing interests

The authors declare that they have no competing interests.

Consent for publication

Consent for publication in the study was obtained.

References

1. Bong MR, Patel V, Chang E, Issack PS, Hebert R, Di Cesare PE. Risks associated with blood transfusion after total knee arthroplasty. J Arthroplasty. 2004;19:281–7.
2. Kalairajah Y, Simpson D, Cossey AJ, Verrall GM, Spriggins AJ. Blood loss after total knee replacement: effects of computer-assisted surgery. J Bone Joint Surg (Br). 2005;87:1480–2.
3. Bierbaum BE, Callaghan JJ, Galante JO, Rubash HE, Tooms RE, Welch RB. An analysis of blood management in patients having a total hip or knee arthroplasty. J Bone Joint Surg Am. 1999;81:2–10.
4. Good L, Peterson E, Lisander B. Tranexamic acid decreases external blood loss but not hidden blood loss in total knee replacement. Br J Anaesth. 2003;90:596–9.
5. Vamvakas EC, Blajchman MA. Transfusion-related mortality: the ongoing risks of allogeneic blood transfusion and the available strategies for their prevention. Blood. 2009;113:3406–17.
6. Georgiadis AG, Muh SJ, Silverton CD, Weir RM, Laker MW. A prospective double-blind placebo controlled trial of topical tranexamic acid in total knee arthroplasty. J Arthroplasty. 2013;28:78–82.
7. Ishida K, Tsumura N, Kitagawa A, Hamamura S, Fukuda K, Dogaki Y, Kubo S, Matsumoto T, Matsushita T, Chin T, et al. Intra-articular injection of tranexamic acid reduces not only blood loss but also knee joint swelling after total knee arthroplasty. Int Orthop. 2011;35:1639–45.
8. Wong J, Abrishami A, El Beheiry H, Mahomed NN, Roderick Davey J, Gandhi R, Syed KA, Muhammad Ovais Hasan S, De Silva Y, Chung F. Topical application of tranexamic acid reduces postoperative blood loss in total knee arthroplasty: a randomized, controlled trial. J Bone Joint Surg Am. 2010;92:2503–13.
9. Alshryda S, Mason J, Vaghela M, Sarda P, Nargol A, Maheswaran S, Tulloch C, Anand S, Logishetty R, Stothart B, et al. Topical (intra-articular) tranexamic acid reduces blood loss and transfusion rates following total knee replacement: a randomized controlled trial (TRANX-K). J Bone Joint Surg Am. 2013;95:1961–8.
10. Konig G, Hamlin BR, Waters JH. Topical tranexamic acid reduces blood loss and transfusion rates in total hip and total knee arthroplasty. J Arthroplasty. 2013;28:1473–6.
11. Gilbody J, Dhotar HS, Perruccio AV, Davey JR. Topical tranexamic acid reduces transfusion rates in total hip and knee arthroplasty. J Arthroplasty. 2014;29:681–4.
12. Gomez-Barrena E, Ortega-Andreu M, Padilla-Eguiluz NG, Perez-Chrzanowska H, Figueredo-Zalve R. Topical intra-articular compared with intravenous tranexamic acid to reduce blood loss in primary total knee replacement: a double-blind, randomized, controlled, noninferiority clinical trial. J Bone Joint Surg Am. 2014;96:1937–44.
13. Sa-Ngasoongsong P, Channoom T, Kawinwonggowit V, Woratanarat P, Chanplakorn P, Wibulpolprasert B, Wongsak S, Udomsubpayakul U, Wechmongkolgorn S, Lekpittaya N. Postoperative blood loss reduction in computer-assisted surgery total knee replacement by low dose intra-articular tranexamic acid injection together with 2-hour clamp drain: a prospective triple-blinded randomized controlled trial. Orthop Rev. 2011;3:e12.
14. Roy SP, Tanki UF, Dutta A, Jain SK, Nagi ON. Efficacy of intra-articular tranexamic acid in blood loss reduction following primary unilateral total knee arthroplasty. Knee surg, sports traumatol, arthroscopy. 2012;20:2494–501.
15. Maniar RN, Kumar G, Singhi T, Nayak RM, Maniar PR. Most effective regimen of tranexamic acid in knee arthroplasty: a prospective randomized controlled study in 240 patients. Clin Orthop Relat Res. 2012;470:2605–12.
16. Seo JG, Moon YW, Park SH, Kim SM, Ko KR. The comparative efficacies of intra-articular and IV tranexamic acid for reducing blood loss during total knee arthroplasty. Knee surg, sports traumatol, arthroscopy. 2013;21:1869–74.
17. American Society of Anesthesiologists Task Force on Perioperative Blood T, Adjuvant T. Practice guidelines for perioperative blood transfusion and adjuvant therapies: an updated report by the American Society of Anesthesiologists Task Force on Perioperative Blood Transfusion and Adjuvant Therapies. Anesthesiology. 2006;105:198–208.
18. Gajdosik RL, Bohannon RW. Clinical measurement of range of motion. Review of goniometry emphasizing reliability and validity. Phys Ther. 1987; 67:1867–72.
19. Russell TG, Jull GA, Wootton R. Can the Internet be used as a medium to evaluate knee angle? Man Ther. 2003;8:242–6.
20. Xu J, Gao W, Ju Y. Tranexamic acid for the prevention of postpartum hemorrhage after cesarean section: a double-blind randomization trial. Arch Gynecol Obstet. 2013;287:463–8.
21. Srivaths LV, Dietrich JE, Yee DL, Sangi-Haghpeykar H, Mahoney Jr D. Oral Tranexamic Acid versus Combined Oral Contraceptives for Adolescent Heavy Menstrual Bleeding: A Pilot Study. J Pediatr Adolesc Gynecol. 2015;28:254–7.
22. Roberts I, Shakur H, Coats T, Hunt B, Balogun E, Barnetson L, Cook L, Kawahara T, Perel P, Prieto-Merino D, et al. The CRASH-2 trial: a randomised controlled trial and economic evaluation of the effects of tranexamic acid on death, vascular occlusive events and transfusion requirement in bleeding trauma patients. Health Technol Assess. 2013;17:1–79.
23. Tang YM, Chapman TW, Brooks P. Use of tranexamic acid to reduce bleeding in burns surgery. J Plast Reconstr Aesthet Surg. 2012;65:684–6.
24. Patel JN, Spanyer JM, Smith LS, Huang J, Yakkanti MR, Malkani AL. Comparison of intravenous versus topical tranexamic acid in total knee arthroplasty: a prospective randomized study. J Arthroplasty. 2014;29:1528–31.
25. Alshryda S, Sarda P, Sukeik M, Nargol A, Blenkinsopp J, Mason JM. Tranexamic acid in total knee replacement: a systematic review and meta-analysis. J Bone Joint Surg (Br). 2011;93:1577–85.
26. Yang ZG, Chen WP, Wu LD. Effectiveness and safety of tranexamic acid in reducing blood loss in total knee arthroplasty: a meta-analysis. J Bone Joint Surg Am. 2012;94:1153–9.
27. Raveendran R, Wong J. Tranexamic acid reduces blood transfusion in surgical patients while its effects on thromboembolic events and mortality are uncertain. Evid Based Med. 2013;18:65–6.

28. Katsumata S, Nagashima M, Kato K, Tachihara A, Wauke K, Saito S, Jin E, Kawanami O, Ogawa R, Yoshino S. Changes in coagulation-fibrinolysis marker and neutrophil elastase following the use of tourniquet during total knee arthroplasty and the influence of neutrophil elastase on thromboembolism. Acta Anaesthesiol Scand. 2005;49:510–6.

29. Reust DL, Reeves ST, Abernathy 3rd JH, Dixon JA, Gaillard 2nd WF, Mukherjee R, Koval CN, Stroud RE, Spinale FG. Temporally and regionally disparate differences in plasmin activity by tranexamic acid. Anesth Analg. 2010;110:694–701.

30. Aguilera X, Martinez-Zapata MJ, Bosch A, Urrutia G, Gonzalez JC, Jordan M, Gich I, Maymo RM, Martinez N, Monllau JC, et al. Efficacy and safety of fibrin glue and tranexamic acid to prevent postoperative blood loss in total knee arthroplasty: a randomized controlled clinical trial. J Bone Joint Surg Am. 2013;95:2001–7.

31. Sarzaeem MM, Razi M, Kazemian G, Moghaddam ME, Rasi AM, Karimi M. Comparing efficacy of three methods of tranexamic acid administration in reducing hemoglobin drop following total knee arthroplasty. J Arthroplasty. 2014;29:1521–4.

17

Risk factors for joint replacement in knee osteoarthritis; a 15-year follow-up study

Flemming K. Nielsen[1*], Niels Egund[1], Anette Jørgensen[2] and Anne Grethe Jurik[1]

Abstract

Background: To evaluate whether clinical, radiographic or MRI findings are associated with long term risk for total knee arthroplasty (TKA) in persons with knee osteoarthritis.

Methods: We performed a follow-up analysis of 100 persons with knee osteoarthritis who participated in a clinical trial between 2000 and 2002. Clinical data as well as radiography and MRI of the inclusion knee were obtained in all participants. Data on TKA procedures were extracted from The Danish National Patient Register. Clinical, radiographic and MRI findings were analyzed for associations with subsequent TKA.

Results: During a mean follow-up period of 15 years, 66% received a TKA in the included knee (target knee); 37% also received a TKA in the other knee. The degree of joint space narrowing was highly associated with subsequent TKA (adjusted odds ratio (OR) 5.0 (95% confidence interval (95% CI) 2.6 – 9.9)) as was a radiological sum score comprising joint space narrowing, osteophytes, subchondral sclerosis and cysts (adjusted OR 1.7 (95% CI 1.3 – 2.1)). MRI detected bone marrow lesions, synovitis and effusion were similarly associated with subsequent TKA with an adjusted OR of 2.3 (95% CI 1.3 – 4.0), 2.8 (95% CI 1.5 – 5.2) and 1.9 (95% CI 1.2 – 3.1), respectively. Increased body mass index (BMI) was not associated with subsequent TKA in the target knee but was associated with TKA in the other knee (OR 2.3 (95% CI 1.2 – 4.3).

Conclusions: Radiographic findings including joint space narrowing and MRI detected bone marrow lesions, synovitis and effusion were all significantly associated with the long term risk of TKA in persons with knee osteoarthritis.

Keywords: Knee osteoarthritis, Radiography, Magnetic resonance imaging, Bone marrow lesion, Synovitis, Joint space narrowing

Background

Worldwide, osteoarthritis (OA) is the most prevalent joint disease and strongly associated with aging and obesity. The knee is the joint most commonly affected by OA with an estimated prevalence of 15% in persons aged 56 to 84 years [1].

The most important risk factors for knee OA include obesity, previous knee injury, and family history of OA [2]. The impact of each factor is debated but obesity is believed to be the most important. Thus, a recent systematic review found that onset of OA knee pain in persons over 50 years of age was related to overweight or obesity in 25% of cases; only 5% were caused by previous knee injury [3].

* Correspondence: flemming.kromann@aarhus.rm.dk
[1]Department of Radiology, Aarhus University Hospital, Noerrebrogade 44, 8000 Aarhus, Denmark
Full list of author information is available at the end of the article

The end stage of OA is characterized by severe pain, disability and joint deformity and total knee arthroplasty (TKA) is often the only effective treatment. A recent study by Weinstein et al. [4] estimated that approximately 52% of adults diagnosed with symptomatic knee OA in the US will undergo TKA. Thus, approximately half of the population with knee OA will not progress to end stage disease and TKA. This has led some to suggest that other factors may be involved in disease manifestation than in disease progression [2, 5].

Conventional radiography is the most commonly used modality for imaging of knee OA although the radiographic changes in knee OA are generally not well correlated with symptoms [6]. However, the radiographic features of OA have been shown to correlate with disease progression and TKA [7, 8], especially the degree of joint space narrowing (JSN) [9]. Magnetic resonance imaging (MRI) offers the ability to visualize all structures in and around the knee, including cartilage, subchondral bone and soft tissue. Specific pathologic findings on MRI, including bone marrow lesions (BMLs) and synovitis, are moderately correlated with pain and have been associated with risk of TKA in studies with short term follow-up [9–12] as well as with progression of JSN [13, 14].

The purpose of our study was to analyze whether clinical, radiographic and MRI findings, including BML and synovitis, correlate with the incidence of TKA during a mean follow-up period of 15 years.

Methods

Data sources

The study was partly based on data from the following Danish registers:

The Danish Civil Registration System, established in 1968, assigns a 10-digit personal identification number to all Danish citizens at birth or immigration. This unique civil registration number can be used across all Danish registers and provide highly reliable data at individual level.

The Danish National Patient Register, established in 1977, includes data on all hospital in-patient contacts. Since 1995, data on out-patient contacts has also been included. Both public and private hospitals are obliged to report discharge diagnoses to the register, which are coded according to the Danish version of the International Classification of Diseases (ICD-10).

Participants

Participants were selected from a previous multi-center, randomized, placebo-controlled double-blind trial including 337 participants comparing five intra-articular injections of Hyalgan® and placebo, respectively [15]. All included participants fulfilled the American College of Rheumatology (ACR) criteria for primary OA [16], had a Lequesne Algofunctional Index score of 10 or more (maximum score 24), a normal C-reactive protein level and e-GFR ≥ 60. The participants entered the study between January 2000 and December 2002. Exclusion criteria were secondary OA, inflammatory joint disease, significant OA symptoms from the other knee, radiographic OA in more than one tibiofemoral compartment, radiographic attrition >5 mm or severe co-morbidity (e.g. cancer and poor general health). One hundred and two participants were enrolled at our institution, constituting the potential study population for the present study.

Baseline radiographs were missing in two, leaving 100 participants with baseline radiographs and clinical data (Fig. 1). MRI was missing in seven participants with tibiofemoral OA, and 10 participants with only patellofemoral OA were excluded from the analyses of MR findings because the MRI protocol did not include an

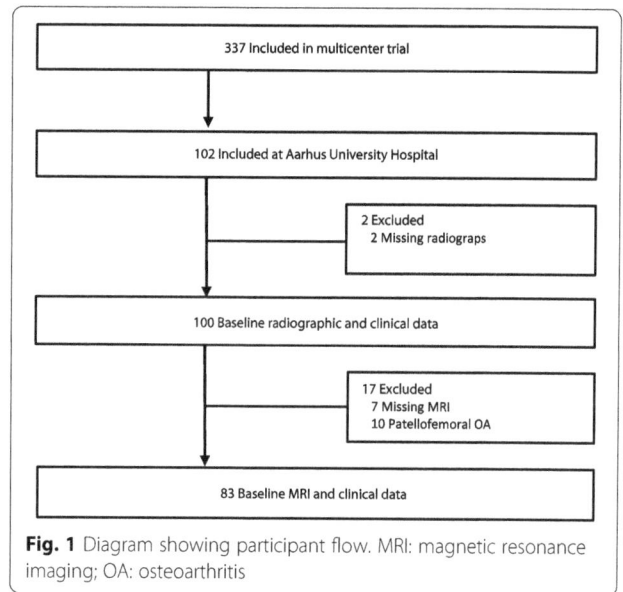

Fig. 1 Diagram showing participant flow. MRI: magnetic resonance imaging; OA: osteoarthritis

axial STIR sequence; thus, the MRI analyses were confined to 83 participants (Fig. 1).

The original study was approved by the Central Denmark Region Committee on Health Research Ethics and was carried out in accordance with the Declaration of Helsinki. Participants gave written informed consent prior to participation, including consent to publish study results and images. Prior to our follow-up study we contacted The Central Denmark Region Committees on Health Research Ethics who waived the need for ethical approval as no human biological material was involved. The study was approved by the Danish Data Protection Agency (1-16-02-126-16).

At inclusion, demographic variables (height and weight) were measured and all participants filled out a Western Ontario and McMaster Universities (WOMAC) questionnaire [17] consisting of the following items: Pain (5 items), stiffness (2 items) and physical function (17 items). Each score was made using a 100 mm Visual Analogue Scale (0 = no pain/stiffness/physical limitation, 100 = extreme pain/stiffness/physical limitation) with the following ranges: pain = 0-500, stiffness = 0-200, physical function = 0-1700, total score = 0-2400. All participants obtained radiography and MRI of the knee.

Imaging

One leg weight-bearing radiographs in 30^0 flexion of both knees were performed in three views: Postero-anterior and lateral views of the tibiofemoral, and axial view of the patellofemoral joint space. The initial lateral radiograph was used as guidance for securing optimal inclination of the lower leg for visualization of the tibiofemoral and patellofemoral joint spaces [18].

MR examinations were performed using a 1.5 Tesla system (Vision, Siemens, Erlangen, Germany) and a transmit receive four-channel knee coil. The examinations consisted of the following sequences: Sagittal STIR, repetition time (TR) = 5000 ms, echo time (TE) = 29 ms, inversion time = 150 ms, field of view (FOV) = 20 cm, slice thickness (ST) = 4.0 mm, interslice gap (IG) = 0.4 mm, matrix = 266 × 512 pixels, one excitation, and acquisition time (AT) 5.26 min; and sagittal and axial T1-weighted sequences. Gadodiamid (Omniscan, GE Healthcare, Norway) was injected at a peripheral intravenous site (0.1 mmol/kg with a maximum of 10 mmol) using a power injector followed by a saline flush. Sagittal and axial T1 fat suppressed contrast enhanced (T1 FS CE) sequences were performed using the following parameters: TR = 860 ms, TE = 20 ms, FOV = 16 cm, ST = 4.0 mm, IG = 0.8 mm, matrix = 512 × 512 pixels, one excitation, AT 7.23 min per sequence. All sagittal images were obtained perpendicular to the line connecting the dorsal aspect of the medial and lateral femoral condyle. Only the sagittal STIR and the sagittal and axial T1 FS CE images were analyzed in the present study.

Follow-up data acquisition

Data on TKA procedures were extracted from the Danish National Patient Register, dividing the study population into a TKA and a non-TKA group.

Image analysis

Radiographs and MR images were separated and anonymized prior to analysis, and readers were blinded to all study information, including outcome.

The radiographic definition of tibiofemoral (TF) OA was confined to visualization of joint space narrowing in either the medial or the lateral TF joint space. Joint space width of the medial TF articulation less than 3 mm was registered as joint space narrowing [19]. In addition, medial TF joint space larger than 3 mm but ≥1 mm reduced compared to the medial TF joint space of the other knee was considered joint space narrowing. Lateral TF joint space narrowing was registered when the joint space width was equal to or less than the medial TF joint space. Patellofemoral OA was registered when the medial and/or the lateral joint space width was less than 5 mm [20].

Radiographic grading was performed by NE and comprised assessment of JSN in the medial and lateral tibiofemoral and patellofemoral articulations according to a modified Ahlbäck grading [21, 22]. Grade 0 = normal joint spaces, grade 0.5 = < 50% JSN, grade 1.0 = > 50%, grade 1.5 = > 75% and grade 2.0 = 100% JSN; grade 3 = 100% JSN and < 5 mm bone attrition. Osteophytes (grades 0-3), subchondral sclerosis (0/1) and subchondral cysts (0/1) were also assessed. A radiographic sum score consisting of the scores for JSN, osteophytes, sclerosis and cysts was calculated.

BMLs at the tibiofemoral articulation were analyzed on the sagittal STIR images using a computer assisted segmentation (CAS) method described previously [23]. In brief, the method was based on pixel segmentation where a signal intensity threshold was calculated in the contralateral femoral condyle and tibial plateau which per definition were unaffected by radiographic OA (see exclusion criteria). The method has proven reliable in detecting even small BMLs compared to manual segmentation [23]. Because of relatively thick slices and interslice gap only three slices could reliably be measured without partial volume interference. The subchondral bone marrow in the affected femoral condyle and tibial plateau was outlined in all slices, excluding areas with partial volume from surrounding soft tissue. All pixels exceeding the threshold value, defined as the mean signal intensity in the radiographically unaffected compartment plus two standard deviations (SDs), were segmented by the CAS program yielding the BML size of the joint compartment relative to the entire bone marrow volume (relative BML).

All BML segmentations were performed twice by a radiological registrar (FKN) with at least three weeks between repeated measurements. Since inter-observer reliability has been high in a previous study [23], only intra-observer analyses were performed in the present study.

The relative BML size was ordered into categories using a 1 - 10 point scale (Grade 1 = 0 - 10% BML; grade 2 = >10 - 20% BML etc.).

Synovitis was assessed and graded according to the methods proposed by Guermazi et al. and Rhodes et al. [24, 25] on the axial and sagittal T1 FS CE images by NE and AGJ. The thickness of the enhanced synovium was measured at six sites, the medial and lateral parapatellar recesses at the level of the proximal half of the patella; the suprapatellar recess 1 – 1.5 cm cranial to the patella; at the ventral intercondylar area and dorsal surfaces of the medial and lateral femoral condyles. Grade 0 = no or patchy thin enhancement; grade 1 = even and continuous thickening of the synovial membrane <2 mm; grade 2 = thickening of the synovial membrane between 2 mm and 4 mm or nodular thickening between 2 mm and 4 mm; grade 3 = even thickening or nodular thickening between 4 mm and 8 mm and grade 4 = > 8 mm thickening. When the synovial space was separated by fluid, the thicknesses of the two adjacent synovial layers were summed. Sites with one synovial layer, e.g. the femoral condyle surfaces, were graded as follows: grade 1 = < 1 mm, grade 2 = 1 – 2 mm, grade 3 = 2 – 4 mm and grade 4 = > 4 mm. The synovitis score was summed over all six sites to one total score (maximum score 24). Effusion was measured in mm as the largest sagittal fluid distension of the suprapatellar recess on the midline sagittal T1 FS CE image. Intra- and inter-observer variation was based on 30 randomly chosen examinations.

Synovitis score was ordered into a five point ordinal scale (Grade 1 = 0 - <5; grade 2 = 5 - <10 etc.), and effusion score into an eight point ordinal scale (the maximum effusion score was 38) (Grade 1 = 0 - <5; grade 2 = 5 - <10 etc.).

Statistical analyses

Data was analyzed using Stata 13.0 (StataCorp, College Station, TX, USA) and Analyse-it software (Analyse-it for Microsoft Excel (version 2.20) Ltd.; 2009).

Baseline characteristics were analyzed descriptively using means and SDs. Associations between baseline factors and any TKA were analyzed using univariate and multivariate logistic regression analyses. Multivariable logistic regression was performed using a single predictor adjusted for other variables (sex, age, body mass index). The extent of any significant association was expressed in odds ratio (OR) with 95% confidence interval (95% CI). Survival analysis comparing the cumulative incidence of TKA over time in relation to JSN, BML, synovitis and effusion was performed using Kaplan-Meier plots [24] and test for significance was performed using Cox proportional hazard ratio, adjusted for sex, age and BMI.

The association between baseline factors and unilateral vs. bilateral TKA was similarly analyzed using univariate and multivariable logistic regression.

Body mass index (BMI) was divided into four categories: Grade 1 (normal) = <25 kg/m^2, Grade 2 (overweight) = 25 - <30 kg/m^2, Grade 3 (obese) = 30 - <35 kg/m^2 and Grade 4 (very obese) = ≥35 kg/m^2.

In case of significant associations using logistic regression the scale used for measurement was ordered into categories using a maximum of 10 points.

Intra-observer reliability for BML measurements and intra- and inter-observer reliability for synovitis and effusion grading was assessed by Bland-Altman analyses, using plots, bias and 95% limits of agreement and by intraclass correlation coefficients.

Results

Baseline characteristics for the 100 participants in the registry study are shown in Table 1. The mean follow-up time was 15.2 years (range 14.2 to 16.4 years). Ninety participants had tibiofemoral OA (80 medial, 10 lateral) and 10 had patellofemoral OA (six medial, four lateral). Baseline demographics of the 17 participants excluded from the MRI analyses due to lack of MRI or patellofemoral OA did not differ from the participants included in the MRI analyses.

A total of 66 participants had undergone TKA in the knee at follow-up; 37 had also obtained TKA in the other knee. There was no significant association between baseline demographics (sex, age, BMI) or Hyalgan treatment and the risk for TKA at follow-up (Table 1). There was a minor, though significant, association between stiffness

Table 1 Baseline characteristics at inclusion and predictors of knee replacement, univariate and multivariate analyses

Variable	Total (n = 100)	Knee replacement Yes (n = 66)	Knee replacement No (n = 34)	Unadjusted OR (95% CI)	p value	Adjusted[a] OR (95% CI)	p value
Female, % (no.)	64% (64)	68% (45)	56% (19)	1.0 (0.9 – 1.0)	0.52		
Age (years), mean (SD)	62.0 (10.4)	61.3 (10.0)	63.4 (10.9)	1.0 (0.9 – 1.0)	0.34		
BMI grade, mean (SD)	2.2 (0.9)	2.2 (0.9)	2.0 (0.9)	1.2 (0.8 – 2.0)	0.41		
WOMAC, mean (SD):							
- Pain	184 (89)	196 (95)	161 (71)	1.0 (1.0 – 1.0)	0.07		
- Stiffness	81 (45)	87(46)	67 (40)	1.3 (1.01 – 1.6)[c]	0.04	1.3 (1.01 – 1.7)[c]	0.04
- Function	657 (319)	692 (332)	588 (281)	1.0 (1.0 – 1.0)	0.13		
- Total	922 (427)	976 (446)	817 (366)	1.0 (1.0 – 1.0)	0.08		
Hyalgan %, (no.)	48% (48)	50% (33)	44% (15)	1.3 (0.6 – 2.9)	0.58		
JSN grade, mean (SD)	1.7 (1.0)	2.0 (0.9)	1.0 (0.8)	3.6 (2.1 - 6.2)	<0.001	5.0 (2.6 - 9.9)	<0.001
Radiological sum score, mean (SD)	5.0 (2.6)	5.8 (2.3)	3.4 (2.5)	1.5 (1.3 - 1.9)	<0.001	1.7 (1.3 - 2.1)	<0.001
BML grade, mean (SD)[b, d]	2.1 (1.4)	2.4 (1.5)	1.4 (0.9)	2.1 (1.2 – 3.7)	0.006	2.3 (1.3 – 4.0)	0.005
Synovitis grade, mean (SD)[b, e]	2.6 (1.0)	2.9 (0.9)	2.0 (1.1)	2.7 (1.5 – 4.7)	0.001	2.8 (1.5 – 5.2)	0.001
Effusion grade, mean (SD)[b, f]	2.4 (1.5)	2.7 (1.6)	1.7 (1.1)	1.9 (1.2 – 3.0)	0.005	1.9 (1.2 – 3.1)	0.006

OR odds ratio, CI confidence interval, No. number, SD standard deviation, BMI body mass index, WOMAC Western Ontario and McMaster Universities OA index, JSN joint space narrowing, BML bone marrow lesion
[a]Adjusted for sex, age and BMI; [b] Based on 83 participants with MRI scans and tibiofemoral osteoarthritis; [c] Logistic regression performed after ordering data into a ten point ordinal scale (Grade 1 = 0 - 10, grade 2 = 11 - 20 etc.); [d] Ordered into a ten point ordinal scale (Grade 1 = 0 - 10% BML, grade 2 = >10 - 20% BML etc.); [e]Ordered into a five point ordinal scale (Grade 1 = 0 - <5; grade 2 = 5 - <10 etc.); [f] Ordered into an eight point ordinal scale (Grade 1 = 0 - < 5; grade 2 = 5 - <10 etc.) (maximum effusion score = 38)

item in WOMAC and TKA (adjusted OR 1.3 (95% CI 1.01 – 1.7)) but not with other WOMAC items.

Significant associations between TKA and JSN (adjusted OR 5.0 (95% CI 2.6 – 9.9)), radiological sum score (adjusted OR 1.7 (95% CI 1.3 – 2.1)), BML (adjusted OR 2.3 (95% CI 1.3 – 4.0)), synovitis (adjusted OR 2.8 (95% CI 1.5 – 5.2)) and effusion (adjusted OR 1.9 (95% CI 1.2 – 3.1)) was observed (Table 1). The Kaplan-Meier time to event analysis illustrates the relation between increasing degrees of JSN, BML, synovitis and effusion and the risk of TKA (Fig. 2). Cox proportional hazard ratio showed a statistically significant hazard ratio for JSN, radiological sum score, BML, synovitis and effusion with the risk for TKA (Table 2).

The 66 participants with TKA at follow-up were compared in relation to unilateral versus bilateral TKA (Table 3); only BMI was associated with the risk of bilateral vs. unilateral TKA (OR 2.3 (95% CI 1.2 – 4.3)).

The intra- and inter-observer agreement for all parameters were good (see Additional files 1, 2, 3 and 4). The intraclass correlation coefficients ranged between 0.88 – 0.99.

Discussion
Our study showed that radiographic findings, specifically the degree of JSN, and MRI detected BML, synovitis and effusion were highly associated with TKA after 15 years of follow-up. Demographic characteristics such as sex, age or BMI were not correlated with the risk for TKA.

There was, however, an association between higher BMI and the risk for bilateral TKA versus unilateral TKA.

The reason for the pronounced association between JSN and TKA could be explained by the surgical criteria for selecting patients with knee OA. According to the Danish national guidelines from 2012, the indications for TKA are primarily based on symptoms and objective findings [26]. It is, however, likely that the surgeon would generally not operate on a knee without radiographic signs of OA, especially JSN. Thus, a relative contra-indication for TKA is absence of or minimal radiologic changes [26]. No formalized Danish guidelines existed before 2012 but a comparison of preoperative knee scores from the Danish Registry of Knee Arthroplasty between 2005 and 2009 revealed no differences in disease severity [27]. Thus, there is no indication that TKA guidelines have changed between 2005 and 2009.

JSN has also previously been shown to be associated with knee OA progression. Oak et al. [28] found that baseline JSN was significantly correlated with worsening of knee osteoarthritis outcome score (KOOS) for pain, KOOS for symptoms and KOOS for quality of life at 4-year follow-up. In a study by Raynauld et al. [9], the degree of JSN was significantly associated with subsequent TKA during a follow-up period of six years.

BML, synovitis and effusion were all significantly associated with the risk of TKA and our results are thus in line with previous studies [9–12, 29]. However, while these studies had a relatively short follow-up period (one to six

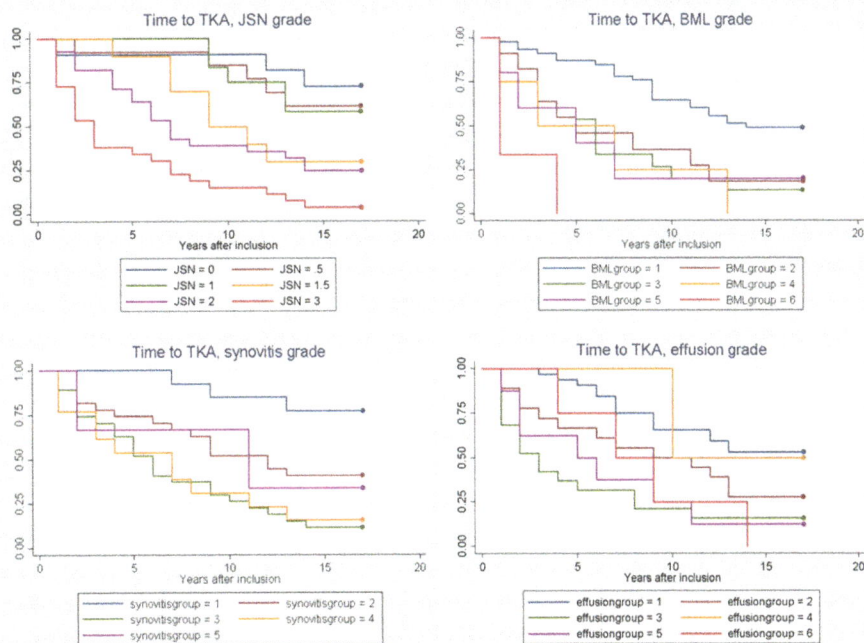

Fig. 2 Kaplan-Meier plot showing the cumulative incidence of TKA in relation to different degrees of JSN, BML, synovitis and effusion. TKA: total knee arthroplasty; JSN: joint space narrowing; BML: bone marrow lesion

Table 2 Cox proportional hazard ratios

Variable	Unadjusted		Adjusted[a]	
	Hazard ratio (95% CI)	p value	Hazard ratio (95% CI)	p value
JSN grade	2.2 (1.7 – 2.9)	<0.001	2.2 (1.7 – 3.0)	<0.001
Total radiological score	1.3 (1.1 – 1.4)	<0.001	1.3 (1.1 – 1.4)	<0.001
BML grade, [b]	1.5 (1.2 – 1.7)	<0.001	1.5 (1.2 – 1.8)	<0.001
Synovitis grade, [c]	1.5 (1.2 – 1.9)	0.001	1.5 (1.2 – 1.9)	0.001
Effusion grade, [d]	1.3 (1.1 – 1.5)	0.002	1.3 (1.1 – 1.5)	0.001

CI confidence interval, *JSN* joint space narrowing, *BML* bone marrow lesion
[a]Adjusted for sex, age and BMI (body mass index); [b] Ordered into a ten point ordinal scale (Grade 1 = 0 - 10% BML, grade 2 = >10 - 20% BML etc.); [c] Ordered into a five point ordinal scale (Grade 1 = 0 - <5; grade 2 = 5 - <10 etc.); [d] Ordered into an eight point ordinal scale (Grade 1 = 0 - <5; grade 2 = 5 - <10 etc.) (maximum effusion score = 38)

years) we showed that BML, synovitis and effusion were associated with long-term risk of TKA and that increasing degree of changes were associated with faster progression to TKA. MRI are not commonly used in the diagnosis of knee OA and the presence or absence of BML, synovitis or effusion are thus not likely to influence the surgeon's decision to perform a TKA. Instead, BML and synovitis have been found associated with symptoms [30–32] and disease progression [33, 34], and our results imply that they play a central role in the disease process.

An association between baseline demographics (age, sex) and TKA at follow-up was not found. Although both age and sex are often highlighted as risk factors for knee OA, neither have consistently been associated with disease progression [7, 35]. Furthermore, we did not find any association between overall WOMAC score

and subsequent TKA. The severity of symptoms and progression of knee OA have been associated in some studies [10, 36], often with a short follow-up. Our study showed that long-term risk of TKA was dependent on the amount of structural changes on radiographs and signs of synovial inflammation or BMLs on MR images.

No significant association was found between baseline BMI and TKA. However, among participants with TKA at follow-up, a higher BMI was associated with an increased risk of bilateral vs. unilateral TKA. Thus, our results suggest that a higher BMI does not increase the risk of TKA in knees with symptomatic OA. However, it seems that an increased BMI predisposes to development of OA in the opposite knee. Other studies have similarly reported that an elevated BMI predisposes to incident but not progression of knee OA [2, 5]. However, based on the amount of available data, we do not believe that we can draw any firm conclusions on this.

Our study has some limitations. The number of participants was limited compared to other longitudinal studies [10]. The absence of an axial STIR sequence implied that we were not able to analyze BML in participants with patellofemoral OA using computer-assisted segmentation. The signal intensity threshold was based on measurements in the contralateral joint compartment that was unaffected by radiographic OA. However, MRI changes, including BMLs, are frequently seen in radiographically normal joints and could affect BML calculations. Great care was therefore taken when outlining regions of interest for threshold calculations in the contralateral joint compartment to avoid areas with any signs of pathologic

Table 3 Baseline characteristics and predictors of unilateral versus bilateral knee replacement, univariate and multivariate analyses

Variable	Total (n = 66)	Knee replacement		Unadjusted		Adjusted[a]	
		Unilateral (n = 29)	Bilateral (n = 37)	OR (95% CI)	p value	OR (95% CI)	p value
Female, % (no.)	68% (45)	76% (22)	62% (23)	1.0 (0.9 – 1.0)	0.24		
Age (years), mean (SD)	61.3 (10.0)	62.9 (11.0)	59.9 (9.0)	0.5 (0.2 – 1.5)	0.23		
BMI, grade, mean (SD)	2.2 (0.9)	1.9 (0.9)	2.5 (0.9)	2.3 (1.2 – 4.3)	0.009		
WOMAC, mean (SD), baseline:							
- Pain	196 (95)	206 (91)	189 (98)	1.0 (1.0 – 1.0)	0.48	1.0 (1.0 – 1.0)	0.42
- Stiffness	87(46)	83 (47)	91 (44)	1.0 (1.0 – 1.0)	0.44	1.0 (1.0 – 1.0)	0.76
- Function	692 (332)	682 (320)	701 (340)	1.0 (1.0 – 1.0)	0.82	1.0 (1.0 – 1.0)	0.69
- Total	976 (446)	970 (420)	981 (465)	1.0 (1.0 – 1.0)	0.92	1.0 (1.0 – 1.0)	0.66
JSN grade, mean (SD)	2.0 (0.9)	1.9 (0.9)	2.1 (0.9)	1.3 (0.8 – 2.3)	0.30	2.2 (1.0 – 4.6)	0.05
Radiological sum score, mean (SD)	5.8 (2.3)	5.4 (2.4)	6.1 (2.2)	1.1 (0.9 – 1.4)	0.26	1.4 (1.0 – 1.9)	0.05
BML grade, mean (SD)[b, c]	2.4 (1.6)	2.5 (1.7)	2.4 (1.5)	1.0 (0.7 – 1.3)	0.82	0.9 (0.6 – 1.3)	0.63
Synovitis grade, mean (SD)[b, d]	2.9 (0.9)	2.8 (1.1)	2.9 (0.7)	1.2 (0.7 – 2.1)	0.61	1.1 (0.6 – 2.1)	0.78
Effusion grade, mean (SD)[b, e]	2.7 (1.6)	2.4 (1.7)	3.0 (1.5)	1.3 (0.9 – 1.8)	0.20	1.2 (0.8 – 1.7)	0.39

OR odds ratio, *CI* confidence interval, *No.* number, *SD* standard deviation, *BMI* body mass index, *WOMAC* Western Ontario and McMaster Universities OA index, *JSN* joint space narrowing, *BML* bone marrow lesion
[a]Adjusted for sex, age and BMI; [b] Based on 56 participants with total knee arthroplasty, accessible MRI scan and tibiofemoral osteoarthritis; [c] Ordered into a ten point ordinal scale (Grade 1 = 0 - 10% BML, grade 2 = >10 - 20% BML etc.); [d] Ordered into a five point ordinal scale (Grade 1 = 0 - <5; grade 2 = 5 - <10 etc.); [e] Ordered into an eight point ordinal scale (Grade 1 = 0 - <5; grade 2 = 5 - <10 etc.) (maximum effusion score = 38)

signal disturbances. Our BMI data was limited to baseline data only and we did not know whether BMI changed from baseline to the time of TKA. Furthermore, other pathologies associated with knee OA, e.g. meniscal or ligamentous damage, were not analyzed.

The strengths of our study were the use of a long follow-up period and a high reliability of registry TKA data. Our synovitis and effusion grading was based on contrast enhanced sequences which have been shown to be superior to fluid sensitive sequences.

Conclusions

In conclusion, we found that radiographic changes associated with knee OA as well as MRI detected BMLs, synovitis and effusion were significantly associated with the risk of TKA in patients with knee OA. Demographic variables including BMI was not associated with TKA in knees already affected by OA. However, an increased BMI was seen in participants who developed knee OA requiring TKA in the opposite knee during follow-up.

Additional files

Additional file 1: Table S1. Observer agreement, BML and synovitis grading, Bland-Altman analyses.

Additional file 2: Table S2. Observer agreement, BML and synovitis grading, Intraclass correlation coefficients.

Additional file 3: Figure S1. Inter-observer synovitis, Bland Altman plot.

Additional file 4: Figure S2. Inter-observer effusion, Bland-Altman plot.

Abbreviations

BMI: Body mass index.; BML: Bone marrow lesion; CAS: Computer assisted segmentation; CI: Confidence interval; JSN: Joint space narrowing; MRI: Magnetic resonance imaging; OA: Osteoarthritis; OR: Odds ratio; SD: Standard deviation; TKA: Total knee arthroplasty; WOMAC: Western Ontario and McMaster Universities OA index

Acknowledgements

We thank Kristian Stengaard-Pedersen for collecting patient material and David Alberg Peters for the development of the software used in BML segmentation.

Funding

The study was financially supported by A.P. Møller og Hustru Chastine McKinney Møllers Fond til Almene Formal by donation of the MR equipment.

Authors´ contributions

FKN, NE and AGJ were all involved in the design and coordination of the study, including data collection and measurement as well as the manuscript preparation. AJ selected the patients and collected clinical data. All authors meet the requirements for authorship including final approval of the manuscript submitted.

Consent for publication

Not applicable.

Competing interests

The authors declare that they have no competing interests.

Author details

[1]Department of Radiology, Aarhus University Hospital, Noerrebrogade 44, 8000 Aarhus, Denmark. [2]Department of Rheumatology, Aarhus University Hospital, Noerrebrogade 44, 8000 Aarhus, Denmark.

References

1. Turkiewicz A, Gerhardsson de Verdier M, Engstrom G, Nilsson PM, Mellstrom C, Lohmander LS, Englund M. Prevalence of knee pain and knee OA in southern Sweden and the proportion that seeks medical care. Rheumatology (Oxford). 2015;54:827–35.
2. Cooper C, Snow S, McAlindon TE, Kellingray S, Stuart B, Coggon D, Dieppe PA. Risk factors for the incidence and progression of radiographic knee osteoarthritis. Arthritis Rheum. 2000;43:995–1000.
3. Silverwood V, Blagojevic-Bucknall M, Jinks C, Jordan JL, Protheroe J, Jordan KP. Current evidence on risk factors for knee osteoarthritis in older adults: a systematic review and meta-analysis. Osteoarthr Cartil. 2015;23:507–15.
4. Weinstein AM, Rome BN, Reichmann WM, Collins JE, Burbine SA, Thornhill TS, Wright J, Katz JN, Losina E. Estimating the burden of total knee replacement in the United States. J Bone Joint Surg Am. 2013;95:385–92.
5. Niu J, Zhang YQ, Torner J, Nevitt M, Lewis CE, Aliabadi P, Sack B, Clancy M, Sharma L, Felson DT. Is obesity a risk factor for progressive radiographic knee osteoarthritis? Arthritis Rheum. 2009;61:329–35.
6. Bedson J, Croft PR. The discordance between clinical and radiographic knee osteoarthritis: a systematic search and summary of the literature. BMC Musculoskelet Disord. 2008;9:116.
7. Chapple CM, Nicholson H, Baxter GD, Abbott JH. Patient characteristics that predict progression of knee osteoarthritis: a systematic review of prognostic studies. Arthritis Care Res (Hoboken). 2011;63:1115–25.
8. Riddle DL, Kong X, Jiranek WA. Factors associated with rapid progression to knee arthroplasty: complete analysis of three-year data from the osteoarthritis initiative. Joint Bone Spine. 2012;79:298–303.
9. Raynauld JP, Martel-Pelletier J, Haraoui B, Choquette D, Dorais M, Wildi LM, Abram F, Pelletier JP, Canadian Licofelone Study Group. Risk factors predictive of joint replacement in a 2-year multicentre clinical trial in knee osteoarthritis using MRI: results from over 6 years of observation. Ann Rheum Dis. 2011;70:1382–8.
10. Roemer FW, Kwoh CK, Hannon MJ, Hunter DJ, Eckstein F, Wang Z, Boudreau RM, John MR, Nevitt MC, Guermazi A. Can structural joint damage measured with MR imaging be used to predict knee replacement in the following year? Radiology. 2015;274:810–20.
11. Scher C, Craig J, Nelson F. Bone marrow edema in the knee in osteoarthrosis and association with total knee arthroplasty within a three-year follow-up. Skelet Radiol. 2008;37:609–17.
12. Tanamas SK, Wluka AE, Pelletier JP, Pelletier JM, Abram F, Berry PA, Wang Y, Jones G, Cicuttini FM. Bone marrow lesions in people with knee osteoarthritis predict progression of disease and joint replacement: a longitudinal study. Rheumatology (Oxford). 2010;49:2413–9.
13. Felson DT, McLaughlin S, Goggins J, LaValley MP, Gale ME, Totterman S, Li W, Hill C, Gale D. Bone marrow edema and its relation to progression of knee osteoarthritis. Ann Intern Med. 2003;139(5 Pt 1):330–6.
14. Edwards MH, Parsons C, Bruyere O, Petit Dop F, Chapurlat R, Roemer FW, Guermazi A, Zaim S, Genant H, Reginster JY, Dennison EM, Cooper C, SEKOIA Study Group. High Kellgren-Lawrence grade and bone marrow lesions predict worsening rates of radiographic joint space narrowing; the SEKOIA study. J Rheumatol. 2016;43:657–65.

15. Jorgensen A, Stengaard-Pedersen K, Simonsen O, Pfeiffer-Jensen M, Eriksen C, Bliddal H, Pedersen NW, Bodtker S, Horslev-Petersen K, Snerum LO, Egund N, Frimer-Larsen H. Intra-articular hyaluronan is without clinical effect in knee osteoarthritis: a multicentre, randomised, placebo-controlled, double-blind study of 337 patients followed for 1 year. Ann Rheum Dis. 2010;69:1097–102.

16. Altman R, Asch E, Bloch D, Bole G, Borenstein D, Brandt K, Christy W, Cooke TD, Greenwald R, Hochberg M. Development of criteria for the classification and reporting of osteoarthritis. Classification of osteoarthritis of the knee. Diagnostic and therapeutic criteria Committee of the American Rheumatism Association. Arthritis Rheum. 1986;29:1039–49.

17. Bellamy N. Western Ontario and McMaster Universities Osteoarthritis Index (WOMAC). 2015. http://www.rheumatology.org/I-Am-A/Rheumatologist/Research/Clinician-Researchers/Western-Ontario-McMaster-Universities-Osteoarthritis-Index-WOMAC. Accessed 08/17 2017.

18. Skou N, Egund N. Patellar position in weight-bearing radiographs compared with non-weight-bearing: significance for the detection of osteoarthritis. Acta Radiol. 2017;58:331–7.

19. Boegard T, Rudling O, Petersson IF, Sanfridsson J, Saxne T, Svensson B, Jonsson K. Postero-anterior radiogram of the knee in weight-bearing and semiflexion. Comparison with MR imaging. Acta Radiol. 1997;38:1063–70.

20. Boegard T, Rudling O, Petersson IF, Sanfridsson J, Saxne T, Svensson B, Jonsson K. Joint-space width in the axial view of the patello-femoral joint. Definitions and comparison with MR imaging. Acta Radiol. 1998;39:24–31.

21. Ahlback S. Osteoarthrosis of the knee. A radiographic investigation. Acta Radiol Diagn (Stockh). 1968;Suppl 277:7–72.

22. Jørgensen A. Knee osteoarthritis hyaluronan treatment, pain modalities and magnetic resonance imaging: ph.D.-thesis. Aarhus, Denmark: Faculty of Health Sciences, University of Aarhus; 2006.

23. Nielsen FK, Egund N, Peters D, Jurik AG. Measurement of bone marrow lesions by MR imaging in knee osteoarthritis using quantitative segmentation methods–a reliability and sensitivity to change analysis. BMC Musculoskelet Disord. 2014;15:447.

24. Guermazi A, Roemer FW, Hayashi D, Crema MD, Niu J, Zhang Y, Marra MD, Katur A, Lynch JA, El-Khoury GY, Baker K, Hughes LB, Nevitt MC, Felson DT. Assessment of synovitis with contrast-enhanced MRI using a whole-joint semiquantitative scoring system in people with, or at high risk of, knee osteoarthritis: the MOST study. Ann Rheum Dis. 2011;70:805–11.

25. Rhodes LA, Grainger AJ, Keenan AM, Thomas C, Emery P, Conaghan PG. The validation of simple scoring methods for evaluating compartment-specific synovitis detected by MRI in knee osteoarthritis. Rheumatology. 2005;44:1569–73.

26. Danish Health Authority. Knee osteoarthritis - national guidelines. 2012. https://sundhedsstyrelsen.dk/da/udgivelser/2012/~/media/CD7B016D7F9C4766A1530172473FD5F2.ashx. Accessed 01/23 2016.

27. Danish Health Authority. Knee osteoarthritis, part 2: Visitation rules and hospital treatment. In: Knæartrose. Del 2: Faglige visitationsretningslinjer. 2011. https://www.sundhed.dk/content/cms/34/75734_kn%C3%A6artrose%2D-del-2-faglige-visitationsretningslinjer.pdf. Accessed 11/15 2016.

28. Oak SR, Ghodadra A, Winalski CS, Miniaci A, Jones MH. Radiographic joint space width is correlated with 4-year clinical outcomes in patients with knee osteoarthritis: data from the osteoarthritis initiative. Osteoarthr Cartil. 2013;21:1185–90.

29. Ayral X, Pickering EH, Woodworth TG, Mackillop N, Dougados M. Synovitis: a potential predictive factor of structural progression of medial tibiofemoral knee osteoarthritis – results of a 1 year longitudinal arthroscopic study in 422 patients. Osteoarthr Cartil. 2005;13:361–7.

30. Felson DT, Chaisson CE, Hill CL, Totterman SM, Gale ME, Skinner KM, Kazis L, Gale DR. The association of bone marrow lesions with pain in knee osteoarthritis. Ann Intern Med. 2001;134:541–9.

31. Barr AJ, Campbell TM, Hopkinson D, Kingsbury SR, Bowes MA, Conaghan PG. A systematic review of the relationship between subchondral bone features, pain and structural pathology in peripheral joint osteoarthritis. Arthritis Res Ther. 2015;17:228.

32. Yusuf E, Kortekaas MC, Watt I, Huizinga TW, Kloppenburg M. Do knee abnormalities visualised on MRI explain knee pain in knee osteoarthritis? A systematic review. Ann Rheum Dis. 2011;70:60–7.

33. Felson D. Association of bone marrow changes with worsening of knee osteoarthritis. Ann Intern Med. 2003;139(5):I33.

34. Conaghan PG, D'Agostino MA, Le Bars M, Baron G, Schmidely N, Wakefield R, Ravaud P, Grassi W, Martin-Mola E, So A, Backhaus M, Malaise M, Emery P,

Dougados M. Clinical and ultrasonographic predictors of joint replacement for knee osteoarthritis: results from a large, 3-year, prospective EULAR study. Ann Rheum Dis. 2010;69:644–7.

35. Bastick AN, Runhaar J, Belo JN, Bierma-Zeinstra SM. Prognostic factors for progression of clinical osteoarthritis of the knee: a systematic review of observational studies. Arthritis Res Ther. 2015;17:152.

36. Holla JF, van der Leeden M, Heymans MW, Roorda LD, Bierma-Zeinstra SM, Boers M, Lems WF, Steultjens MP, Dekker J. Three trajectories of activity limitations in early symptomatic knee osteoarthritis: a 5-year follow-up study. Ann Rheum Dis. 2014;73:1369–75.

18

Effect of local infiltration analgesia, peripheral nerve blocks, general and spinal anesthesia on early functional recovery and pain control in unicompartmental knee arthroplasty

M. T. Berninger[1,2]* (iD), J. Friederichs[2], W. Leidinger[3], P. Augat[4,5], V. Bühren[2], C. Fulghum[1] and W. Reng[1]

Abstract

Background: The aim of the study was to analyze the effect of local infiltration analgesia (LIA), peripheral nerve blocks, general and spinal anesthesia on early functional recovery and pain control in primary unicompartmental knee arthroplasty (UKA).

Methods: Between January 2016 until August 2016, 134 patients underwent primary UKA and were subdivided into four groups according to their concomitant pain and anesthetic procedure with catheter-based techniques of femoral and sciatic nerve block (group GA&FNB, $n = 38$) or epidural catheter (group SP&EPI, $n = 20$) in combination with general anesthesia or spinal anesthesia, respectively, and LIA combined with general anesthesia (group GA&LIA, $n = 46$) or spinal anesthesia (group SP&LIA, $n = 30$). Outcome parameters focused on the evaluation of pain (NRS scores), mobilization, muscle strength and range of motion up to 7 days postoperatively. The cumulative consumption of (rescue) pain medication was analyzed.

Results: The LIA groups revealed significantly lower (about 50%) mean NRS scores (at rest) compared to the catheter-based groups at the day of surgery. In the early postoperative period, the dose of hydromorphone as rescue pain medication was significantly lower (up to 68%) in patients with SP&EPI compared to all other groups. No significant differences could be detected with regard to grade of mobilization, muscle strength and range of motion. However, there seemed to be a trend towards improved mobilization and muscle strength with general anesthesia and LIA, whereof general anesthesia generally tended to ameliorate mobilization.

Conclusions: Except for a significant lower NRS score at rest in the LIA groups at day of surgery, pain relief was comparable in all groups without clinically relevant differences, while the use of opioids was significantly lower in patients with SP&EPI. A clear clinically relevant benefit for LIA in UKA cannot be stated. However, LIA offers a safe and effective treatment option comparable to the well-established conventional procedures.

Keywords: Local infiltration analgesia, Femoral nerve block, Unicompartmental knee arthroplasty, Epidural catheter, General anesthesia, Spinal anesthesia

* Correspondence: Markus.Berninger@bgu-murnau.de
[1]endogap, Joint Replacement Institute, Garmisch-Partenkirchen Medical Center, Auenstr. 6, 82467 Garmisch-Partenkirchen, Germany
[2]Department of Trauma Surgery, BG Trauma Center Murnau, Prof.-Küntscher Str. 8, 82418 Murnau, Germany
Full list of author information is available at the end of the article

Background

Anteromedial knee osteoarthritis is a distinct clinicopathological entity which often leads to disabling pain and limitation of range of motion [1]. If conservative treatment fails, unicompartmental knee arthroplasty (UKA) is a good treatment option achieving good-to-excellent results and a 10-year survivorship up to 96% [2]. Compared with total knee arthroplasty (TKA), benefits of UKA include joint and bone preservation by replacing only one compartment and preservation of the other intact weight-bearing compartment as well as the anterior and posterior cruciate ligaments. This contributes to reducing intraoperative blood loss and postoperative pain for early rehabilitation. The unicompartmental implants are less bulky and allow for almost normal knee kinematics. All in all, UKA allows patients a faster return to a more functional level than TKA [3–5]. However, although unicompartmental arthroplasty with a minimally invasive technique results in less operative trauma, moderate to severe pain postoperatively remains a common problem, which restricts early mobilization and functional recovery.

Along with UKA, minimally invasive surgery became more and more popular in the early 1990s [6]. Besides a more soft tissue sparing surgical approach, minimally invasive surgery includes a faster recovery with a greater range of motion and less peri- and postoperative pain. This, however, also requires improvements in the postoperative care of physical therapy, the anesthetic techniques and postoperative pain management being significant contributors to an accelerated recovery and pain-free result. This led to the introduction of a perioperative multimodal approach to pain management including modified analgesic techniques of peripheral and epidural nerve blocks and local intraarticular injections [7]. Catheter-based techniques as femoral nerve blocks (FNB) usually result in a sufficient pain relief [8]. However, the catheter themselves limit the patients´ ability to ambulate in the immediate post-operative period until the catheters are removed after some days. Furthermore, the motor impairment, quadriceps weakness, and risk of nerve injury can lead to a longer usage of knee immobilizer or crutches to avoid falls in the intermediate postoperative period [9, 10].

As an alternative method for multimodal, postoperative pain management, local infiltration analgesia (LIA) around the soft tissues of the knee joint gained increasing interest in recent years with excellent pain relief and absent muscle weakness [11]. This led to many studies comparing LIA with peripheral nerve blocks showing comparable results with regard to the postoperative pain [12–14] with slight advantages of the LIA technique in the early postoperative period [15, 16]. Data comparing LIA with continuous epidural analgesia are limited and favor LIA over continuous epidural analgesia [17–19]. However, all these studies have in common, that they are performed with patients who have received a TKA.

In literature, there are only a few trials, which described the LIA technique in UKA. In preliminary trials, Beard et al. [20] and Reilley et al. [21] tested the LIA technique in unicompartmental arthroplasty and presented promising results in terms of patient satisfaction and pain relief. Essving et al. showed a significantly shorter median hospital stay, lower postoperative pain (at rest and with movement) within the first day and lower morphine consumption in the LIA group compared to a control group which received saline instead [22]. However, the LIA mixture or saline was injected both intraoperatively and 21 h postoperatively via an intraarticular catheter. Therefore, an interpretation of the results is difficult.

In literature, there is no study analyzing the effect of LIA, (peripheral) catheter-based techniques and their combination with general or spinal anesthesia on pain control, mobilization, muscle strength and range of motion for up to 7 days postoperatively in one patient collective of UKA. Therefore, the aim of the study was to analyze the effect of these different peri- and postoperative anesthetic therapies on early functional recovery and pain control in primary UKA.

Methods

Patients

One hundred thirty four patients were treated for medial knee osteoarthritis with UKA between January and August 2016 and were included for this retrospective analysis. The inclusion criterion was primary medial knee osteoarthritis. Patients were excluded if they had significant patellofemoral or lateral osteoarthritis, secondary arthritis due to rheumatoid arthritis or trauma, osteonecrosis or revision surgery. Patient demographics and clinical data are shown in Table 1. Depending on the anesthetic procedure and the peri–/postoperative pain management, patients were divided into 4 groups as follows: 38 patients received general anesthesia in combination with a FNB and sciatic nerve block (GA&FNB), 20 patients spinal anesthesia combined with epidural anesthesia (SP&EPI), 46 patients general anesthesia and LIA (GA&LIA) and 30 patients spinal anesthesia and LIA (SP&LIA).

This study was performed in conformity with the Declaration of Helsinki and was approved by the Ethics Committee of the Bavarian State Chamber of Physicians (ID: 2017–109).

Anesthetic techniques

After induction of general anesthesia, patients allocated to group GA&FNB had a FNB catheter inserted with real-time monitored ultrasound imaging. A total of 20 ml of 0.1% ropivacaine was injected around the

Table 1 Patients demographics and clinical data

	GA&FNB	SP&EPI	GA&LIA	SP&LIA
Patients	$n = 38$	$n = 20$	$n = 46$	$n = 30$
Gender	f = 20; m = 18	f = 12; m = 8	f = 23; m = 23	f = 10; m = 20
Age	68 ± 9.0	70 ± 9.2	68 ± 9.4	69 ± 8.4
Piritramide	OP: $n = 14$ (36.8%): 10.7 mg ± 5.8	OP: n = 2 (10%): 8.3 mg ± 1.1	OP: $n = 29$ (63.0%): 8.1 mg ± 4.5	OP: n = 3 (10.0%): 7.5 mg ± 0.0
	Day 1: n = 4 (10.5%): 9.4 mg ± 3.8	Day 1: -	Day 1: n = 2 (4.4%): 7.5 mg ± 0.0	Day 1: n = 4 (13.3%): 9.4 mg ± 3.8
	Day 2: n = 3 (7.9%): 7.5 mg ± 0.0	Day 2: -	Day 2: -	Day 2: -
Implant fixation	cementless: $n = 20$ (52.6%)	cementless: $n = 11$ (55.0%)	cementless: $n = 23$ (50.0%)	cementless: $n = 16$ (53.3%)
	hybrid $n = 10$ (26.3%)	hybrid $n = 5$ (25.0%)	hybrid $n = 9$ (19.6%)	hybrid n = 5 (16.7%)
	cemented $n = 8$ (21.1%)	cemented n = 4 (20.0%)	cemented n = 14 (30.4%)	cemented n = 9 (30.0%)
Salvage pain management	n = 1 (2.6%)	n = 1 (2.6%)	n = 1 (2.6%)	–
	→PCIA: n = 1	→PCIA: n = 1 →3in1: $n = 1$ →G.A.: n = 1	→3in1: n = 3 →PCIA: n = 1	
LIA	–	–	100 ml	100 ml
Dexamethasone	–	–	15.4 mg ± 3.1	16.6 mg ± 2.1

femoral nerve; additionally ultrasound-guided sciatic nerve block with 20 ml of 0.1% ropivacaine was established as single shot block. Postoperatively, 0.2% ropivacaine was continuously infused at the rate of 3 ml/h for 3 days through the femoral catheter.

In group SP&EPI, a catheter was preoperatively sited at the cranial lumbar vertebrae.

combined with a spinal anesthesia (1 ml of 0.5% bupivacaine and 10 µg sufentanil in the subarachnoid space) in a single needle technique. After recovery from spinal anesthesia under the level L3, an initial 10 ml bolus containing 0.5% bupivacaine, 0.6 µg/ml sufentanil and saline was introduced. Thereafter, patients were self-medicated with a bolus of 4 ml via a patient-controlled epidural anesthesia (PCEA) system with a lockout of 20 min. PCEA was discontinued three days after surgery.

Local infiltration analgesia (LIA)
In the LIA groups, 100 ml of 0.2% ropivacaine without any additional components were intraoperatively administered by the surgeon periarticularly in the soft tissues according to the injection technique popularized by Kerr and Kohan [11]. During the beginning of the narcosis, 0,2 mg/kg dexamethasone was injected intravenously. All infiltration was done using 25-ml syringes and 10-cm-long 19-G spinal needles. The LIA solution was administered after completion of all femoral and tibial osteotomy steps, immediately before cement fixation of the tibial component. The LIA solution was systematically injected into the tissues around the knee joint according to a standardized protocol: in the medial and lateral tibial and femoral periosteum as well as medial

and lateral posterior articular capsule, and in the subcutaneous tissue, in the Hoffa fat pad and finally intraarticularly after capsular suture.

Surgery
All surgeries were performed by three senior surgeons. Intra-operatively, single-shot cefazolin 2 g (or clindamycin 600 mg in case of incompatibility of penicillin) for infection prophylaxis was given to all patients. The surgeries were performed with a standard minimal invasive midline vertical incision and medial parapatellar approach; the patella was removed laterally but not dislocated or everted. A tourniquet was inflated to 250 mmHg at the beginning of the surgery and deflated after removal of the surgical dressings. In all cases, the Oxford® Partial Knee System (Zimmer Biomet, Warsaw, IN, USA) was used. Implants were fixated cementless, hybrid cemented (cemented tibial and cementless femoral component) or fully cemented depending on bone stock and age (see Table 1). Bone resections and implant insertion were performed according to the manufacturers manual.

Postoperative pain management and care
Postoperative management was identical in all groups. After surgery, every patient was given a peripheral pain medicament (WHO grade I, e.g. paracetamol, metamizole, ibuprofen or diclofenac) for about 2 weeks to relieve pain and low molecular weight heparins subcutaneously for about 2 weeks to prevent deep vein thrombosis. The cumulative doses of rescue analgesia (hydromorphone p.o. or piritramide i.v.) were also registered.

Postoperative physiotherapy was started immediately after surgery in a progressive manner and all patients received physiotherapy daily. A specially trained pain service regularly visited all patients twice a day for the first four postoperative days.

Outcome measures

Self-reported pain scores in terms of numeric rating scores (NRS) at rest and with activity (0 = no pain; 10 = worst pain) from day of surgery until postoperative day 4 were collected and analyzed. For evaluation of functional outcomes, grade of mobilization ranging from values of 1 to 6 according to our institutional grading system of mobilization was analyzed: 1 = bedridden, 2 = sitting, 3 = standing, 4 = walking in room, 5 = walking on the floor, 6 = walking stairs. Furthermore, muscle strength according to the British medical research council (M0/5-M5/5) and passive range of motion (degrees of extension and flexion) were examined. Functional outcomes of mobilization, muscle strength and range of motion were documented daily from pre-operative day until postoperative day 7, respectively. The patients' medical files were also studied for potential analgesic technique-related and surgery-related complications within the first 7 days, such as rates of neurologic events, cardiovascular events, falls, knee joint infections, prosthesis loosening, or revision surgery. All data were collected from the patients' medical records and nurses' observational charts.

Data analysis

Statistical analysis was performed with SPSS statistical software 20.0 (SPSS for Windows, ver. 20.0; SPSS, Chicago, IL, USA). Descriptive statistics were calculated for all variables of interest. Continuous measures such as age were summarized using means and standard deviations whereas categorical measures were summarized using counts and percentages.

The Kruskal-Wallis test was used for analysis of one nominal variable and one ranked variable. In a further detailed analysis, post-hoc comparisons of factor-level combinations were conducted by use of Mann-Whitney-U test, depending on previous (overall) significance testing. In this explorative study, no adjustment of the alpha-error level was conducted.

Results

Baseline characteristics of patients were comparable among all groups (Table 1). No patient suffered from chronic pain in daily life with use of opioids prior to the surgery. Approximately 50% of the implants were fixated cementless while the other 50% included hybrid cemented (cemented tibial and cementless femoral component) or fully cemented implant fixation.

Pain exacerbation after surgery due to insufficient pain relief (NRS > 7) with the current anesthetic technique led to another analgesic technique. In GA&FNB, one patient received a patient-controlled intravenous analgesia (PCIA) with an initial bolus of 4 mg piritramide followed by an optional bolus of 2 mg piritramide with a lockout of 10 min. In SP&EPI, 3 patients (15.0%) were converted to PCIA ($n = 1$), secondary application of a FNB (n = 1) and to general anesthesia ($n = 1$). In GA&LIA, 4 patients (8.7%) were changed to FNB ($n = 3$) and PCIA (n = 1). These patients were excluded from analysis. In SP&LIA, a modification of anesthetic regime was not necessary for any patient. No analgesic technique-related and surgery-related complication was encountered in any group within the first postoperative 7 days. At the day of surgery, the demand for piritramide was significantly higher (51% vs. 10%; $p < 0.05$) in groups with general anesthesia compared to spinal anesthesia. All LIA patients received 100 ml of the LIA mixture with 15.4 mg ± 3.1 (GA&LIA) and 16.6 mg ± 2.1 (SP&LIA) dexamethasone, respectively.

Pain

At the day of surgery, the NRS scores at rest of the LIA groups were statistically significant lower (GA&LIA: 1.0 ± 1.0; SP&LIA: 0.8 ± 1.3) compared to the catheter-based groups (GA&FNB: 1.9 ± 2.2; SP&EPI: 1.7 ± 1.2; $p < 0.05$) (Fig. 1). At any further time point, the NRS scores did not show any significant differences ($p > 0.05$). The values of the LIA groups slightly increased at day 1 while the catheter-based groups showed almost constant pain values at the day of surgery and day 1. Afterwards, a gradual reduction of pain values was detectable.

The development of the NRS scores with activity was comparable among groups (p > 0.05) (Fig. 1). In comparison with the NRS scores at rest, SP&EPI showed an almost constant pain score during these days. The NRS value of GA&LIA was the lowest of all groups at the day of surgery (2.2 ± 1.2); however, the pain nearly doubled at postoperative day 1 (4.1 ± 2.2) to diminish again at day 2 (3.0 ± 1.9), which was similar in SP&LIA (day 1: 3.9 ± 2.2; day 2: 3.1 ± 1.4).

At the day of surgery as well as at postoperative days 1, 2 and 3, the doses of hydromorphone were on average 38 to 68% lower in SP&EPI compared to all other groups ($p < 0.05$) (Fig. 2). The dose of hydromorphone seemed to slightly increase in all groups on postoperative day 1 in order to gradually fall afterwards.

Mobilization

Upon analyzing the grade of mobilization, no significant differences among the groups at any time point were observed (Fig. 3). All patients with general anesthesia were able to stand up (values≥3) at the day of surgery (GA&FNB:

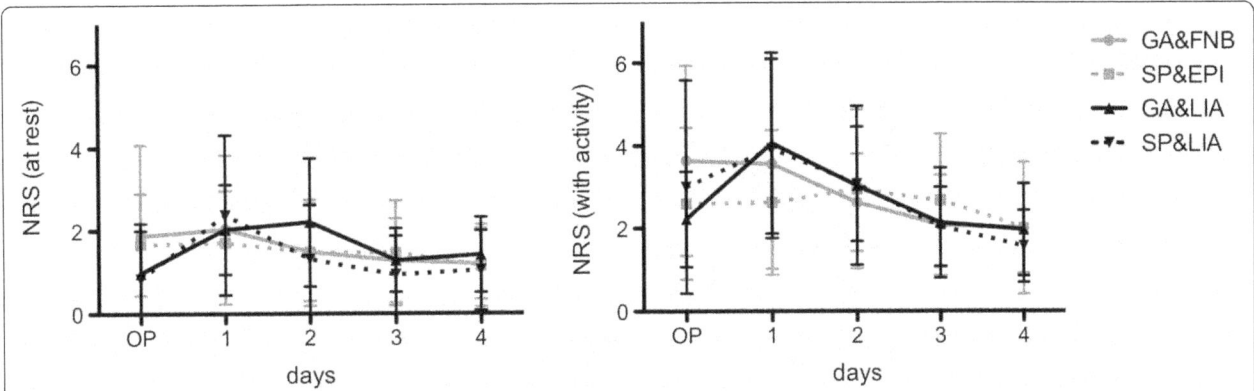

Fig. 1 Numeric Rating Scores at rest (left) and with activity (right) are presented for day of surgery (OP) and postoperative days 1 to 4

3.0 ± 1.3; GA&LIA: 3.2 ± 1.0) while patients with spinal anesthesia showed non-significantly (p = 0.121) lower values (SP&EPI: 1.8 ± 1.0; SP&LIA: 2.7 ± 1.0) and reached full standing as recently as on postoperative day 1. From day 2 on, all patients were able to walk in the room or even on the floor (values≥4) and the slight differences in mobilization among the groups were diminished. Overall, GA&LIA still tended to achieve a slightly accelerated and earlier mobilization compared to all other groups, particularly at the day of surgery with on average 21% higher grade of mobilization while at later time points this trend diminished to about 6% (p > 0.05).

Muscle strength
There were no significant differences (p > 0.05) among the groups with respect to muscle strength (M0/5-M5/5) (Fig. 4). At the day of surgery, all patients showed reduced strength and the knee joint could only be moved without examiner's resistance (GA&FNB: 3.1 ± 0.7; SP&EPI: 3.0 ± 0; GA&LIA: 3.6 ± 0.9; SP&LIA: 3.2 ± 1.0). From day 3 on, muscle strength increased daily and the

knee joint could be moved against resistance (values> 4 in all groups). GA&LIA seemed to show ameliorated muscle strength in the early postoperative period. Afterwards, the spinal anesthesia groups revealed comparably higher values (p > 0.05).

Range of motion
The mean range of motion (flexion and extension of the knee joint) was similar within the groups (Fig. 5). At the day of surgery, the LIA groups showed a non-significantly improved flexion (GA&LIA: 64.4° ± 38.2° and SP&LIA: 50.8° ± 19.6°) compared to the catheter-based groups (GA/FNB: 45.7° ± 11.3° and SP&EPI: 40.0° ± 0°). Afterwards, these slight differences diminished and the flexion gradually increased while extension decreased. Considering all groups, all patients reached 80° of flexion at day 5.

Discussion
In recent years, several studies described the benefit of LIA as an alternative analgesic procedure in TKA [15, 16, 23, 24]; studies in UKA are rare [20–22]. While

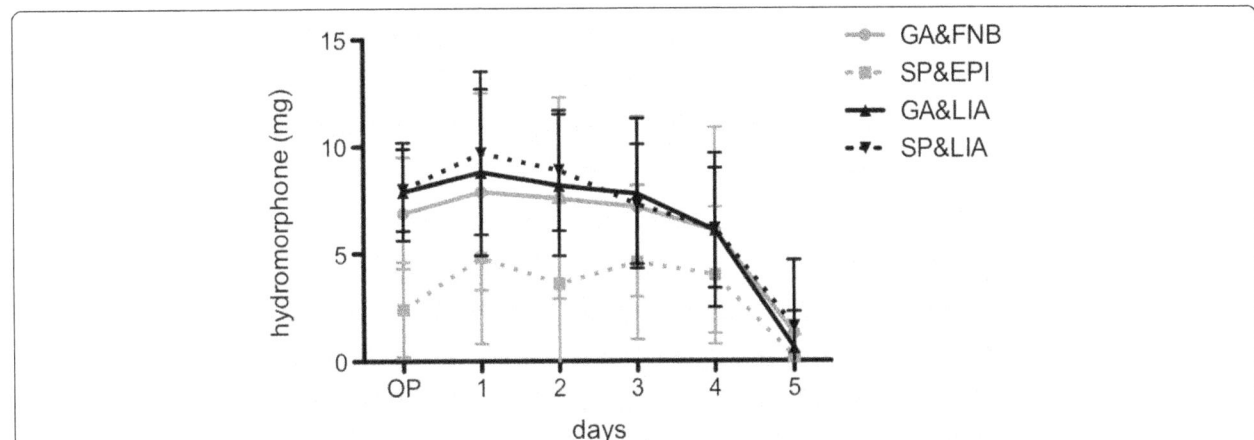

Fig. 2 The cumulative dose of hydromorphone (in mg) for all groups at day of surgery until postoperative days 4 is shown

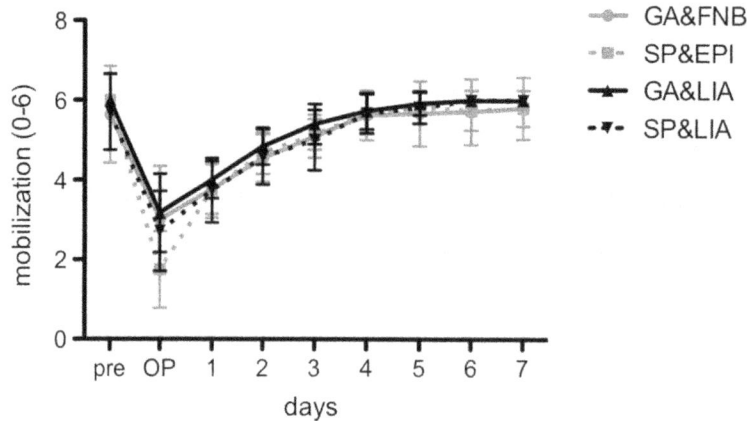

Fig. 3 The grade of mobilization (0 to 6) revealed a gradual increase after surgery until postoperative day 7

Beard et al. [20] and Reilley et al. [21] revealed encouraging results of patient satisfaction and pain relief, Essving et al. particularly showed lower postoperative pain at rest and with movement within the first day and lower morphine consumption in the LIA group [22]. The authors compared the results to a control group, which received saline. However, both were injected intraoperatively and, additionally, 21 h postoperatively via an intraarticular catheter.

At the day of surgery, the LIA technique revealed about 50% lower mean NRS values at rest (0.9 ± 0.1) compared to the catheter-based groups (1.8 ± 0.1). However, even when being statistically significant these findings are not clinically relevant because the differences are too marginal to reach a clinical impact. At postoperative day 1, pain values of NRS scores with activity in LIA with general or spinal anesthesia, respectively, nearly doubled to decrease again at day 2 indicating a pain exacerbation at day 1. A slight increase of the dose of hydromorphone was also visible at day 1. However, the results of the significant differences in the

dose of hydromorphone in patients with SP&EPI within the early postoperative days may be very well of clinical relevance; alone by the not negligible side effects including nausea, dizziness and constipation [25], which can restrict early mobilization, particularly in elderly patients. In the early postoperative period, the dose of hydromorphone was the lowest (up to 68%) in SP&EPI compared to all others. This is a clear advantage of this analgesic treatment in UKA in our patient collective. In a study analyzing fast-track recovery by use of general and spinal anesthesia, Munk et al. described a high level of pain during the first postoperative night and the next day [26]. At the day after surgery, patients needed 10 mg opioid (oxycodone), which was comparable with our result with mean hydromorphone of 9.3 mg at postoperative day 1 in the LIA groups. It is questionable if patients with this high need of opioid usage should be discharged at day after surgery as performed in the study of Munk. The authors, however, also stated that due to this high level of pain and use of strong opioids in the initial period after surgery, there is no recommendation

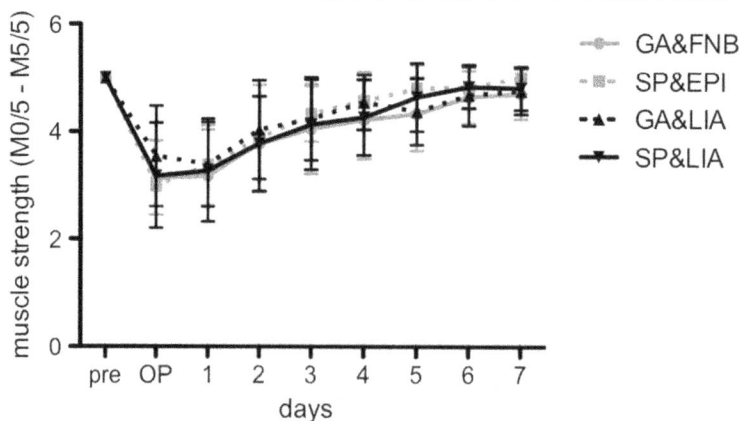

Fig. 4 The grade of muscle strength according to the British medical research council (M0/5-M5/5) after surgery until postoperative day 7 is shown

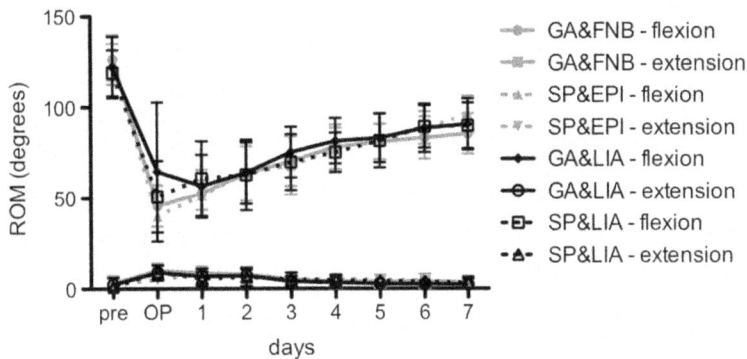

Fig. 5 Degrees of range of motion (flexion and extension) of all groups from preoperative day to postoperative day 7 are presented

for UKA in an outpatient procedure unless perioperative analgesia is improved. The use of opioids need a strict surveillance and we therefore strongly do not support a discharge before opioids have been decreased significantly.

Interestingly, we did not find any significant differences in terms of mobilization, muscle strength or range of motion. It is well known, that UKA resulted in improved and faster postoperative knee function compared to TKA [3–5]. The effect of changing perioperative analgesic strategies in UKA might be too small to further improve these functional outcome parameters. Our results only showed a trend towards improved mobilization and muscle strength with the combination of general anesthesia and LIA, whereof general anesthesia generally tended to ameliorate mobilization. An advantage of general anesthesia in terms of functional parameters compared to spinal anesthesia is not surprising since the continuous epidural infiltration of anesthetics for three days, of course, affects muscle strength and thereby, decreases function.

Finally, it is up to the treating surgeon to choose a procedure, which is individually and thoroughly adapted to the patient. It is important to obtain a detailed medical history and clinical examination upon meeting the patient including analysis of the individual sense of pain and knee function. It has to be considered individually whether the advantage of spinal anesthesia and epidural catheter in terms of comparably lower dose of opioids predominantly exceeds the slightly poorer function. Patients with good preoperative knee function and muscle strength may physically and mentally benefit from decreased pain postoperatively by use of spinal anesthesia; while patients who predominantly suffer from functional restrictions rather than chronic knee pain might be more satisfied with LIA.

Originally, Kerr and Kohan described the LIA mixture as a combination of ropivacaine 2 mg/ml, ketorolac 30 mg and adrenaline 10 mg/ml that is infiltrated in different layers of the joint in volumes of 150–170 ml for TKA [11]. However, in subsequent years different

mixtures, containing among others opioids and steroids, non-steroidal anti-inflammatory drugs, morphine, and epinephrine have been used in addition to local anesthetics without reaching a consensus on a certain dose or drug combination [27–31]. As local anesthetics both bupivacaine and ropivacaine are regularly used for LIA in clinic. Thereby, ropivacaine offers a long-acting profile with reduced cardiotoxicity compared to bupivacaine and intrinsic vasoconstrictor properties [32].

In the present study, we only used 100 ml of 0.2% ropivacaine for infiltration for several reasons. In knee arthroplasty, chondrolysis due to injected local anesthetics is mainly of concern after UKA, since there is still healthy cartilage remaining in the joint. With numerous studies demonstrating chondrotoxicity of local anesthetics in human and animal joints, it is very important to understand the molecular mechanisms and clinical effects of these medications on chondrocytes including decreased cell metabolism, increased apoptosis, necrosis and morphologic tissue degeneration and thereby, the risk for early osteoarthritis [33–36].

The chondrotoxic effects occur dose- and time-dependent [37–39]. In literature, there is no study that could show a significant chondrotoxic effect with low concentrations of bupivacaine (0.0625%) or ropivacaine (0.1 and 0.2%) [33]. Higher concentrations, however, led to a significant chondrocyte cell death [40–42]. Piper et al. compared the in vitro toxicity of bupivacaine and ropivacaine in human articular chondrocytes and showed that 0.5% ropivacaine is significantly less toxic than 0.5% bupivacaine in both intact human articular cartilage and chondrocyte culture [35]. In the study of Grishko et al., exposure of primary human chondrocytes to single-dose ropivacaine (0.5 and 0.2%) did not affect chondrocyte viability after 24 h [41]. However, after 5 days, a significant decrease of viable cells at all concentrations of lidocaine, bupivacaine, and ropivacaine analyzed, were detected, except for 0.2% ropivacaine. In UKA, Essving et al. also did not see any clinical evidence of chondrolysis during the

6 months of follow up after LIA with high-dose ropivacaine (400 mg) [43]. In terms of clinical use, we conclude in accordance with the current literature that ropivacaine at very low concentrations should be preferably used over bupivacaine [33].

Furthermore, a direct linear relationship of increasing cell death with increasing duration of exposure has been described in prior studies [38, 44, 45]. Long-term exposure is promoted by continuous intraarticular application of local anesthetics. Several studies described the continuous LIA in order to prolong its effect by use of e.g. infusion pumps [46, 47]. The results are varying: In a randomized double-blind study, Ali et al. did not show any clinically relevant effect on VAS pain, analgesic consumption, range of motion or length of hospital stay with continuous intraarticular analgesia after TKA [48]. However, a higher risk of wound-healing complications including deep infections was described [48, 49]. In another study comparing single-injection and continuous LIA, continuous infiltration resulted in prolonged superior analgesia and was associated with better functional recovery and patient satisfaction [50]. In terms of accelerated chondrotoxicity and risk for infection after prolonged exposure, we recommend avoiding using continuous infiltration or even additional single shots after some hours.

There are some limitations that pertain to that study. Due to its retrospective design, the study was not blinded or randomized, which may have introduced reporting bias. Furthermore, the choice of anesthesia by the patient might have induced some selection bias, although the group characteristics appeared to be identical among the four groups. Although it was a retrospective investigation, the strengths of the study include a large number of patients managed according to clear inclusion and exclusion criteria. The surgical and anesthetic procedures followed a consistent standard-treatment protocol in the same hospital by the same surgeons with extensive surgical experience in the treatment of UKA and its concomitant analgesic procedures.

Conclusions

In conclusion, the findings from this study suggest a slight but clinically not relevant advantage of the LIA groups in the early postoperative period in terms of mobilization, muscle strength and range of motion. In general, pain relief was similar in all groups, with exception of a significant lower NRS score at rest in the LIA groups at day of surgery. The use of rescue pain medication was significantly lower in patients with SP&EPI. A clear clinically relevant benefit for LIA in UKA can not be stated. Preoperative information including knee function and pain status should be considered for each patient individually before choosing a multimodal perioperative analgesia protocol. In UKA, infiltration of a local anesthetic offers a safe and effective treatment option comparable to the well-established conventional procedures.

Abbreviations
FNB: femoral nerve block; GA&FNB: General anesthesia and femoral nerve block (+sciatic nerve block); GA&LIA: General anesthesia and local infiltration analgesia; LIA: local infiltration analgesia; NRS: Numeric rating scale; OP: Operation (day of surgery); PCIA: Patient-controlled intravenous analgesia; SNB: Sciatic nerve block; SP&EPI: Spinal anesthesia and epidural catheter; SP&LIA: Spinal anesthesia and local infiltration analgesia; TKA: Total knee arthroplasty; UKA: Unicompartmental knee arthroplasty

Acknowledgments
The authors thank the research assistants (Steffen Klingbeil and Dr. Isabella Klöpfer-Krämer), Christa Gerhäußer and the whole (pain) nursing staff as well as the physiotherapy department for their support.

Authors' contributions
MTB, JF, PA and WR drafted the manuscript and contributed to the acquisition of data, analysis, and interpretation of data. PA helped with the statistical analysis of the data. MTB, WL and CF participated in conception, design and coordination. WR and VB supervised the whole study and helped to finalize the manuscript. All authors read and approved the final manuscript.

Consent for publication
Not applicable.

Competing interests
The authors declare that they have no competing interests.

Author details
[1]endogap, Joint Replacement Institute, Garmisch-Partenkirchen Medical Center, Auenstr. 6, 82467 Garmisch-Partenkirchen, Germany. [2]Department of Trauma Surgery, BG Trauma Center Murnau, Prof.-Küntscher Str. 8, 82418 Murnau, Germany. [3]Department of Anesthesiology and Intensive Care, Garmisch-Partenkirchen Medical Center, Auenstr. 6, 82467 Garmisch-Partenkirchen, Germany. [4]Institute of Biomechanics, BG Trauma Center Murnau, Prof.-Küntscher Str. 8, 82418 Murnau, Germany. [5]Institute of Biomechanics, Paracelsus Medical University, Strubergasse 21, 5020 Salzburg, Austria.

References
1.   White SH, Ludkowski PF, Goodfellow JW. Anteromedial osteoarthritis of the knee. J Bone Joint Surg Br. 1991;73(4):582–6.

2. Pandit H, Jenkins C, Gill HS, Barker K, Dodd CA, Murray DW. Minimally invasive Oxford phase 3 unicompartmental knee replacement: results of 1000 cases. J Bone Joint Surg Br. 2011;93(2):198–204.

3. Lombardi AV Jr, Berend KR, Walter CA, Aziz-Jacobo J, Cheney NA. Is recovery faster for mobile-bearing unicompartmental than total knee arthroplasty? Clin Orthop Relat Res. 2009;467(6):1450–7.

4. Walton NP, Jahromi I, Lewis PL, Dobson PJ, Angel KR, Campbell DG. Patient-perceived outcomes and return to sport and work: TKA versus mini-incision unicompartmental knee arthroplasty. J Knee Surg. 2006;19(2):112–6.

5. Liddle AD, Judge A, Pandit H, Murray DW. Adverse outcomes after total and unicompartmental knee replacement in 101,330 matched patients: a study of data from the National Joint Registry for England and Wales. Lancet. 2014;384(9952):1437–45.

6. Repicci JA, Eberle RW. Minimally invasive surgical technique for unicondylar knee arthroplasty. J South Orthop Assoc. 1999;8(1):20–7. discussion 27

7. Tria AJ, Scuderi GR. Minimally invasive knee arthroplasty: an overview. World J Orthop. 2015;6(10):804–11.

8. Chan EY, Fransen M, Parker DA, Assam PN, Chua N. Femoral nerve blocks for acute postoperative pain after knee replacement surgery. Cochrane Database Syst Rev. 2014;5:CD009941.

9. Ilfeld BM, Duke KB, Donohue MC. The association between lower extremity continuous peripheral nerve blocks and patient falls after knee and hip arthroplasty. Anesth Analg. 2010;111(6):1552–4.

10. Pelt CE, Anderson AW, Anderson MB, Van Dine C, Peters CL. Postoperative falls after total knee arthroplasty in patients with a femoral nerve catheter: can we reduce the incidence? J Arthroplast. 2014;29(6):1154–7.

11. Kerr DR, Kohan L. Local infiltration analgesia: a technique for the control of acute postoperative pain following knee and hip surgery: a case study of 325 patients. Acta Orthop. 2008;79(2):174–83.

12. Emerson RH Jr, Barrington JW, Olugbode O, Lovald S, Watson H, Ong K. Femoral nerve block versus long-acting wound infiltration in Total knee arthroplasty. Orthopedics. 2016;39(3):e449–55.

13. Albrecht E, Guyen O, Jacot-Guillarmod A, Kirkham KR. The analgesic efficacy of local infiltration analgesia vs femoral nerve block after total knee arthroplasty: a systematic review and meta-analysis. Br J Anaesth. 2016; 116(5):597–609.

14. McDonald DA, Deakin AH, Ellis BM, Robb Y, Howe TE, Kinninmonth AW, Scott NB. The technique of delivery of peri-operative analgesia does not affect the rehabilitation or outcomes following total knee arthroplasty. Bone Joint J. 2016;98-B(9):1189–96.

15. Yun XD, Yin XL, Jiang J, Teng YJ, Dong HT, An LP, Xia YY. Local infiltration analgesia versus femoral nerve block in total knee arthroplasty: a meta-analysis. Orthop Traumatol Surg Res. 2015;101(5):565–9.

16. Moghtadaei M, Farahini H, Faiz SH, Mokarami F, Safari S. Pain Management for Total Knee Arthroplasty: single-injection femoral nerve block versus local infiltration analgesia. Iran Red Crescent Med J. 2014;16(1):e13247.

17. Spreng UJ, Dahl V, Hjall A, Fagerland MW, Raeder J. High-volume local infiltration analgesia combined with intravenous or local ketorolac +morphine compared with epidural analgesia after total knee arthroplasty. Br J Anaesth. 2010;105(5):675–82.

18. Andersen KV, Bak M, Christensen BV, Harazuk J, Pedersen NA, Soballe K. A randomized, controlled trial comparing local infiltration analgesia with epidural infusion for total knee arthroplasty. Acta Orthop. 2010;81(5):606–10.

19. Binici Bedir E, Kurtulmus T, Basyigit S, Bakir U, Saglam N, Saka G. A comparison of epidural analgesia and local infiltration analgesia methods in pain control following total knee arthroplasty. Acta Orthop Traumatol Turc. 2014;48(1):73–9.

20. Beard DJ, Murray DW, Rees JL, Price AJ, Dodd CA. Accelerated recovery for unicompartmental knee replacement–a feasibility study. Knee. 2002;9(3):221–4.

21. Reilly KA, Beard DJ, Barker KL, Dodd CA, Price AJ, Murray DW. Efficacy of an accelerated recovery protocol for Oxford unicompartmental knee arthroplasty–a randomised controlled trial. Knee. 2005;12(5):351–7.

22. Essving P, Axelsson K, Kjellberg J, Wallgren O, Gupta A, Lundin A. Reduced hospital stay, morphine consumption, and pain intensity with local infiltration analgesia after unicompartmental knee arthroplasty. Acta Orthop. 2009;80(2):213–9.

23. Andersen LO, Husted H, Kristensen BB, Otte KS, Gaarn-Larsen L, Kehlet H. Analgesic efficacy of subcutaneous local anaesthetic wound infiltration in bilateral knee arthroplasty: a randomised, placebo-controlled, double-blind trial. Acta Anaesthesiol Scand. 2010;54(5):543–8.

24. Niemelainen M, Kalliovalkama J, Aho AJ, Moilanen T, Eskelinen A. Single periarticular local infiltration analgesia reduces opiate consumption until 48

hours after total knee arthroplasty. A randomized placebo-controlled trial involving 56 patients. Acta Orthop. 2014;85(6):614–9.

25. Benyamin R, Trescot AM, Datta S, Buenaventura R, Adlaka R, Sehgal N, Glaser SE, Vallejo R. Opioid complications and side effects. Pain Physician. 2008; 11(2):S105–20.

26. Munk S, Dalsgaard J, Bjerggaard K, Andersen I, Hansen TB, Kehlet H. Early recovery after fast-track Oxford unicompartmental knee arthroplasty. 35 patients with minimal invasive surgery. Acta Orthop. 2012;83(1):41–5.

27. Christensen CP, Jacobs CA, Jennings HR. Effect of periarticular corticosteroid injections during total knee arthroplasty. A double-blind randomized trial. J Bone Joint Surg Am. 2009;91(11):2550–5.

28. Joo JH, Park JW, Kim JS, Kim YH. Is intra-articular multimodal drug injection effective in pain management after total knee arthroplasty? A randomized, double-blinded, prospective study. J Arthroplasty. 2011;26(7):1095–9.

29. Pang HN, Lo NN, Yang KY, Chong HC, Yeo SJ. Peri-articular steroid injection improves the outcome after unicondylar knee replacement: a prospective, randomised controlled trial with a two-year follow-up. J Bone Joint Surg Br. 2008;90(6):738–44.

30. Ng YC, Lo NN, Yang KY, Chia SL, Chong HC, Yeo SJ. Effects of periarticular steroid injection on knee function and the inflammatory response following Unicondylar knee arthroplasty. Knee Surg Sports Traumatol Arthrosc. 2011;19(1):60–5.

31. McCarthy D, Iohom G. Local infiltration analgesia for postoperative pain control following Total hip arthroplasty: a systematic review. Anesthesiol Res Pract. 2012;2012:709531.

32. Fenten MG, Bakker SM, Touw DJ, van den Bemt BJ, Scheffer GJ, Heesterbeek PJ, Stienstra R. Pharmacokinetics of 400 mg ropivacaine after periarticular local infiltration analgesia for total knee arthroplasty. Acta Anaesthesiol Scand. 2017;61(3):338–45.

33. Kreuz PC, Steinwachs M, Angele P. Single-dose local anesthetics exhibit a type-, dose-, and time-dependent chondrotoxic effect on chondrocytes and cartilage: a systematic review of the current literature. Knee Surg Sports Traumatol Arthrosc. 2017;26(3):819–30.

34. Breu A, Scheidhammer I, Kujat R, Graf B, Angele P. Local anesthetic cytotoxicity on human mesenchymal stem cells during chondrogenic differentiation. Knee Surg Sports Traumatol Arthrosc. 2015;23(4):937–45.

35. Piper SL, Kim HT. Comparison of ropivacaine and bupivacaine toxicity in human articular chondrocytes. J Bone Joint Surg Am. 2008;90(5):986–91.

36. Anderson SL, Buchko JZ, Taillon MR, Ernst MA. Chondrolysis of the glenohumeral joint after infusion of bupivacaine through an intra-articular pain pump catheter: a report of 18 cases. Arthroscopy. 2010;26(4):451–61.

37. Chu CR, Coyle CH, Chu CT, Szczodry M, Seshadri V, Karpie JC, Cieslak KM, Pringle EK. In vivo effects of single intra-articular injection of 0.5% bupivacaine on articular cartilage. J Bone Joint Surg Am. 2010;92(3):599–608.

38. Chu CR, Izzo NJ, Papas NE, Fu FH. In vitro exposure to 0.5% bupivacaine is cytotoxic to bovine articular chondrocytes. Arthroscopy. 2006;22(7):693–9.

39. Dragoo JL, Korotkova T, Kim HJ, Jagadish A. Chondrotoxicity of low pH, epinephrine, and preservatives found in local anesthetics containing epinephrine. Am J Sports Med. 2010;38(6):1154–9.

40. Chu CR, Izzo NJ, Coyle CH, Papas NE, Logar A. The in vitro effects of bupivacaine on articular chondrocytes. J Bone Joint Surg Br. 2008;90(6):814–20.

41. Grishko V, Xu M, Wilson G, AWt P. Apoptosis and mitochondrial dysfunction in human chondrocytes following exposure to lidocaine, bupivacaine, and ropivacaine. J Bone Joint Surg Am. 2010;92(3):609–18.

42. Breu A, Rosenmeier K, Kujat R, Angele P, Zink W. The cytotoxicity of bupivacaine, ropivacaine, and mepivacaine on human chondrocytes and cartilage. Anesth Analg. 2013;117(2):514–22.

43. Essving P, Axelsson K, Otterborg L, Spannar H, Gupta A, Magnuson A, Lundin A. Minimally invasive surgery did not improve outcome compared to conventional surgery following unicompartmental knee arthroplasty using local infiltration analgesia: a randomized controlled trial with 40 patients. Acta Orthop. 2012;83(6):634–41.

44. Anz A, Smith MJ, Stoker A, Linville C, Markway H, Branson K, Cook JL. The effect of bupivacaine and morphine in a coculture model of diarthrodial joints. Arthroscopy. 2009;25(3):225–31.

45. Lo IK, Sciore P, Chung M, Liang S, Boorman RB, Thornton GM, Rattner JB, Muldrew K. Local anesthetics induce chondrocyte death in bovine articular cartilage disks in a dose- and duration-dependent manner. Arthroscopy. 2009;25(7):707–15.

46. Rasmussen S, Kramhoft MU, Sperling KP, Pedersen JH. Increased flexion and reduced hospital stay with continuous intraarticular morphine and ropivacaine after primary total knee replacement: open intervention study of efficacy and safety in 154 patients. Acta Orthop Scand. 2004;75(5):606–9.

47. Keijsers R, van den Bekerom M, van Delft R, van Lotten M, Rademakers M, Nolte PA. Continuous local infiltration analgesia after TKA: a meta-analysis. J Knee Surg. 2016;29(4):310–21.

48. Ali A, Sundberg M, Hansson U, Malmvik J, Flivik G. Doubtful effect of continuous intraarticular analgesia after total knee arthroplasty: a randomized double-blind study of 200 patients. Acta Orthop. 2015;86(3):373–7.

49. Sun XL, Zhao ZH, Ma JX, Li FB, Li YJ, Meng XM, Ma XL. Continuous local infiltration analgesia for pain control after Total knee arthroplasty: a meta-analysis of randomized controlled trials. Medicine (Baltimore). 2015;94(45):e2005.

50. Zhang S, Wang F, Lu ZD, Li YP, Zhang L, Jin QH. Effect of single-injection versus continuous local infiltration analgesia after total knee arthroplasty: a randomized, double-blind, placebo-controlled study. J Int Med Res. 2011; 39(4):1369–80.

19

Comparison of oral versus intra-articular tranexamic acid in enhanced-recovery primary total knee arthroplasty without tourniquet application

Duan Wang[1†], Hui Zhu[2,3†], Wei-Kun Meng[1†], Hao-Yang Wang[1†], Ze-Yu Luo[1], Fu-Xing Pei[1], Qi Li[1*] and Zong-Ke Zhou[1*] (ID)

Abstract

Background: Although randomized controlled trials have confirmed oral tranexamic acid (TXA) can provide similar blood-sparing efficacy compared with intravenous (IV) TXA in total knee arthroplasty (TKA), some concerns do remain about thromboembolic events after such systemic administration. Many studies have confirmed that intra-articular (IA) application of TXA can show similar blood-saving efficacy with minimal levels of systemic absorption compared with IV TXA. However, it remains unclear whether the efficacy and safety of oral TXA administration is equal to or less than that of IA administration in TKA without the use of a tourniquet and drain. Thus, this study was to verify non-inferior efficacy and safety of oral TXA compared with IA TXA in primary TKA.

Methods: A double-blind, randomized, controlled trial was performed to compare three oral doses of TXA (2 g of TXA 2 h before incision, and 1 g of TXA 6 and 12 h after surgery, respectively) with IA TXA (3 g of TXA in 100 mL of saline solution). One hundred forty-seven patients scheduled for TKA were randomized to one of the two interventions. The primary outcome was total blood loss. The secondary outcomes included reduction of hemoglobin concentration, clinical outcomes, blood coagulation values, thromboembolic complications, and transfusion rates.

Results: The mean total blood loss was 788.8 mL in the oral TXA group compared with 872.4 mL in the IA TXA group, with no statistical significance ($p > 0.05$). There were no significant differences in reduction of hemoglobin level, blood coagulation level, and clinical outcomes. The transfusion rates were 4% in oral group and 5% IA group, respectively. Also, no significant differences were identified in thromboembolic complications.

Conclusion: Oral TXA according to the described protocol demonstrated non-inferiority for primary TKA, with no safety concerns and a greatly reduced cost, compared with the IA TXA. This randomized controlled trial supports the oral administration of TXA in TKA.

Keywords: Total knee arthroplasty, Tranexamic acid, Oral, Intra-articular, Blood loss

* Correspondence: liqimm@yahoo.com; zongkehx@163.com
†Equal contributors
[1]Department of Orthopedics, West China Hospital/West China School of Medicine, Sichuan University, 37# Wuhou Guoxue road, Chengdu 610041, People's Republic of China
Full list of author information is available at the end of the article

Background

Total knee arthroplasty (TKA) is viewed as one of the most successful orthopedic surgeries that relieves pain and improves function but is associated with excessive perioperative blood loss that might lead to anemia and blood transfusions [1–4]. Allogeneic transfusion may result in several undesirable adverse events, but not limited to, including infection, heart failure, immunologic reaction, and myocardial infarction, and as a consequence involve increased morbidity and mortality and additional health care costs [5–7]. Based on a multimodal fast-track methodology at many institutions, numerous blood-saving strategies have been suggested to successfully reduce surgery-related blood loss and minimize the risk of post-operative transfusions, such as perioperative blood salvage, autologous blood transfusion, intraoperative hypotensive anesthesia, application of cryotherapy, and use of pharmacologic antifibrinolytics such as tranexamic acid (TXA) [8–11].

Tranexamic acid, an antifibrynolitic medication, can prevent plasminogen activation by blocking the lysine binding site of plasminogen and inhibiting the formation of plasmin, and thereby promote coagulation process [12, 13]. TXA can be administered either intravenously (IV), intra-articularly (IA), or orally in the setting of TKA. Oral administration of TXA had beneficial blood- and cost-saving effect, as confirmed in some randomized controlled trials (RCT), and also reduced transfusions without increased risk of thromboembolic complications compared with placebo [14, 15]. Compared with oral or IV TXA, the IA TXA can provide a maximum concentration of TXA in surgical site and thereby a prolonged effect to reduce postoperative blood loss, but is associated with minimal levels of systemic absorption, which may increase safety. Numerous RCTs [16, 17] and meta-analyses [18] showed valid evidence favoring the effectiveness of various dosages and routes of IA TXA in reducing blood loss and allogeneic transfusion requirements in TKA.

Recent RCTs and meta-analyses have confirmed that oral TXA showed similar blood-sparing efficacy, at a greatly reduced cost, compared with IV TXA [19, 20]. In spite of the potential cost-saving benefits of oral TXA, some concerns do remain about thromboembolic events after systemic administration in high-risk patient population [21]. Many studies have shown the non-inferiority of IV compared with IA TXA regarding both blood loss and thromboembolic complications. However, it is not clear whether the efficacy and safety of oral TXA administration is equal to or less than that of IA administration.

Some studies have demonstrated that tourniquet application may be related to tissue damage, severe thigh pain, and delayed rehabilitation [22]. In view of these concerns, no tourniquet was applied during the perioperative period at our institution. However, little is known about the efficacy and safety of oral TXA when tourniquet is not utilized in the knee surgery due to the substantial effect of tourniquet-related fibrinolysis on bleeding kinetics.

Thus, the objective of our prospective, randomized, double-blind trial, conducted in an enhanced recovery setup at our institution, was to assess the efficacy and safety of oral administration of three doses compared with IA administration of 3 g of TXA in the setting of primary unilateral TKA, with no tourniquet and drain. We hypothesized that oral TXA would be equivalent to IA TXA in reduction of blood loss and transfusion rates without increased thromboembolic complications.

Methods

This prospective, randomized, controlled trial was conducted at the Department of Joint Surgery in West China Hospital, Sichuan University. Approval was obtained from the Institutional Review Board (No. 201302008), and written informed consent and research authorizations were obtained from all participants. The trial was registered in the Chinese Clinical Trial Registry.

From March 2017 to July 2017, all patients (aged 18 year. or older) with primary osteoarthritis scheduled for undergoing primary unilateral TKA were screened for enrollment. All perioperative managements of TKA were conducted based on a well-established multimodal enhanced-recovery strategy, including pain control [23–25], blood-saving management [26], and early ambulation [27, 28]. The exclusion criteria were secondary osteoarthritis (i.e., rheumatoid arthritis, post-septic arthritis, or post-traumatic arthritis), known allergy to TXA, a history of arterial or venous thromboembolic disease (i.e. deep venous thrombosis (DVT), or pulmonary embolism (PE)), a history of major comorbidities (i.e. severe pulmonary disease, severe renal insufficiency, hepatic failure, or severe stroke), a history of hematopoietic or hemophilia disease or active cancer, participation in another clinical trial during the last year, pregnancy, and alcohol abuse. These patients were also excluded if they declined to participate or refused to receive blood products.

Drug delivery and randomization

Recruited patients were randomly allocated to two interventions (i.e., oral-only or IA-only) based on a computer-generated randomization list, which was generated with use of Randomization.com.

Group 1 (Oral TXA)

Patients assigned to the oral group were given 2 g of TXA (4 tablets of 500 mg) by oral bolus appropriately 2 h before incision as a preoperative dose. A postoperative dose of 1 g was repeated 6 and 12 h after surgery, respectively. Also, the oral group received 100 mL of an intra-articular placebo solution (0.9% physiological saline solution) in a manner identical to the application of the solution in the IA group. Pharmacokinetic studies have demonstrated that 2 g oral TXA reaches therapeutic concentration after approximately 2 to 3 h and remains above the effective levels required to inhibit fibrinolysis for 6 h after such administration [29, 30].

Group 2 (IA TXA)

Patients assigned to the IA group received an intra-articular administration of 100 mL of saline solution containing a 3-g dose of TXA on the basis of previous study of topical TXA in TKA showing high efficacy for reducing bleeding with this dosage and concentration [31, 32]. IA TXA (topical study medication) was administered at two points: (1) after all components were cemented and the joint was thoroughly irrigated, half of the volume (50 mL of 1.5-g TXA solution) was applied to soak the open joint surface and tissue for 5 min; (2) the remaining half was administered using a needle to achieve tissue impregnation before capsule closure [32–34]. Moreover, the IA group was given small placebo pills identical to oral TXA in appearance and quantity with no active ingredient 2 h before incision, 6 and 12 h after surgery, respectively.

One experienced surgeon responsible for all TKAs enrolled all participants, and a research personnel prepared patient assignments, recorded practical details, and rechecked inclusion criteria. The randomization assignments were placed into sequentially numbered opaque sealed envelopes, which were kept by a certificated research pharmacist and were inaccessible through the investigation period. An envelope was opened on the day of surgery, and the appropriate study drug and placebo preparations were handled by a research pharmacist not involved in patient care to ensure identical appearance. The patients, trial participants, anesthesiologists, health-care providers, outcome assessors, and data collectors were blinded to allocation and route of TXA administration.

Surgical procedure and postoperative management

At our institution, the TKA was conducted by the same senior orthopaedic surgeons (XXX) under general anesthesia with a standard medial para-patellar approach. All prostheses were fixed with cement, and patella resurface technique was used in all patients.

All patients received multimodal analgesia consisting of adductor canal block (20 ml 5 g/L ropivacaine and 0.1 mg adrenaline) and periarticular multi-site infiltration (70 ml 2.5 g/L ropivacaine and 0.1 mg adrenaline) [35]. All patients also received a standard analgesia peri-

operatively [23, 24]. Antibiotic prophylaxis in all patients was administered intravenously with 1.5 g of cefuroxime half an hour before surgery. No tourniquet, intra-articular drainage tube, and pressure dressing were applied in all patients in our center [22, 36].

Thromboembolism prophylaxis protocol

Patients received standard venous thromboembolism prophylaxis based on individualized protocol at our institution, including mechanical and chemical thromboprophylaxis. Patients were given mechanical prophylaxis by means of an intermittent inflatable lower-extremity pump on the first day after surgery, and lower-extremity strength training and passive and active physiotherapy were performed under the supervision of a professional physiotherapist. As for chemical prophylaxis, patients received low-molecular-weight heparin (LMWH; Clexane, Sanofi-Aventis, France, 2000 IU) administered subcutaneously appropriately 8 h after surgery and followed by 4000 IU once a day during hospitalization. Rivaroxaban (10 mg, Xarelto, Bayer, Germany) was administered orally once a day for 10 days after discharge if no bleeding events occurred.

Blood transfusion protocol

Participants were also received the standard practice of blood-transfusion protocol at our institution, which was consistent with the perioperative transfusion guidelines of Chinese Ministry of Health. Blood products were transfused if the hemoglobin (Hb) level < 7 g/dL in patients who were asymptomatic or if Hb level between 7 and 10 g/dL in patients who developed concomitant clinical symptoms (anemia or myocardial ischemia) or if a patient with any anemia-related organ dysfunction regardless of Hb level.

Outcome assessment

The primary outcome was total blood loss. The estimated blood loss was calculated applying the Gross formula [37]:

$$\text{Total blood loss} = \text{PBV} \times (\text{Hct}_{pre}\text{-Hct}_{post})/\text{Hct}_{ave}$$

$\text{PBV} = \text{patient's blood volume}$

$\text{Hct}_{pre} = \text{the initial preoperative hematocrit level}$

$\text{Hct}_{post} = \text{the hematocrit level on the morning of the third postoperative day}$

$\text{Hct}_{ave} = \text{the average of the Hct}_{pre}\text{and Hct}_{post}$

The PBV was assessed according to the formula of Nadler et al. [38]: PBV (mL) = k_1 x height (m) + k_2 x weight (kg) + k_3; $k_1 = 0.3669$, $k_2 = 0.03219$, and $k_3 = 0.6041$ for men; $k_1 = 0.3561$, $k_2 = 0.03308$, and $k_3 =$

0:1833 for women. If a reinfusion or an allogenic transfusion was performed, the volume transfused should be added when calculating total blood loss.

The secondary outcomes included Hb, reduction of Hb concentration, platelet concentration, hematocrit level, coagulation indicators (i.e., prothrombin time, INR, and activated partial thromboplastin time) on postoperative day (POD) 3, intraoperative blood loss, and amount of IV fluid. Other secondary outcomes included postoperative knee function (i.e., the range of motion and knee society score), pain score, quality of recovery (QoR-40), thromboembolic complications occurring ≤90 days after surgery, surgical site infection, transfusion rates, and number of blood units transfused.

The active range of motion of the knee was measured with use of a standard clinical goniometer in a supine position before surgery and on postoperative 1 and 3 months. By the measurement of suction drains contents and surgical swabs, intraoperative blood loss was evaluated [39]. All patients were examined daily for clinical symptoms of DVT during hospitalization, including pain, swelling, tenderness, superficial venous engorgement, and Homan's sign in the thigh or calf. When a patient has any suspicious symptom of DVT, a diagnostic Doppler ultrasound was applied to exam both lower limbs by senior ultrasound physicians. All adverse events or thromboembolic events were noted during the first 3 months after surgery. All patients stayed in the hospital for a minimum of 3 days.

Statistical analysis and sample size
Statistical analyses were conducted using SPSS version 21.0 (SPSS Inc., Chicago, IL) software. A two-sided P value of less than 0.05 was generally considered statistically significant for all comparisons. Distributions of demographic data, preoperative laboratory values, surgical data, knee function, and primary and secondary outcomes were assessed with summary statistics, including measures of central tendency (means and standard deviations) for quantitative data and numbers and percentages for qualitative data. Independent t-test was used to compare the normal distributed continuous variables, and Wilcoxon Mann-Whitney U test was applied to analyze non-normal distribution or unequal variables. Pearson chi-square test or Fisher exact test was used for categorical variables. Before breaking the randomization code, statistical analyses were conducted blinded.

The sample-size estimate was determined based on the primary outcome (i.e., total blood loss). Sample size calculations were based on the preliminary data with a minimally clinically important difference of 10% and standard deviation of 15%. Based on the abovementioned information, sample size estimation at an alpha (two-tailed) of 0.05, power of 90%, and standard effect

size of 0.65 indicated that 62 patients were required for each arm. To compensate for the expected dropouts (20%), 75 patients per group were planned to include in this study.

Results
Patients
During the recruitment period from March 2017 to July 2017, 238 patients scheduled for primary unilateral total knee arthroplasty were screened for participation in this trial. Eighty-eight patients were excluded for the following reasons: 71 were ineligible based on our exclusion criteria, 10 declined to participate, and 7 were excluded due to other reasons (Fig. 1). The remaining 150 patients underwent randomization to receive study medication. Three patients were excluded for various reasons, including tourniquet application (one patient), medication preparation not in time (one), and withdrew consent (one) (Fig. 1). Thus, a total of 147 eligible participants were randomized to receive oral TXA ($n = 74$) or IA TXA ($n = 73$) (Fig. 1). No patient was lost or excluded during follow-up.

No significant differences between the allocation groups were identified with respect to demographic data, perioperative surgical characteristics (i.e., operative time), preoperative Caprini score (i.e., evaluation of individual patients regarding DVT risk based on comorbidities and risk factors), knee function, and preoperative laboratory values (Table 1). The follow-up duration was 3 months after surgery.

Blood loss
The calculated blood loss (primary outcome) was 788.8 ± 349.1 mL in the oral group and 872.4 ± 393.1 mL in the IA group ($p = 0.21$), respectively, with no significant difference between the groups. Regarding secondary outcomes, there were no differences among the groups in terms of intraoperative blood loss ($p = 0.58$) and the amount of postoperative IV fluids on POD 1 ($p = 0.18$) (Table 2).

Postoperative laboratory values and clinical outcomes
No difference between the two groups was identified regarding Hb level on POD 3 (Table 2). The reduction of Hb concentration on POD 3 were 2.2 ± 0.9 g/dL in oral group and 2.4 ± 1.1 g/dL in IA group, respectively, with no significant difference. Also, there were no significant differences identified regarding platelet count, hematocrit level, and red blood cell count on POD 3. In addition, blood coagulation values were similar between the groups (Table 2).

Moreover, knee range of motion and knee society score were similar among the groups at the three-month follow-up visit. Similarly, postoperative pain declined

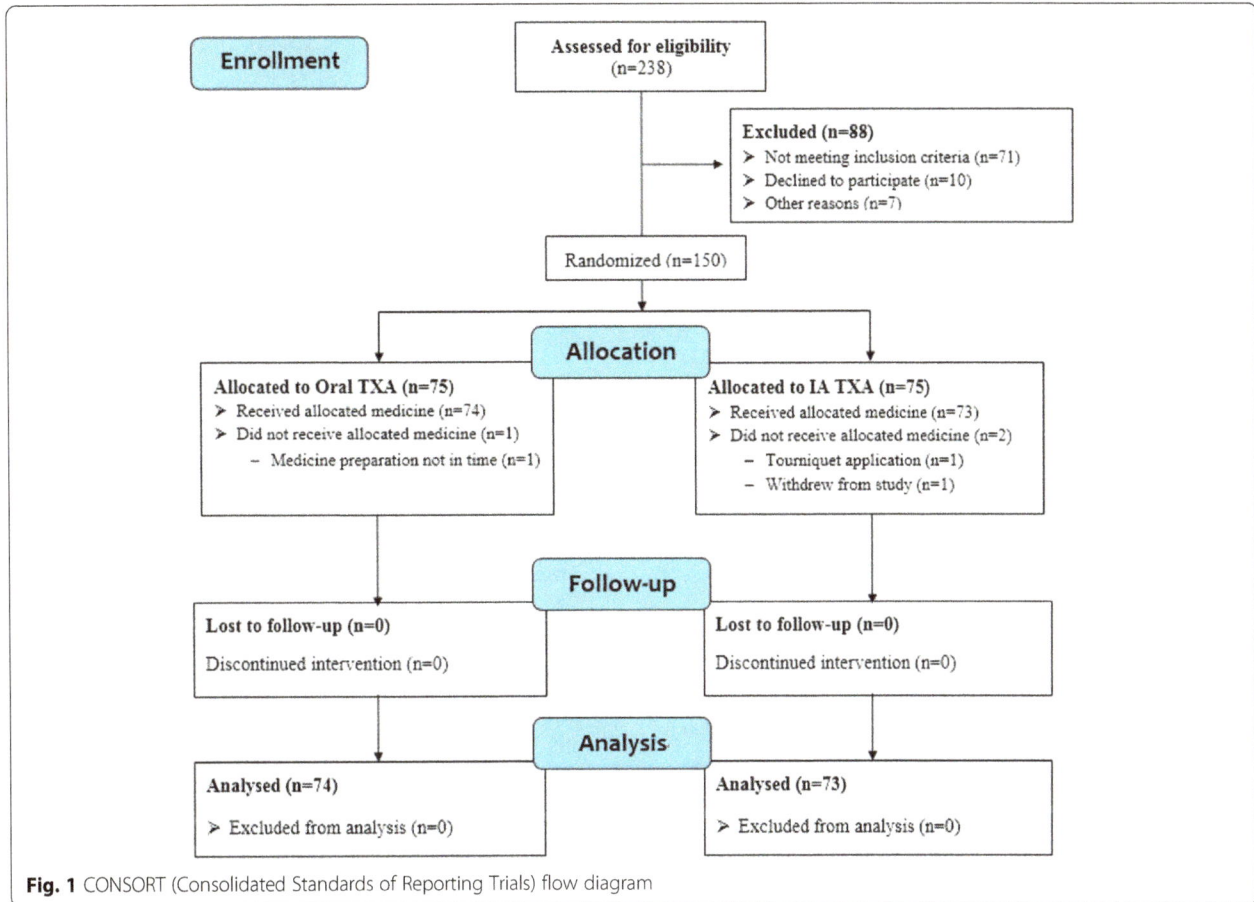

Fig. 1 CONSORT (Consolidated Standards of Reporting Trials) flow diagram

daily, and no significant difference was identified between groups at any follow-up point. When it comes to the severity of the knee swelling, there was no difference between the two groups at postoperative 3 months (Table 3). Moreover, there was no significant intergroup difference observed in terms of QoR-40 during the three-month follow-up visit (Table 3).

Blood transfusion

Seven patients received allogeneic blood transfusion due to a postoperative Hb of < 7 g/dL, including three patients (4%) in the oral group and four (5%) in the IA group, respectively, with no significant intergroup difference (Table 2). Similarly, there were no differences regarding the number of units of packed red blood cells transfused.

Postoperative complications

The frequency of DVT manifestations did not differ significantly between the groups, with 1 case in the oral group compared with none in the IA group. The diagnose of DVT was confirmed by Doppler ultrasonography. However, this patient showed no DVT-related clinical symptoms and was discharged and managed

based on usual thromboembolism prophylaxis protocol at our center (Table 3) [32]. No superficial vein thrombosis and PE occurred in any group.

There was one adverse event in the oral group (one wound secretion) and one in the IA group (one hematoma), respectively. No superficial infection and gastric hemorrhage occurred in either group during follow-up period (Table 3). All adverse events were successfully resolved.

Discussion

Growing evidence has confirmed the efficacy of TXA in reducing blood loss and transfusion rates without additional complications [40, 41]. Our study was conducted to compare the effects of TXA regarding blood loss, transfusions and thromboembolic events, when administered by oral or IA modalities. Several studies have compared the efficacy of oral and IV use of TXA in TKA, while others have compared the effects of IA and IV administration of TXA. The present study was the first that we know of to evaluate two different routes of TXA administration in an enhanced-recovery setup without use of a tourniquet

Table 1 Baseline characteristics and intraoperative demographics

Variable	Oral TXA Group (N = 74)	IA TXA Group (N = 73)	P value
Patient characteristics			
Age (yr)[b]	65.0 ± 13.1	63.6 ± 11.5	0.51
Gender (Female/Male)[a]	58/16	56/17	0.81
Height (m)[b]	1.5 ± 0.1	1.6 ± 0.2	0.39
Weight (kg)[b]	62.7 ± 11.1	62.9 ± 9.5	0.86
BMI (kg/m^2)[b]	25.1 ± 4.1	25.5 ± 3.7	0.52
Operated side (L/R)[a]	47/27	43/30	0.57
ASA classification[a]			
I	15 (20%)	12 (16%)	0.79
II	49 (66%)	52 (71%)	
III	10 (14%))	9 (10%)	
IV	0 (0%)	0 (0%)	
Caprini score[b]	8.2 ± 0.9	8.4 ± 1.1	0.27
Preop. laboratory values[b]			
Hemoglobin (g/dL)	13.4 ± 1.3	13.3 ± 1.2	0.40
Hematocrit (L/L)	0.41 ± 0.04	0.41 ± 0.03	0.24
Platelet count (×10^9/L)	186.4 ± 53.6	189.1 ± 59.1	0.77
Red blood cell count (× 10^{12}/L)	4.5 ± 0.5	4.5 ± 0.4	0.63
Prothrombin time (s)	11.6 ± 0.8	11.7 ± 0.9	0.39
INR	0.9 ± 0.1	1.0 ± 0.2	0.28
APTT (s)	27.2 ± 3.4	28.2 ± 3.6	0.10
Fibrinogen (g/L)	2.9 ± 0.9	2.7 ± 0.8	0.24
D-Dimer (mg/L)	0.93 ± 1.1	1.0 ± 1.3	0.68
FDP (mg/L)	2.7 ± 2.1	2.9 ± 3.4	0.62
Surgical data			
Operative time (min)[b]	66.3 ± 10.9	68.8 ± 12.8	0.20
Preop. knee function[b]			
QoR-40	150.9 ± 4.5	151.1 ± 5.0	0.89
ROM	91.8 ± 16.9	92.1 ± 16.7	0.91
KSS	45.4 ± 10.3	47.1 ± 9.5	0.29
Pain VAS score	6.1 ± 1.8	6.2 ± 1.9	0.78
Knee circumference (cm)[b]			
Upper pole of patella	39.9 ± 3.7	39.7 ± 5.5	0.89
Lower pole of patella	33.2 ± 2.8	32.7 ± 3.1	0.25

ASA American Society of Anesthesiologists, *PBV* patient's blood volume, *INR* international normalized ratio, *APTT* activated partial thromboplastin time, *FDP* fibrinogen degradation product, *ROM* range of motion, *KSS* knee society score, *BMI* body mass index, *VAS* visual analogue scale, *QoR-40* quality of recovery-40
[a]Data are presented as number of patients with percentage
[b]Data are presented as Mean ± standard deviation

Table 2 Perioperative outcomes regarding blood loss

Variable	Oral TXA Group	IA TXA Group	P value
Primary outcome			
Total blood loss (mL)[b]	788.8 ± 349.1	872.4 ± 393.1	0.21
Secondary outcomes			
Intro-operative blood loss (mL)[b]	143.1 ± 25.4	145.6 ± 28.7	0.58
Postop. IV fluid amount (mL)[b]	2729.9 ± 366.5	2818.1 ± 419.2	0.18
Blood transfusion (U)[a]	7	9	0.73
Transfusion rate (%)[a]	3 (4%)	4 (5%)	0.69
Postop. laboratory values at 72 h[b]			
Hemoglobin (g/dL)	11.2 ± 1.3	10.9 ± 1.2	0.22
Reduction of hemoglobin (g/dL)	2.2 ± 0.9	2.4 ± 1.1	0.66
Hematocrit (L/L)	0.34 ± 0.04	0.32 ± 0.03	0.20
Red blood cell count (·×10^{12}/L)	3.6 ± 0.4	3.5 ± 0.4	0.37
Platelet count (×10^9/L)	165.8 ± 53.2	162.2 ± 57.7	0.70
Prothrombin time (s)	11.7 ± 1.3	12.0 ± 1.3	0.17
INR	0.9 ± 0.1	0.9 ± 0.6	0.76
APTT (s)	30.8 ± 5.0	31.4 ± 3.8	0.38
Fibrinogen (g/L)	4.5 ± 1.0	4.4 ± 1.3	0.67
D-Dimer (mg/L)	3.4 ± 2.2	3.2 ± 1.9	0.60
FDP (mg/L)	9.2 ± 6.4	9.1 ± 8.0	0.96

TXA tranexamic acid, *INR* international normalized ratio, *APTT* activated partial thromboplastin time, *FDP* fibrinogen degradation product
[a]Data are presented as number of patients with percentage
[b]Data are presented as Mean ± standard deviation

There are several limitations in our study. First, this trial had no placebo group, because the efficacy of TXA has been confirmed in many studies. In addition, the study patients receiving no TXA would be exposed to risks of no beneficial effects of TXA administration, such as reduction in blood loss and the need for transfusions, which may raise ethical issues. Second, we excluded patients undergoing bilateral or revision knee arthroplasty due to much larger blood loss compared with primary TKA; thus, our findings may not be suitable for these patients. Third, the duration of follow-up (3 months) may be short in this study; however, it was adequate to observe associated adverse reactions in three-month follow-up period, as the biological half-life of an intravenous TXA dose is 1.9 to 2.7 h, 90% of which was excreted within 24 h. In addition, blood coagulation concentrations were also monitored for the risk of thrombogenesis postoperatively, which did not differ between groups. The finding was consistent with the previous study [42]. Fourth, no blood analyses were conducted to estimate serum tranexamic acid levels, and thus no

and postoperative drains in TKA. The major finding of this study was that oral administration of three doses of TXA was not inferior to IA administration of 3-g dose with respect to blood loss.

Table 3 Postoperative outcomes regarding complications and knee function

Variable	Oral TXA Group	IA TXA Group	P value
Postop. Complications (%)[a]	2 (2.7%)	1 (1.3%)	0.76
DVT	1	0	0.51
PE	0	0	–
Superficial infection	0	0	–
Hematoma	0	1	0.50
Wound secretion	1	0	0.51
Gastric hemorrhage	0	0	–
Postop. knee function[b]			
QoR-40[b]			
1 M	181.9 ± 5.4	183.4 ± 6.6	0.11
3 M	189.4 ± 5.9	190.1 ± 3.4	0.34
ROM [b]			
1 M	113.9 ± 8.7	112.6 ± 8.2	0.37
3 M	122.4 ± 10.4	124.4 ± 9.13	0.17
Pain score[b]			
POD 1	4.2 ± 2.3	4.5 ± 1.5	0.39
POD 3	2.4 ± 1.4	2.6 ± 1.5	0.37
3 M	1.4 ± 1.1	1.3 ± 1.2	0.71
KSS [b]	84.6 ± 4.8	85.9 ± 7.1	0.18
Knee circumference (cm)[b]			
Upper pole of patella	41.2 ± 3.2	41.8 ± 6.0	0.46
Lower pole of patella	35.5 ± 2.4	36.0 ± 3.2	0.28
All cause 30-day mortality[a]	0	0	–
All cause 90-day readmission[a]	0	0	–

ROM range of motion, QoR-40 quality of life-40, DVT deep vein thrombosis, PE pulmonary embolism, KSS knee society score

[a]Data are presented as number of patients with percentage

[b]Data are presented as Mean ± standard deviation

toxicity-related information can be provided after such TXA administration following TKA. Fifth, some confounding issues, such as complexity of surgical techniques and extent of soft tissue release, may have a substantial effect on the postoperative blood loss. However, these effects may be negligible due to the randomization design.

Tranexamic acid, an antifibrinolytic agent, can inhibit fibrinolysis though competitively inhibiting plasminogen activation and blocking the binding of plasminogen to fibrin and thereby prevent bleeding. At our institution, retrospective studies containing thousands of patients undergoing TKA revealed no increase in thromboembolic events rates [43]. TXA can be administered intravenously, intra-articularly, and orally. However, the majority of prior studies focused on IV or IA modalities of administration in TKA. However, concerns about the safety of IV and oral administration of TXA and the risk of thromboembolic events still remain for high-risk

patient population, who has a history of a thromboembolic event, acute myocardial infarction, or ischemic cerebrovascular accident. In view of these safety concerns, topical application of TXA may be a safer route of administration to reduce postoperative bleeding without increasing the hypercoagulable state associated with knee surgery. IA use of TXA in surgical site can directly target the site of bleeding, achieve surgical hemostasis, and thereby inhibit local activation of fibrinolysis stimulated by surgical site. Also, high topical TXA dose can lead to greater thrombus formation and lower time to vascular occlusion, and result in enhanced microvascular hemostasis with low systemic absorption and less systemic side effects.

However, the dosage and concentration of TXA solution used in topical application show no clear-cut guidelines in studies. Existing data on clinical efficacy and safety of topical TXA administration compared with placebo in TKA have been confirmed in many RCTs with various dosages (1.5 to 3 g) and topical routes of administration (Table 4). Some studies demonstrated that IA delivery of > 2-g TXA can effectively reduce blood loss and transfusion requirements [44]. Moreover, a recent meta-analysis has confirmed that topical administration of > 2-g TXA is a safe and simple alternative for patients with high risk of thromboembolic complications [45]. At our institution, a well-conducted RCT by Yue et al. has demonstrated that a high dose (3 g) of topical TXA appears to represent an effective and safe way to stop bleeding and transfusions [31]. Also, Huang et al. has demonstrated that a regimen with combined topical high-concentration TXA solution (1.5 g TXA diluted in 50 mL normal saline) and 1.5 g of IV TXA was effective in reducing the blood loss. This trial is a continuation of these previous studies, and compares efficacy of topical dose of 3 g of TXA with multiple doses of oral TXA administration.

Data on comparison of the effectiveness of oral TXA administration and placebo on blood loss, reduction of Hb, and transfusions are summarized in Table 4. Although oral application of TXA was effective in reducing blood loss, as also confirmed in a recent meta-analysis [46], to our knowledge, limited research has been conducted on the route of the less expensive oral form of TXA administration in TKA. A 4-armed RCT by Zohar included four treatment groups (i.e., IV TXA, oral TXA, IV plus oral TXA, and placebo) and demonstrated that oral application of TXA (1 g before surgery and repeat every 6 h for the next 18 h) was superior to IV TXA administration due to significant difference in blood savings and ease of oral drug administration [15]. Fillingham et al. performed a RCT containing only 71 patients with the treatment groups of IV TXA and oral TXA. They found that a single gram of oral TXA 2 h

Table 4 Overview of relevant randomized controlled trial regarding Oral and IA administration of TXA compared with placebo in total knee arthroplasty

Authors	Year	Dosing regimens	No. of patients		Reduced blood loss	Reduction of Hb	Increased complications	Reduced transfusion
			TXA	Control				
Oral administration								
Zohar et al.	2004	1 g oral TXA before surgery, 6 h, 12 h, and 18 h	20	20	Significant	NA	NS	Significant
Charoencholvanich et al.	2011	10 mg/kg before deflation; 0.5 g oral TXA for 5 days	50	50	Significant	Significant	NS	Significant
Alipour et al.	2013	1 g oral TXA before surgery, 6 h, 12 h, and 18 h	26	27	Significant	NA	NS	NA
Lee et al.	2017	1 g oral TXA 2 h before surgery, 6 and 12 h	95	95	Significant	Significant	NS	NA
Yuan et al.	2017	20 mg/kg oral TXA 2 h before surgery; 2 g oral TXA 12 h postoperatively	140	140	NA	Significant	NS	NA
IA administration								
Wong et al. (1)	2010	1.5 g/100 mL after cement	33	35	Significant	Significant	NS	NS
Wong et al. (2)	2010	3 g/100 mL after cement	31	35	Significant	Significant	NS	NS
Ishida et al.	2011	2 g/20 mL at closure	50	50	NA	NA	NS	NS
Sa-Ngasoongsong et al.	2011	0.25 g/25 mL at closure	24	24	Significant	Significant	NS	Significant
Onodera et al.	2012	1 g/50 mL after closure	50	50	Significant	Significant	NS	NS
Roy et al.	2012	0.5 g/5 mL	25	25	NA	Significant	NS	NS
Alshryda et al.	2013	1 g/50 mL at closure	79	78	Significant	Significant	NS	Significant
Georgiadis et al.	2013	2 g/75 mL	50	51	Significant	Significant	NS	NS
Sa-Ngasoongsong et al. (1)	2013	0.25 g/25 mL after closure	45	45	Significant	Significant	NS	NS
Sa-Ngasoongsong et al. (2)	2013	0.5 g/25 mL after closure	45	45	Significant	Significant	NS	NS
Martin et al.	2014	2 g/100 mL prior to closure	25	25	NA	Significant	NS	NA
Lin et al.	2015	1 g/20 mL prior to closure	40	40	Significant	Significant	NS	Significant
Wang et al.	2015	0.5 g/10 mL prior to closure	30	30	Significant	Significant	NS	Significant
Yang et al.	2015	0.5 g/20 mL prior to closure	40	40	Significant	Significant	NS	Significant
Maniar et al.	2012	3.0 g/100 mL before deflation for 5 mins	40	40	Significant	NA	NS	NS
Seo et al.	2013	1.5 g/100 mL	50	50	Significant	NS	NS	Significant
Sarzaeem et al. (1)	2014	3.0 g TXA/100 mL before suturing	50	50	NA	NS	NS	NS
Sarzaeem et al. (2)	2014	1.5 g TXA/100 mL after closure	50	50	NA	Significant	NS	NS
Aguilera et al.	2015	1.0 g/10 mL after cement	50	50	Significant	NS	NS	NS
Cavusoglu et al.	2015	2.0 g/100 mL before closure	20	20	NA	NA	NS	NA
Digas et al.	2015	2.0 g TXA after closure	30	30	Significant	NS	NS	NS
Oztas et al.	2015	2.0 g TXA	30	30	Significant	NA	NS	Significant
Drosos et al.	2016	1.0 g/30 mL	30	30	Significant	NS	NS	Significant
Keyhani et al.	2016	1.5 g/50 mL before closure; 1.5 g/50 mL after closure	40	40	Significant	Significant	NS	NS
Tzatzairis et al.	2016	1.0 g/100 mL after closure	40	40	Significant	Significant	NS	Significant
Prakash et al. (1)	2017	3 g/50 ml prior to closure	50	50	NA	NA	NS	NS
Prakash et al. (2)	2017	3 g/50 ml after closure	50	50	NA	NA	NS	NS
Song et al.	2017	3 g/50 ml after closure	50	50	Significant	Significant	NS	NS

Table 4 Overview of relevant randomized controlled trial regarding Oral and IA administration of TXA compared with placebo in total knee arthroplasty (Continued)

Authors	Year	Dosing regimens	No. of patients		Reduced blood loss	Reduction of Hb	Increased complications	Reduced transfusion
			TXA	Control				
Stowers et al.	2017	1.5 g TXA	59	21	Significant	NA	NS	NS
Ugurlu et al.	2017	1.5 g/50 mL before closure; 1.5 g/50 mL after closure	42	41	NA	Significant	NS	NS
Yuan et al.	2017	3 g/60 ml after closure	140	140	NA	Significant	NS	Significant

NA not available, NS not significant

before incision can provide an equivalent reduction in Hb level and blood loss in comparison with IV medicine administration [47]. In spite of the blood-sparing efficacy and potential cost-saving benefits of oral TXA, some concerns do remain about thromboembolic complications after oral administration in high-risk patient population. In addition, a tourniquet and postoperative drain were applied as a standard practice in the abovementioned studies. Thus, it remains unclear whether the efficacy and safety of oral TXA is equal to or less than that of IA TXA in TKA without a tourniquet and drain.

Some drainage-related factors, such as the gradually declining hematocrit in drain output and residual blood in the drain, could have an effect on the accuracy of blood loss measurement [48]. A RCT conducted by Wang et al. [36] demonstrated that the postoperative drainage provided no clear benefits in blood loss, knee function, and early recovery in primary TKA. Moreover, Huang et al. performed a RCT of application of tourniquet in TKA at our institution and reported that tourniquet application may cause muscle damage and delay strength recovery [22]. Also, a recent meta-analysis has confirmed that tourniquet could increase the risk of thromboembolic events [49]. Some RCTs have demonstrated that the lack of tourniquet did not affect the tibial cement mantle thickness [50] and short-term fixation [51]. Thus, the tourniquet and postoperative drain were not applied after surgery routinely. The tourniquet-related fibrinolysis may have a substantial effect on bleeding kinetics, which is related to the assessment of the effect of oral TXA administration when a tourniquet is not utilized in the procedure.

Although our trial had a similar goal of comparing oral and other routes of TXA administration as the above-mentioned studies, we assessed the efficacy of perioperative standardized oral TXA versus IA TXA alone for unilateral TKA, conducted in a fast-track setup, without the use of a tourniquet and postoperative drains. The dosing and timing of oral regimes were based on pharmacokinetic and serum studies, and therapeutic levels can be maintained for approximately 12 h after surgery, which covers the most period of postoperative hyperfibrinolysis. The major finding of our study was that oral TXA

administration provided an equivalent blood-saving benefit when compared with IA administration of 3 g of TXA.

Blood-conservation strategy during "enhanced recovery" knee replacement, as part of multimodal protocol, has substantially affected costs by decreasing the incidence of morbidity and mortality, transfusion-associated complications, and hospital stay. The finding was supported by a retrospective economic analysis of TXA application, which indicated $879 direct savings per joint surgery with use of TXA [52]. Moreover, a retrospective analysis by Irwin et al. [29] contained 2698 patients undergoing total joint arthroplasty and demonstrated that the patients receiving the substituted 2-g oral TXA bolus had a lower risk of blood transfusion, with great cumulative savings (£29,788), when in comparison with 15-mg/kg IV administration. Retrospective clinical and cost-benefit evaluation of IA TXA administration have shown an estimated cost savings of $1500 per patient with decreased transfusion costs [53]. A RCT by Kayupov et al. reported that an appropriate oral dose can save $33 to $94 compared with an equivalent dose depending on the TXA formulation and administration route selected [20]. In China, more than 200,000 primary TKAs were conducted annually. Considering aging population and longer life expectancy, the number of TKAs will increase dramatically over time [54]. Thus, a transition to oral TXA may lead to great cost savings per year for health-care system.

No significant differences identified in transfusion rates and thromboembolic complications (i.e., DVT and PE) in this current study. However, there is substantial evidence supporting the safety of oral and IA application of TXA with no additional thromboembolic complications. In our study, there was no significant differences between the two groups regarding knee function and quality of life, which were tested with use of range of motion, knee society score, pain score, and QoR-40 measures after surgery.

Conclusions

This prospective randomized controlled trial in the setting of total knee arthroplasty using a fast-track protocol, with no tourniquet and postoperative drain, demonstrated that oral administration of TXA (2-g TXA before incision and 1 g TXA every 6 h for 12 h after surgery) provided an equivalent blood-saving benefit compared with 3 g of IA TXA administration with great cost savings and no increased thrombo-embolic events.

Abbreviations
IA: Intra-articular; IV: Intravenous; RCT: Randomized controlled trials; TKA: Total knee arthroplasty; TXA: Tranexamic acid

Acknowledgements
We would like to thank the relevant staff for guidance and assistance for their support and collaboration in our hospital.

Funding
No funding was obtained for this study.

Authors' contributions
ZKZ, FXP, and QL conceived and designed this study; DW, HZ, WKM, and HYW collected the data; DW, HYW, DW, and ZYL performed the statistical analysis; HYW and DW prepared tables 1–4; DW, HYW, and ZYL prepared figure 1; DW, WKM, and HYW wrote the manuscript; DW, QL, HZ, and ZKZ revised this manuscript. All authors reviewed the final manuscript. All authors agree to be accountable for all aspects of the work.

Consent for publication
Not applicable.

Competing interests
The authors declare that they have no competing interests.

Author details
[1]Department of Orthopedics, West China Hospital/West China School of Medicine, Sichuan University, 37# Wuhou Guoxue road, Chengdu 610041, People's Republic of China. [2]Out-patient department, West China Second University Hospital, Sichuan University, Chengdu 610041, People's Republic of China. [3]Key Laboratory of Birth Defects and Related Disease of Woman and Children (Ministry of Education), West China Second University Hospital, Sichuan University, Chengdu 610041, People's Republic of China.

References
1. Bierbaum BE, Callaghan JJ, Galante JO, Rubash HE, Tooms RE, Welch RB. An analysis of blood management in patients having a total hip or knee arthroplasty. J Bone Joint Surg Am. 1999;81(1):2–10.
2. Bong MR, Patel V, Chang E, Issack PS, Hebert R, Di Cesare PE. Risks associated with blood transfusion after total knee arthroplasty. J Arthroplast. 2004;19(3):281–7.
3. Freedman J, Luke K, Monga N, Lincoln S, Koen R, Escobar M, et al. A provincial program of blood conservation: the Ontario Transfusion Coordinators (ONTraC). Transfus Apher Sci. 2005;33(3):343–9.
4. Good L, Peterson E, Lisander B. Tranexamic acid decreases external blood loss but not hidden blood loss in total knee replacement. Br J Anaesth. 2003;90(5):596–9.
5. Blajchman MA, Beckers EA, Dickmeiss E, Lin L, Moore G, Muylle L. Bacterial detection of platelets: current problems and possible resolutions. Transfus Med Rev. 2005;19(4):259–72.

6. Fuller AK, Uglik KM, Savage WJ, Ness PM, King KE. Bacterial culture reduces but does not eliminate the risk of septic transfusion reactions to single-donor platelets. Transfusion. 2009;49(12):2588–93.
7. Kirksey M, Chiu YL, Ma Y, Della Valle AG, Poultsides L, Gerner P, et al. Trends in in-hospital major morbidity and mortality after total joint arthroplasty: United States 1998-2008. Anesth Analg. 2012;115(2):321–7.
8. Leigheb M, Pogliacomi F, Bosetti M, Boccafoschi F, Sabbatini M, Cannas M, et al. Postoperative blood salvage versus allogeneic blood transfusion in total knee and hip arthroplasty: a literature review. Acta Biomed. 2016;87(Suppl 1):6–14.
9. Markert SE. The use of cryotherapy after a total knee replacement: a literature review. Orthop Nurs. 2011;30(1):29–36.
10. Sharrock NE, Salvati EA. Hypotensive epidural anesthesia for total hip arthroplasty: a review. Acta Orthop Scand. 1996;67(1):91–107.
11. Themistoklis T, Theodosia V, Konstantinos K, Georgios DI. Perioperative blood management strategies for patients undergoing total knee replacement: where do we stand now? World J Orthop. 2017;8(6):441–54.
12. Astedt B. Clinical pharmacology of tranexamic acid. Scand J Gastroenterol Suppl. 1987;137:22–5.
13. Okamoto S, Hijikata-Okunomiya A, Wanaka K, Okada Y, Okamoto U. Enzyme-controlling medicines: introduction. Semin Thromb Hemost. 1997;23(6):493–501.
14. Alipour M, Tabari M, Keramati M, Zarmehri AM, Makhmalbaf H. Effectiveness of oral tranexamic acid administration on blood loss after knee artroplasty: a randomized clinical trial. Transfus Apher Sci. 2013;49(3):574–7.
15. Zohar E, Ellis M, Ifrach N, Stern A, Sapir O, Fredman B. The postoperative blood-sparing efficacy of oral versus intravenous tranexamic acid after total knee replacement. Anesth Analg. 2004;99(6):1679–83. table of contents
16. Goyal N, Chen DB, Harris IA, Rowden NJ, Kirsh G, MacDessi SJ. Intravenous vs intra-articular tranexamic acid in total knee arthroplasty: a randomized, double-blind trial. J Arthroplast. 2017;32(1):28–32.
17. Tzatzairis TK, Drosos GI, Kotsios SE, Ververidis AN, Vogiatzaki TD, Kazakos KI. Intravenous vs topical tranexamic acid in total knee arthroplasty without tourniquet application: a randomized controlled study. J Arthroplast. 2016;31(11):2465–70.
18. Sun X, Dong Q, Zhang YG. Intravenous versus topical tranexamic acid in primary total hip replacement: a systemic review and meta-analysis. Int J Surg. 2016;32:10.
19. Luo ZY, Wang HY, Wang D, Zhou K, Pei FX, Zhou ZK. Oral vs intravenous vs topical tranexamic acid in primary hip arthroplasty: a prospective, randomized, double-blind, controlled study. J Arthroplast. 2018;33(3):786–93.
20. Kayupov E, Fillingham YA, Okroj K, Plummer DR, Moric M, Gerlinger TL, et al. Oral and intravenous tranexamic acid are equivalent at reducing blood loss following total hip arthroplasty: a randomized controlled trial. J Bone Joint Surg Am. 2017;99(5):373–8.
21. Wong J, Abrishami A, El Beheiry H, Mahomed NN, Roderick Davey J, Gandhi R, et al. Topical application of tranexamic acid reduces postoperative blood loss in total knee arthroplasty: a randomized, controlled trial. J Bone Joint Surg Am. 2010;92(15):2503–13.
22. Huang ZY, Pei FX, Ma J, Yang J, Zhou ZK, Kang PD, et al. Comparison of three different tourniquet application strategies for minimally invasive total knee arthroplasty: a prospective non-randomized clinical trial. Arch Orthop Trauma Surg. 2014;134(4):561–70.
23. Lei YT, Xu B, Xie XW, Xie JW, Huang Q, Pei FX. The efficacy and safety of two low-dose peri-operative dexamethasone on pain and recovery following total hip arthroplasty: a randomized controlled trial. Int Orthop. 2017;42(3):499–505.
24. Li D, Yang Z, Xie X, Zhao J, Kang P. Adductor canal block provides better performance after total knee arthroplasty compared with femoral nerve block: a systematic review and meta-analysis. Int Orthop. 2015;40(5):925–33.
25. Xu B, Ma J, Huang Q, Huang ZY, Zhang SY, Pei FX. Two doses of low-dose perioperative dexamethasone improve the clinical outcome after total knee arthroplasty: a randomized controlled study. Knee Surg Sports Traumatol Arthrosc. 2017;472(1):169–74.
26. Ma J, Huang Z, Shen B, Pei F. Blood management of staged bilateral total knee arthroplasty in a single hospitalization period. J Orthop Surg Res. 2014;9:116.
27. Wang D, Yang Y, Li Q, Tang SL, Zeng WN, Xu J, et al. Adductor canal block versus femoral nerve block for total knee arthroplasty: a meta-analysis of randomized controlled trials. Sci Rep. 2017;7:40721.
28. Zeng WN, Zhou K, Zhou ZK, Shen B, Yang J, Kang PD, et al. Comparison between drainage and non-drainage after total hip arthroplasty in Chinese subjects. Orthop Surg. 2014;6(1):28–32.

29. Irwin A, Khan SK, Jameson SS, Tate RC, Copeland C, Reed MR. Oral versus intravenous tranexamic acid in enhanced-recovery primary total hip and knee replacement: results of 3000 procedures. Bone Joint J. 2013;95-b(11):1556–61.
30. Pilbrant A, Schannong M, Vessman J. Pharmacokinetics and bioavailability of tranexamic acid. Eur J Clin Pharmacol. 1981;20(1):65–72.
31. Yue C, Kang P, Yang P, Xie J, Pei F. Topical application of tranexamic acid in primary total hip arthroplasty: a randomized double-blind controlled trial. J Arthroplast. 2014;29(12):2452–6.
32. Huang Z, Ma J, Shen B, Pei F. Combination of intravenous and topical application of tranexamic acid in primary total knee arthroplasty: a prospective randomized controlled trial. J Arthroplast. 2014;29(12):2342–6.
33. Gomez-Barrena E, Ortega-Andreu M, Padilla-Eguiluz NG, Perez-Chrzanowska H, Figueredo-Zalve R. Topical intra-articular compared with intravenous tranexamic acid to reduce blood loss in primary total knee replacement: a double-blind, randomized, controlled, noninferiority clinical trial. J Bone Joint Surg Am. 2014;96(23):1937–44.
34. Nielsen CS, Jans O, Orsnes T, Foss NB, Troelsen A, Husted H. Combined intra-articular and intravenous tranexamic acid reduces blood loss in total knee arthroplasty: a randomized, double-blind, placebo-controlled trial. J Bone Joint Surg Am. 2016;98(10):835–41.
35. Li D, Tan Z, Kang P, Shen B, Pei F. Effects of multi-site infiltration analgesia on pain management and early rehabilitation compared with femoral nerve or adductor canal block for patients undergoing total knee arthroplasty: a prospective randomized controlled trial. Int Orthop. 2017;41(1):75–83.
36. Wang D, Xu J, Zeng WN, Zhou K, Xie TH, Chen Z, et al. Closed suction drainage is not associated with faster recovery after total knee arthroplasty: a prospective randomized controlled study of 80 patients. Orthop Surg. 2016;8(2):226–33.
37. Gross JB. Estimating allowable blood loss: corrected for dilution. Anesthesiology. 1983;58(3):277–80.
38. Nadler SB, Hidalgo JH, Bloch T. Prediction of blood volume in normal human adults. Surgery. 1962;51(2):224–32.
39. Zhou K, Wang H, Li J, Wang D, Zhou Z, Pei F. Non-drainage versus drainage in tourniquet-free knee arthroplasty: a prospective trial. ANZ J Surg. 2017;87:1048.
40. Wang CG, Sun ZH, Liu J, Cao JG, Li ZJ. Safety and efficacy of intra-articular tranexamic acid injection without drainage on blood loss in total knee arthroplasty: a randomized clinical trial. Int J Surg. 2015;20:1–7.
41. Yang Y, Lv YM, Ding PJ, Li J, Ying-Ze Z. The reduction in blood loss with intra-articular injection of tranexamic acid in unilateral total knee arthroplasty without operative drains: a randomized controlled trial. Eur J Orthop Surg Traumatol. 2015;25(1):135–9.
42. Jansen AJ, Andreica S, Claeys M, D'Haese J, Camu F, Jochmans K. Use of tranexamic acid for an effective blood conservation strategy after total knee arthroplasty. Br J Anaesth. 1999;83(4):596–601.
43. Xie J, Ma J, Kang P, Zhou Z, Shen B, Yang J, et al. Does tranexamic acid alter the risk of thromboembolism following primary total knee arthroplasty with sequential earlier anticoagulation? A large, single center, prospective cohort study of consecutive cases. Thromb Res. 2015;136(2):234–8.
44. Prakash J, Seon JK, Park YJ, Jin C, Song EK. A randomized control trial to evaluate the effectiveness of intravenous, intra-articular and topical wash regimes of tranexamic acid in primary total knee arthroplasty. J Orthop Surg (Hong Kong). 2017;25(1):2309499017693529.
45. Shin YS, Yoon JR, Lee HN, Park SH, Lee DH. Intravenous versus topical tranexamic acid administration in primary total knee arthroplasty: a meta-analysis. Knee Surg Sports Traumatol Arthrosc. 2016;25(11):3585–595.
46. Zhang LK, Ma JX, Kuang MJ, Zhao J, Wang Y, Lu B, et al. Comparison of oral versus intravenous application of tranexamic acid in total knee and hip arthroplasty: a systematic review and meta-analysis. Int J Surg. 2017;45:77–84.
47. Fillingham YA, Kayupov E, Plummer DR, Moric M, Gerlinger TL, Della Valle CJ. The James A. Rand Young Investigator's Award: a randomized controlled trial of oral and intravenous tranexamic acid in total knee arthroplasty: the same efficacy at lower cost? J Arthroplast. 2016;31(9 Suppl):26–30.
48. Quinn M, Bowe A, Galvin R, Dawson P, O'Byrne J. The use of postoperative suction drainage in total knee arthroplasty: a systematic review. Int Orthop. 2015;39(4):653–8.
49. Zhang W, Li N, Chen S, Tan Y, Al-Aidaros M, Chen L. The effects of a tourniquet used in total knee arthroplasty: a meta-analysis. J Orthop Surg Res. 2014;9(1):13.
50. Pfitzner T, von Roth P, Voerkelius N, Mayr H, Perka C, Hube R. Influence of the tourniquet on tibial cement mantle thickness in primary total knee arthroplasty. Knee Surg Sports Traumatol Arthrosc. 2014;24(1):96–101.
51. Ledin H, Aspenberg P, Good L. Tourniquet use in total knee replacement does not improve fixation, but appears to reduce final range of motion: a randomized RSA study involving 50 patients. Acta Orthop. 2012;83(5):499–503.
52. Gillette BP, Maradit Kremers H, Duncan CM, Smith HM, Trousdale RT, Pagnano MW, et al. Economic impact of tranexamic acid in healthy patients undergoing primary total hip and knee arthroplasty. J Arthroplast. 2013;28(8 Suppl):137–9.
53. Chimento GF, Huff T, Ochsner JL Jr, Meyer M, Brandner L, Babin S. An evaluation of the use of topical tranexamic acid in total knee arthroplasty. J Arthroplast. 2013;28(8 Suppl):74–7.
54. Dai K-R, Li H-W, Yan M-N. Twenty-year accelerated development of artificial joints in China. Chin J Joint Surg. 2015;9(6):691–4.

20

Outcomes and early revision rate after medial unicompartmental knee arthroplasty: prospective results from a non-designer single surgeon

Jonathan R. B. Hutt[1], Avtar Sur[1]*(iD), Hartej Sur[1], Aine Ringrose[1] and Mark S. Rickman[2]

Abstract

Background: This prospective study evaluates outcomes and reoperation rates for unicompartmental knee arthroplasty (UKA) from a single non-designer surgeon using relatively extended criteria of degenerative changes of grade 2 or above in either or both non-operated compartments.

Methods: 187 consecutive medial mobile bearing UKA implants were included after history, clinical assessment and radiological evaluation. 91 patients had extended clinical outcomes. Post-operative assessment included functional scoring with the Oxford Knee Score (OKS) and radiographic review. Survivorship curves were constructed using the life-table method, with 95% confidence intervals calculated using Rothman's equation. Separate endpoints were examined: revision for any reason and revision for confirmed loosening.

Results: The mean follow-up was 3.5 years. The pre-operative OKS improved from a mean of 21.2 to 38.9 (Mann-Whitney U Test, $p = < 0.001$). Twelve Patients required further operations including 9 revisions. No patients developed deep infection and no surviving implants were loose radiographically. Survivorship at 7 years with endpoints of re-operation, revision and aseptic loosening at surgery or radiographically was 88.4% (95% CI 79.6–93.7), 93.1% (95% CI 85.5–96.9) and 97.3% (95% CI 91.2–99.2) respectively. The presence of pre-operative mild contralateral tibiofemoral or any extent of patellofemoral joint degeneration was of no consequence.

Discussion: The indications for UKA are being expanded to include patients with greater deformity, more advanced disease in the patellofemoral joint and even certain features in the lateral compartment indicative of an anteromedial pattern of osteoarthritis (OA). However, much of the supporting literature remains available only from designer centres. This study represents a group of patients with what we believe to be wider indications, along with decisions to treat made on clinical grounds and radiographs alone.

Conclusion: This study shows comparable clinical outcomes of UKA for extended indications from a high volume, high-usage non-designer unit.

Keywords: Unicompartmental, Arthroplasty, Outcomes, Survivorship, Indications

* Correspondence: avtarsur@doctors.org.uk
[1]Department of Trauma and Orthopaedics, St George's University Hospitals
NHS Foundation Trust, London, UK
Full list of author information is available at the end of the article

Background

The Oxford unicompartmental knee arthroplasty (UKA) (Biomet, Warsaw, Indiana) is a well-established implant and reports from the designer centre demonstrate good results for the medial UKA out into the second decade [1] and into the midterm for its lateral counterpart [2]. Whilst the initial indications were relatively narrow, increased experience has led to an expansion of potential inclusion criteria, particularly with regard to the level of deformity and disease presence elsewhere in the knee [3–5]. The performance of the Oxford UKA in the wider orthopaedic community has been variable, with units reporting conflicting results, some equally favourable [6–10], and others less so [11–14]. Much of the concern regarding UKA in general has come from the analysis of registry data. The Australian, the New Zealand and the UK implant registries all report higher revision rates for unicompartmental prostheses [15–17]. There is a debate as to what registry data can reveal about the success of an implant or technique, and analysis of published literature on the subject will be biased by numerous reports from the designing centre [18–20]. As such, reports from surgeons independent of such centres add valuable information on outcomes from the use of implants by the wider orthopaedic community.

Between 2005 and 2013, the senior author implanted 187 consecutive UKAs in 173 patients, a caseload of 23 per year. During the same period, the senior author performed 604 TKAs, and 12 lateral UKAs. 14 bilateral UKA procedures were performed sequentially. This corresponds to a usage of 30% in keeping with recommendations that 30% of a surgeon's total knee arthroplasties should be UKAs to achieve optimum results [7, 21, 22].

The aim of this study was to prospectively evaluate the early outcomes and revision rate from a single high volume non-designer practice of unicompartmental knee replacement as well as the effect of using relatively extended criteria with regards to other compartments in the knee.

Methods

Patients presenting to the senior author with symptomatic knee arthritis are evaluated for their suitability for UKA as follows: The history and clinical examination focuses on presence of isolated unicompartmental knee pain severe enough to justify joint replacement and anterior cruciate ligament (ACL) integrity. Clinical evidence of sagittal instability and the presence of inflammatory disease remain absolute contraindications to UKA. Maximum acceptable pre-operative deformity is 15 degrees of varus that is correctable to neutral and 10 degrees of fixed flexion. No patients have been refused UKA based on BMI. Radiographic evaluation is with standing AP and Rosenberg views along with standard lateral and skyline views. The presence of bone-on-bone contact was considered an indication to proceed with UKA. Stress radiographs and MRI scans are not used. Evidence of mild disease of the contralateral compartment, for example marginal osteophytes, is not considered a contra-indication in the setting of minimal joint space narrowing. Degeneration of the patellofemoral joint (PFJ) is considered irrelevant unless pain is wholly anterior, and specifically worse on stairs than with simple walking. No arthroscopic examinations are performed solely to evaluate the knee for decision-making purposes. For this study, both the patellofemoral and contralateral tibiofemoral compartment were evaluated on pre-operative radiographs according to the Kellgren-Lawrence grading. We considered patients with evidence of degenerative change of grade 2 or above in either or both non-operated compartments to have relatively extended indications for UKA. At surgery, ACL integrity is assessed clinically with examination under anaesthesia (EUA) and direct inspection and the lateral compartment is also directly inspected. Intra-operative findings of patellofemoral joint degeneration, whatever the severity, are not considered a contraindication to UKA. Within the time frame of the study, no patients were converted to TKR based on concerns with ACL integrity at operation. Three patients scheduled for a UKA received a TKA due to significant lateral disease that was not identified on pre-operative radiographs. Surgical technique was per manufacturer guidelines using a tourniquet and thigh support with free draping of the limb using the described minimally invasive approach [23]. All patients underwent a standardized post-operative recovery physiotherapy programme of immediate full weight bearing, range of motion and strengthening exercises without restrictions. Post-operative review was at 6 weeks, 6 months and then annually, including functional scoring with the Oxford Knee Score (OKS) and radiographs with standard AP standing and lateral views. All patients were followed prospectively and reviewed by independent examiners. For this study, patients undergoing combined UKA and ACL reconstruction have been excluded.

Statistical analysis

Data was tested for normality using D'Agostino's K^2 test. Pre-and post-operative OKS were thus compared using the Mann-Whitney U-test with significance set at $p < 0.05$. Correlations for age and BMI used Spearman's rank test. Complication rates for extended indications were compared using Fisher's exact test. Survivorship curves were constructed using the life-table method, with 95% confidence intervals calculated using Rothman's equation [24, 25]. Separate endpoints were examined: revision for any reason and revision for confirmed

Table 1 Cohort Demographics

	UKA Patients
Number	187
M:F	92:95
Mean BMI, Range	29.7 (17.9–45.1)
Mean Age at Surgery / Years, Range	64.2 (49–84)
Mean Follow-up / Years, Range	3.6 (0.5–8)

loosening. Patients who died or were lost to follow-up were treated as censored data.

All procedures performed in studies involving human participants were in accordance with the ethical standards of the Clinical Research Facility of St George's Hospital.

All patients provided written informed consent to their data being part of this study as part of their surgical consent.

Results

Between 2005 and 2013, the senior author implanted 187 consecutive UKAs in 173 patients. During the same period, the senior author performed 604 TKAs, and 12 lateral UKAs. 14 bilateral UKA procedures were performed sequentially. Patient demographics are shown in Table 1. The mean overall follow-up was 3.5 years. 5 patients died from unrelated causes, all with well-functioning implants. 7 patients (3.7%) were lost to follow-up and proved untraceable. 2 had data at 6 months, whilst 5 had no follow-up data available. The pre-operative OKS improved from a mean of 21.2 to 38.9 (Fig. 1, p = < 0.001). There was no correlation between the post-op OKS and either age (*p* = 0.88) or BMI (*p* = 0.47).

Twelve patients required 13 further operations. Two required bearing revision after dislocation within 6 months. One of these was later revised at 7 yrs. for progression of osteoarthritis (OA) in the lateral compartment, whilst the other had no further problems. Four patients had revision to total knee arthroplasty (TKA)

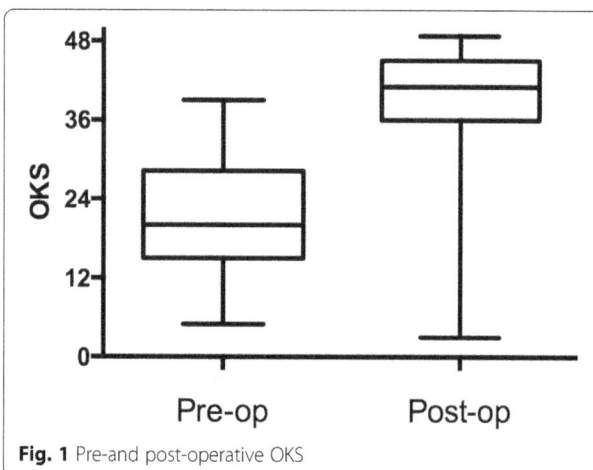

Fig. 1 Pre-and post-operative OKS

for pain alone, without evidence of component loosening at surgery. Three patients had revision for femoral component loosening, all with single peg components. Two were converted to TKA and 1 had a revision of the UKA femoral component alone to a twin peg design. One patient was revised to a TKA for progression of arthritis following multiple haemarthroses for a familial bleeding disorder. Two further patients had additional lateral compartment and patellofemoral arthroplasty respectively without revision of the original UKA. No patients developed deep infection and no surviving implants were loose radiographically.

Survivorship at 7 years with endpoints of re-operation, revision and aseptic loosening at surgery or radiographically was 88.1% (95% CI 79.1–93.5), 92.9% (95% CI 85.1–96.8) and 97.3% (95% CI 90.9–99.2) respectively. All revisions were included for the re-operation endpoint. Only operations where the UKA implant was removed or replaced were included for the revision endpoint. The full survivorship curves and confidence intervals for the three outcomes are shown in Fig. 2a-c. The complete life tables for each outcome including confidence intervals and effective number at risk each year are provided in Additional file 1.

Effect of degeneration in other compartments

96 patients (51%) had no pre-operative extended indications, compared with 91 (49%) who did. The outcomes for patients with extended indications in various combinations are set out in Table 2. The extended indications group had a significantly higher OKS (*p* = 0.01), a difference which remained significant for any case with PFJ degeneration (p = 0.01) or with isolated PFJ degeneration (*p* = 0.05). However, as the differences are less than 5 points, an accepted minimally important clinical difference for the OKS, this may not translate into clinical significance. No other comparisons reached statistical significance; importantly, patients without extended indications did not demonstrate superior post-operative outcomes when compared with any subgroups of patients with extended indications including those with a PFJ grade of 3 or 4 (*p* = 0.15). Only one patient with extended indications had a revision to a TKA for arthritis progression – this was the patient with a familial bleeding disorder. Overall, patients with extended indications had significantly lower rates of re-operation and revision (*p* = 0.003).

Discussion

The indications for UKA are being expanded to include patients with greater deformity, more advanced disease in the patellofemoral joint and even certain features in the lateral compartment indicative of an anteromedial pattern of OA [3–5]. However, much of the supporting literature remains available only from designer centres.

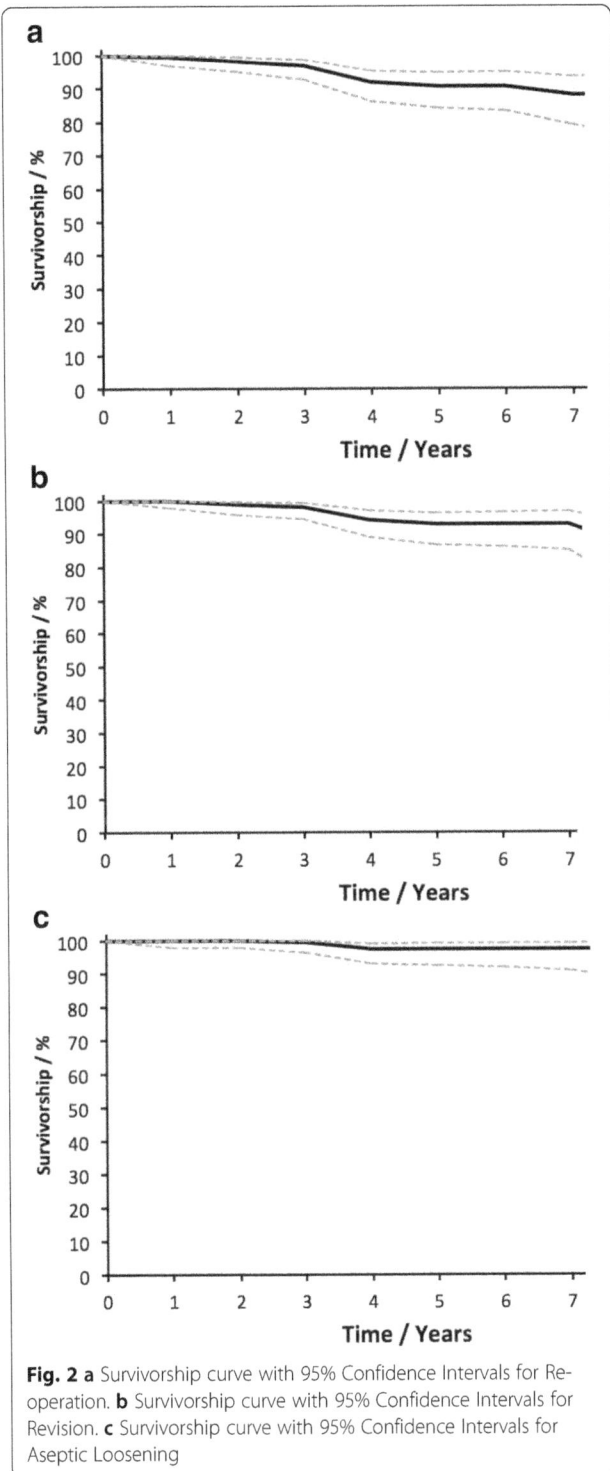

Fig. 2 a Survivorship curve with 95% Confidence Intervals for Re-operation. **b** Survivorship curve with 95% Confidence Intervals for Revision. **c** Survivorship curve with 95% Confidence Intervals for Aseptic Loosening

Table 2 Outcomes for Extended Indications

	Number of Patients	Mean Post-op OKS	Re-operation, Revision or Aseptic Loosening
No Extended Indications	96	37.6	12
Either Extended Indication	91	40.3	1
PFJ +/− Lateral grade > 2	93	40.2	0
Lateral +/− PFJ grade > 2	27	40.8	0
Isolated PFJ grade > 2	64	40.1	0
Isolated Lateral grade > 2	3	44.0	1
PFJ Grade III/IV	39	39.5	0

period, the senior author performed 604 TKAs, and 12 lateral UKAs. 14 bilateral UKA procedures were performed sequentially. This corresponds to a usage of 30% in keeping with recommendations that 30% of a surgeon's total knee arthroplasties should be UKAs to achieve optimum results Despite the broad criteria and the fact that the senior author receives patients from other consultants in the hospital for consideration of UKA, the ratio of UKA:TKA for patients presenting with symptomatic knee arthrosis in the period of this study was approximately 1:3.

Nine UKA implants have been revised so far, and we are not aware of any currently at risk. Four revisions were for unexplained but persistent medial pain. All were uncomplicated revisions to a TKA using simple primary implants and no obvious cause for pain was identified in any case. Whilst 3 patients have gone on to a reasonable result, one continues to have unexplained pain. None of these patients had extended indications as we have defined. Three femoral components were revised for aseptic loosening. All were of the single peg design, which has been noted in the past to be associated with an incidence of early loosening [26]. One was revised to a twin peg design and continues to function well (recent OKS 47), whilst the other 2 cases were revised to total knee arthroplasty, with satisfactory outcomes. During this series of patients, the twin-peg design for the femoral component became available. Within the literature there are no reports of femoral loosening issues for this iteration. Similarly, there were no failures of the twin peg femoral component in this series. It is possible therefore that these 3 revisions could have been avoided with the use of the newer design implants.

There were 2 bearing dislocations; one undoubtedly due to surgical error, with residual cement at the back of the tibial component leading to anterior dislocation in full flexion. At revision, an identical bearing was replaced after removal

This study represents a group of patients with what we believe to be wider indications, along with decisions to treat made on clinical grounds and radiographs alone. Only very rarely was the procedure changed based on intra-operative findings.

The senior author implanted 187 consecutive UKAs in 173 patients, a caseload of 23 per year. During the same of the errant cement. The second dislocation occurred for no clear reason and was revised to a bearing 1 mm thicker; this patient is currently functioning extremely well (2-year OKS 48). The dislocation rate of 1% is in line with other published rates in the literature and remains a potential complication of any mobile bearing UKA design.

Two cases went on to have further compartments replaced – one patellofemoral at 40 months and one lateral at 32 months after UKA. If anything, this represents a failure of patient selection, necessitating a further operation a moderate time after the primary surgery with a rate of 1%. Patient selection and indeed implant selection in any orthopaedic surgery is complex and often difficult, and no selection process will be perfect. By narrowing the inclusion criteria for UKA this 1% failure rate could be lowered, but perhaps not eradicated due to natural variances. There were no deep infections in this series, and this is consistent with other reports of low infection rates for UKA in comparison with TKA [27–29].

For any new orthopaedic implant, favourable results would be expected from developing centres, and whilst it might be rational to assume that similar outcomes will not be achieved by the wider surgical community, our series forms part of a growing number of independent reports of good results and favourable revision rates [6, 7, 9, 10]. There are also reports from other units with less success [11–14], but the main contrast comes from concerns raised primarily by registry data [30]. Inevitably the performance of an implant is dependent on the technique used to implant it, and studies have demonstrated the effect of a significant learning curve for UKA [31–34] with some authors advocating minimum numbers to be undertaken in order to maintain competence [7].

Strengths of the study that should be noted are the series does not include the learning curve of the senior author, with more than 50 procedures being carried out as a registrar and fellow, but all cases carried out as a consultant are included with a usage of 30% as recommended for optimal results.

Limitations include the difficulty to quantify the effect of a single surgeon's ability to master a new technique. Undoubtedly many surgeons never get over this learning curve before abandoning the technique in favour of either osteotomy or total knee arthroplasty, which will affect global outcomes. Ultimately, the fate of UKA may depend on whether there is any clinical benefit for the patients. Level one evidence on this issue is on the way [30].

Conclusions

In conclusion, we have shown comparable clinical outcomes and survivorship of the medial Oxford UKA when used with wider indications in a large cohort of patients. Our all cause revision survivorship rate of 93%

at 7 years is similar to figures reported from systematic reviews of registry data which show an all cause revision rate for total knee replacement of 6% at 5 years and 12% at 10 years [35]. In addition, the use of extended indications in this series has not had a detrimental effect on post-operative outcomes or re-operation or revision rates. We believe this data justifies the continued use of UKA at our institution within our current indications and serves to highlight the importance of practice analysis by individual surgeons of techniques that might be controversial in the wider orthopaedic literature.

Funding
No funding was received for this study.

Authors' contributions
JH was involved in data analysis and drafting the manuscript. AR and HS were involved in data acquisition. AS was involved in data acquisition and preparation for submission. MR was the operating surgeon and was involved in the acquisition and interpretation of the data. All authors read and approved the final manuscript.

Competing interests
The authors declare that they have no competing interests.

Author details
[1]Department of Trauma and Orthopaedics, St George's University Hospitals NHS Foundation Trust, London, UK. [2]Department of Orthopaedics and Trauma, The University of Adelaide and Royal Adelaide Hospital, Adelaide, Australia.

References
1. Pandit H, Hamilton TW, Jenkins C, et al. The clinical outcome of minimally invasive phase 3 Oxford unicompartmental knee arthroplasty: a 15-year follow-up of 1000 UKAs. Bone Jt J. 2015;97-B(11):1493–500. https://doi.org/10.1302/0301-620X.97B11.35634.
2. Weston-Simons JS, Pandit H, Kendrick BJL, et al. The mid-term outcomes of the Oxford domed lateral unicompartmental knee replacement. Bone Jt J. 2014;96:59–64.
3. Beard DJ, Pandit H, Gill HS, et al. The influence of the presence and severity of pre-existing patellofemoral degenerative changes on the outcome of the Oxford medial unicompartmental knee replacement. J Bone Joint Surg Br. 2007;89:1597–601. https://doi.org/10.1302/0301-620X.89B12.19259.
4. Kendrick BJL, Rout R, Bottomley NJ, et al. The implications of damage to the lateral femoral condyle on medial unicompartmental knee replacement. J Bone Joint Surg Br. 2010;92:374–9. https://doi.org/10.1302/0301-620X.92B3.23561.
5. Murray DW, Pandit H, Weston-Simons JS, et al. Does body mass index affect the outcome of unicompartmental knee replacement? Knee. 2013;20:461–5. https://doi.org/10.1016/j.knee.2012.09.017
6. Emerson RH, Alnachoukati O, Barrington J, Ennin K. The results of Oxford unicompartmental knee arthroplasty in the United States: a mean ten-year survival analysis. Bone Joint J. 2016;98-B(10 Supple B):34–40.
7. Hamilton TW, Rizkalla JM, Kontochristos L, et al. The interaction of caseload and usage in determining outcomes of Unicompartmental knee arthroplasty: a meta-analysis. J Arthroplast. 2017;32(10):3228–37.e2. https://doi.org/10.1016/j.arth.2017.04.063 .

8. Streit MR, Walker T, Bruckner T, et al. Mobile-bearing lateral unicompartmental knee replacement with the Oxford domed tibial component: an independent series. J Bone Joint Surg Br. 2012;94:1356–61.

9. Yoshida K, Tada M, Yoshida H, et al. Oxford phase 3 unicompartmental knee arthroplasty in Japan–clinical results in greater than one thousand cases over ten years. J Arthroplast. 2013;28:168–71. https://doi.org/10.1016/j.arth.2013.08.019.

10. Lyons MC, MacDonald SJ, Somerville LE, et al. Unicompartmental versus Total knee arthroplasty database analysis: is there a winner? Clin Orthop Relat Res. 2012;470:84–90. https://doi.org/10.1007/s11999-011-2144-z.

11. Kort NP, van Raay JJAM, Cheung J, et al. Analysis of Oxford medial unicompartmental knee replacement using the minimally invasive technique in patients aged 60 and above: an independent prospective series. Knee Surg Sports Traumatol Arthrosc Off J ESSKA. 2007;15:1331–4. https://doi.org/10.1007/s00167-007-0397-6.

12. Mercier N, Wimsey S, Saragaglia D. Long-term clinical results of the Oxford medial unicompartmental knee arthroplasty. Int Orthop. 2010;34:1137–43. https://doi.org/10.1007/s00264-009-0869-z.

13. Schroer WC, Barnes CL, Diesfeld P, et al. The Oxford Unicompartmental knee fails at a high rate in a high-volume knee practice. Clin Orthop Relat Res. 2013;471:3533–9. https://doi.org/10.1007/s11999-013-3174-5.

14. Zermatten P, Munzinger U. The Oxford II medial unicompartmental knee arthroplasty: an independent 10-year survival study. Acta Orthop Belg. 2012;78:203–9.

15. NZ Joint Registry. https://nzoa.org.nz/nz-joint-registry. Accessed 4 Aug 2014.

16. UK National Joint Registry. http://www.njrcentre.org.uk/njrcentre/default.aspx. Accessed 25 July 2014.

17. Australian National Joint Registry. https://aoanjrr.sahmri.com/en. Accessed 25 July 2014.

18. Labek G, Sekyra K, Pawelka W, et al. Outcome and reproducibility of data concerning the Oxford unicompartmental knee arthroplasty: a structured literature review including arthroplasty registry data. Acta Orthop. 2011;82:131–5. https://doi.org/10.3109/17453674.2011.566134.

19. Goodfellow JW, O'Connor JJ, Murray DW. A critique of revision rate as an outcome measure: re-interpretation of knee joint registry data. J Bone Joint Surg Br. 2010;92:1628–31. https://doi.org/10.1302/0301-620X.92B12.25193.

20. Konan S, Haddad FS. Joint registries: a Ptolemaic model of data interpretation? Bone Jt J. 2013;95-B:1585–6. https://doi.org/10.1302/0301-620X.95B12.33353.

21. Liddle AD, Pandit H, Judge A, Murray DW. Optimal usage of unicompartmental knee arthroplasty: a study of 41,986 cases from the National Joint Registry for England and Wales. Bone Jt J. 2015;97-B(11):1506–11. https://doi.org/10.1302/0301-620X.97B11.35551.

22. Liddle AD, Pandit H, Judge A, Murray DW. Effect of surgical caseload on revision rate following Total and Unicompartmental knee replacement. J Bone Joint Surg Am. 2016;98(1):1–8. https://doi.org/10.2106/JBJS.N.00487.

23. Oxford Knee Operative Technique. http://www.biomet.se/resource/17723/Oxford%20ST.pdf. Accessed 25 July 2014.

24. Carr AJ, Morris RW, Murray DW, Pynsent PB. Survival analysis in joint replacement surgery. J Bone Joint Surg Br. 1993;75:178–82.

25. Rothman KJ. Estimation of confidence limits for the cumulative probability of survival in life table analysis. J Chronic Dis. 1978;31:557–60.

26. White SH, Roberts S, Jones PW. The twin peg Oxford partial knee replacement: the first 100 cases. Knee. 2012;19:36–40. https://doi.org/10.1016/j.knee.2010.12.006.

27. Pandit H, Jenkins C, Gill HS, et al. Minimally invasive Oxford phase 3 unicompartmental knee replacement RESULTS OF 1000 CASES. J Bone Joint Surg Br. 2011;93:198–204.

28. Furnes O, Espehaug B, Lie SA, et al. Failure mechanisms after unicompartmental and tricompartmental primary knee replacement with cement. J Bone Joint Surg Am. 2007;89:519–25. https://doi.org/10.2106/JBJS.F.00210.

29. Jamsen E, Furnes O, Engesaeter LB, et al. Prevention of deep infection in joint replacement surgery. Acta Orthop. 2010;81:660–6. https://doi.org/10.3109/17453674.2010.537805

30. Beard D, Price A, Cook J, et al. Total or partial knee arthroplasty trial-TOPKAT: study protocol for a randomised controlled trial. Trials. 2013;14:292.

31. Rees JL, Price AJ, Beard DJ, et al. Minimally invasive Oxford unicompartmental knee arthroplasty: functional results at 1 year and the effect of surgical inexperience. Knee. 2004;11:363–7. https://doi.org/10.1016/j.knee.2003.12.006.

32. Hamilton WG, Ammeen D, Engh Jr CA, Engh GA. Learning curve with minimally invasive Unicompartmental knee arthroplasty. J Arthroplast. 2010;25:735–40. https://doi.org/10.1016/j.arth.2009.05.011.

33. Robertsson O, Knutson K, Lewold S, Lidgren L. The routine of surgical management reduces failure after unicompartmental knee arthroplasty. J Bone Joint Surg Br. 2001;83:45–9.

34. Badawy M, Espehaug B, Indrekvam K, et al. Higher revision risk for unicompartmental knee arthroplasty in low-volume hospitals. Acta Orthop. 2014;85:342–7. https://doi.org/10.3109/17453674.2014.920990.

35. Labek G, Thaler M, Janda W, et al. Revision rates after total joint replacement. Cumulative results from Worldwide Joint Register Datasets. J Bone Joint Surg Br. 2011;93-B:293–7. https://doi.org/10.1302/0301-620X.93B3.25467.

21

A case of bilateral revision total knee arthroplasty using distal femoral allograft–prosthesis composite and femoral head allografting at the tibial site with a varus-valgus constrained prosthesis: ten-year follow up

Sung-Hyun Lee[1], Sung-Hyun Noh[1], Keun-Churl Chun[1], Joung-Kyue Han[2] and Churl-Hong Chun[1*]

Abstract

Background: We report the successful use of allograft–prosthesis composite (APC) and structural femoral head allografting in the bilateral reconstruction of large femoral and tibial uncontained defects during revision total knee arthroplasty (RTKA).

Case presentation: A 67-year-old female with degenerative arthritis underwent bilateral total knee arthroplasty (TKA) using the Press Fit Condylar (PFC) modular knee system at our clinic in March, 1996. At 8 years postoperatively, the patient presented with painful, bilateral varus knees, with swelling, limited passive range of motion (ROM), and severe instability. We treated to reconstruct both knee using a femoral head allograft at the tibial site, a structural distal femoral allograft at the femoral site, and a varus-valgus constrained (VVC) prosthesis with cement. At the 10-year follow up, we found no infection, graft failure, loosening of implants, in spite of using massive bilateral structural femoral head allografts in RTKA.

Conclusion: The use of APC enabled a stable and durable reconstruction in this uncommon presentation with large femoral bone deficiencies encountered during a RTKA.

Keywords: APC, Structural allograft, RTKA, Bilateral knee

Background

Bone loss in revision total knee arthroplasty (RTKA) presents a significant surgical challenge because of the need to maintain proper alignment while establishing a stable bone-implant interface. The management of femoral and tibial bone loss is crucial for a successful RTKA, and the severity and location of bony defects determine the optimal type of reconstruction. Options for reconstruction of large defects include metal augments, custom prostheses, massive autogenous bone-grafts and massive allografts [1].

Allografts provide a biological solution, with the advantage of easy fashioning to fit irregular defects, and restore bone stock at a relatively low cost. Allograft–prosthesis composite (APC) are useful for implants when extensive bone loss is present, and are recommended for tibial plateau or femoral metaphyseal deficiency, according to Engh and Parks [2]. The majority of knee surgeons prefer metal augmentation, rotational hinge, and megaprosthesis when extensive bone loss occurs after TKA, but APC is used in this study.

We report a successful case of consecutive bilateral RTKAs using APC for the distal femur and structural femoral head allografting for the proximal tibia in the reconstruction of large femoral and tibial uncontained defects.

---
* Correspondence: cch@wku.ac.kr; cch@wonkwang.ac.kr
[1]Department of Orthopedic Surgery, School of Medicine, Wonkwang University Hospital, Muwang-ro 895, Iksan, Jeollabuk-do, South Korea
Full list of author information is available at the end of the article

Case presentation

A 67-year-old female with degenerative arthritis underwent bilateral total knee arthroplasty (TKA) using the Press Fit Condylar (PFC) modular knee system (PFC™, Johnson & Johnson Professional Inc., Raynham, MA, USA) at our clinic in March, 1996 (Fig. 1a, b). Normal rehabilitation processes were followed after surgery and the patient was able to walk with normal gait and without complications.

At 8 years postoperatively, the patient presented with painful, bilateral varus knees, with swelling, limited passive range of motion (ROM) (right knee: 0–45°, left knee: 0–90°), and severe instability. The patient was unable to walk and presented in a wheelchair. Anteroposterior and lateral radiographs revealed severe osteolytic bone defects in both the femoral and tibial aspects, along with primary total knee prosthesis and dissociation and subluxation of bilateral implants (Fig. 1c). Moreover, there were severe osteolytic lesions around the femoral prosthesis and along the femoral shaft on computed tomography (Fig. 1d). Preoperative bone scan and laboratory data rulled out infection. We decided to reconstruct the left knee first, using a femoral head allograft at the tibial site, a structural distal femoral allograft at the femoral site, and a varus-valgus constrained (VVC) prosthesis (NexGen LCCK, Zimmer, Warsaw, IN, USA) with cement. Determining the size of the APC to use prior to surgery is a very important and was measured using templating on the previous radiographs. The size of the structural distal femoral allograft was determined using a templating technique before surgery.

In order to prevent a skin problem, an anterior midline incision was performed over the previous incision. A medial parapatellar arthrotomy was performed, and hypertrophic synovium was excised from the suprapatellar recess and internal and lateral gutters. The hypertrophic synovium was removed thoroughly to prevent later inflammation or dissociation. Then, the patella was everted, and the knee was flexed to 90°. During surgery, soft tissues and attached bones were preserved except hypertrophic synovium. Operative findings showed hypertrophic villous synovium, loosening of prosthesis (Fig. 2a), and wearing of tibial (Fig. 2b) and patellar polyethylene (Fig. 2c). Debridement revealed about 10 cm of extensive, anterior distal femoral cortical bone loss (Fig. 2d) and an uncontained type III defect of the entire femoral condyle (Fig. 2e). In addition, the proximal tibia had a massive, uncontained type IIA defect, according to the Anderson Orthopaedic Research Institute classification (Fig. 2f).

A fresh-frozen femoral head allograft was used to fill in the proximal tibial bone loss and restore the tibial joint line; 10 mm medial and lateral proximal tibial metal blocks were used for reinforcement. In order to implant the femoral head allograft, cortical bone and cartilage were removed until cancellous bone was exposed (Fig. 3a). Next, the shape and size of the graft and bone defect sites were designed (Fig. 3b). The surface of the femoral head allograft was removed using a bone mill (Fig. 3c). The reaming exposed a trabecular structure that rapidly unites with host bone by ingrowth of woven bone, and provided an ideal surface for interdigitation of cement between the graft and implant. Bone lost in the proximal tibia and sclerotic areas was trimmed to an appropriate size, taking care not to damage cortical bone with the acetabular reamer. Allogeneic bone was designed to be 1 to 2 mm larger than the implant, allowing for impaction during implantation (Fig. 3d). The allograft was resected along the tibial surface (Fig. 3e) and

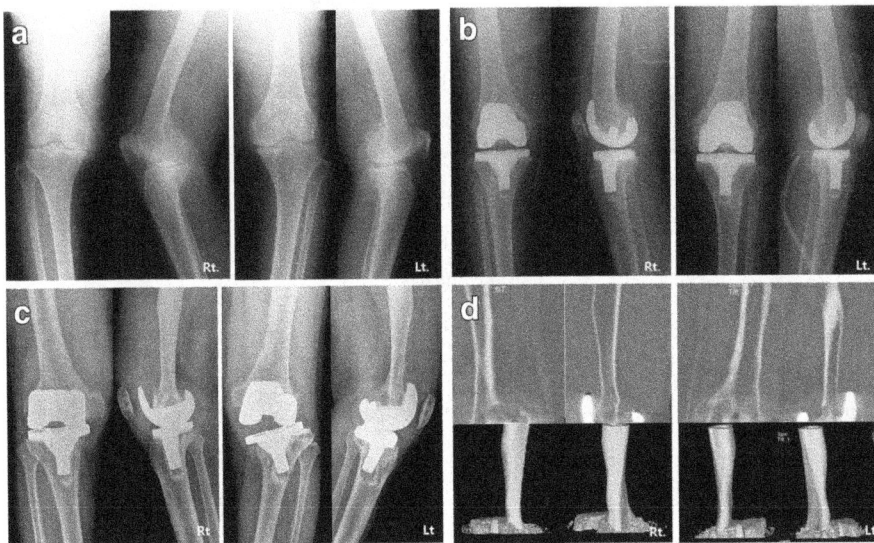

Fig. 1 a Pre- and **b** postoperative radiographs of primary bilateral TKA; **c** 8-year postoperative radiographs showing extensive osteolysis on both femoral and tibial sides; **d** computed tomography of both knees showing smooth bony erosion on the anterior aspect of the both distal femur

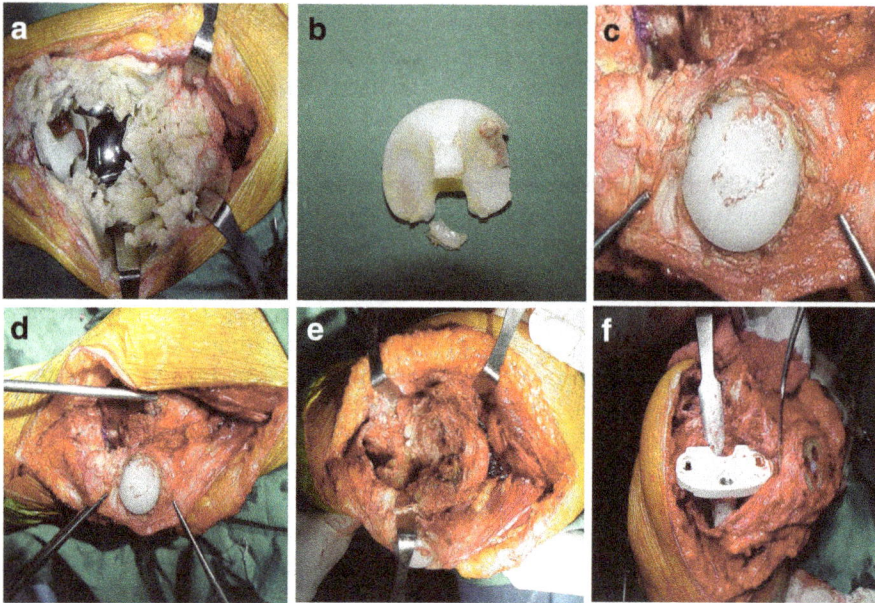

Fig. 2 Intraoperative photographs. **a** Hypertrophic villous synovium, **b** extensive wear, delamination and deformation of the polyethylene insert distributed asymmetrically over the medial and lateral sides, **c** patellar polyethylene wear, **d** extensive bone loss in the anterior distal femur, **e** uncontained bone defect of the entire distal femoral condyle, **f** uncontained bone defect of the proximal tibia

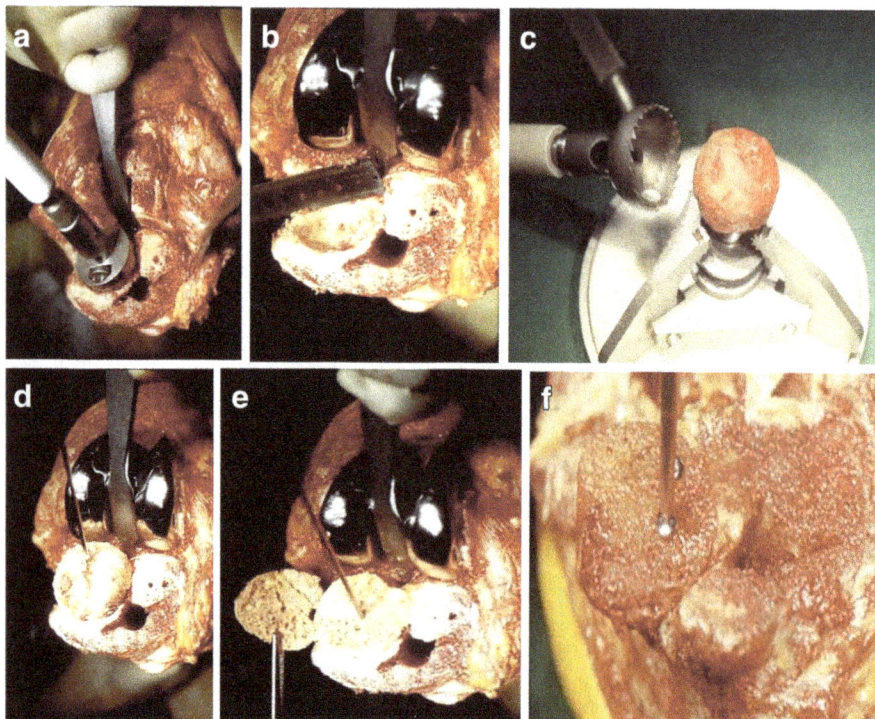

Fig. 3 Surgical procedures on the tibial side. **a** Removal of sclerotic areas using acetabular reamer, **b** checking the defect size, **c** denuding femoral head cartilage using milling system, **d** impaction of femoral head allograft, **e** allograft resection along the tibial surface, **f** allogenic bone grafting and fixation with screws

internal fixation was performed using a screw (Fig. 3f); the screw was completely inserted vertically under the prosthesis to avoid contact with the prosthesis.

At another table, allografts were resected to match the prosthesis, and the grafted portions were designed in a step-cut to structurally stabilize the graft (Fig. 4a). Similarly, the host bone was designed to be step-cut to engage the allografts. Implants were inserted and allografts were attached to the host bone to confirm flexion and extension intervals, rotational alignment, and overall basic alignment. Soft tissue balance was performed to make the flexion and extension gap equal. After the trial, the cement is used to locate the prosthesis in structural allogeneic bone. Cement was used only between the constrained condylar knee stem and structural allogeneic bone, not between structural allogeneic bone and host bone. Once the cement had set, the construct was implanted with the full assembly, matching the two step-cuts. The residual host femur, with its ligaments and other soft tissues attached, was wrapped around the allograft host junction to serve as a living bone graft. Then, APC was fixed with cerclage cable (Dall-Miles®Cable System, Stryker, Mahwah, NJ, USA) (Fig. 4b, c). Using metal plates or screws can create many holes and lead to fractures. Step-cut resection and press-fit fixation were adequate to secure the allogenic bone. The extensor mechanism alignment and tracking were checked, and the wound was closed in layers. A Robert-Jones dressing was used after surgery. Post op radiographs showed no specific findings (Fig. 5a). Quadriceps strengthening and continuous passive motion exercises were started 2 days after surgery. No weight-bearing was allowed for 6 weeks, followed by 6 weeks of partial weight-bearing with crutches and a brace, then full weight-bearing with a walker starting at 12 weeks postoperatively.

After 6 weeks right revision TKA was performed using NexGen LCCK with the same technique. Rehabilitation for the right knee was similar to that for the left knee. No signs of complications were found in follow-up examinations and post-operative radiological examinations as of February 2016 (Fig. 5b, c). The patient walked with full weight-bearing and had complete incorporation of allograft and host bone, with no signs of osteolysis. Active ROM was 0–90° in the left knee and 0–100° in the right knee. At the postoperative HSS score increased from 25/38 to 80/86. The patient is in satisfactory condition and had a in normal daily life.

Discussion and conclusions

In this case, our patient presented with a unique problem, having severe bone loss in the both femoral and tibial aspects of both knees. Bone loss found during RTKA is caused by several causes, including; malalignment, insufficient soft tissue balance, improper cement use, asymmetric load due to improper prosthesis design, and foreign body

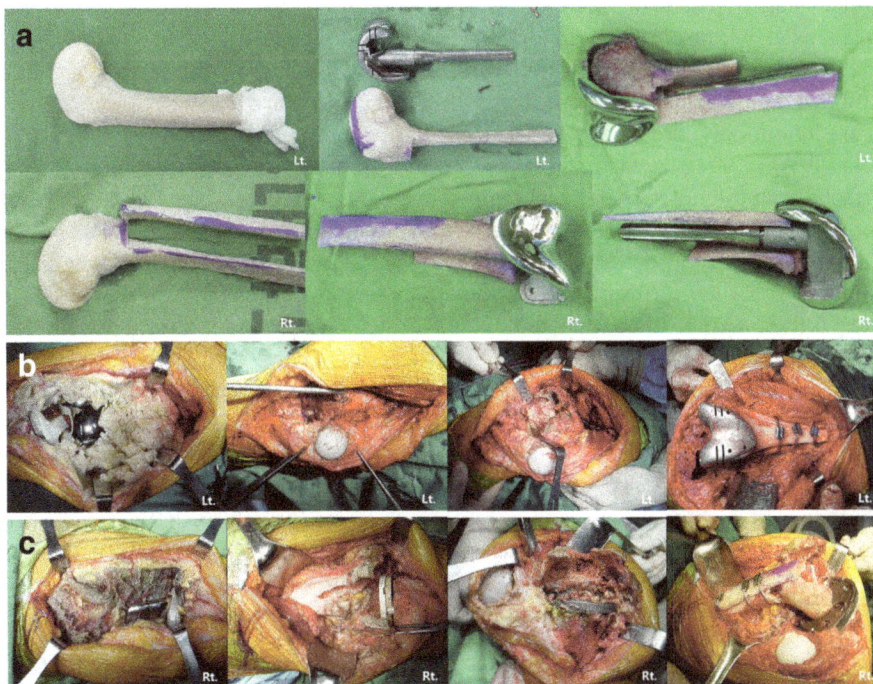

Fig. 4 Surgical procedures on the femoral side. **a** Step-cut prepared distal femoral allografts and prepared composite distal femoral allograft with LCCK implant, using APC (allograft–prosthesis composite). **b** After extensive removal of the hypertrophic synovium of the left knee, extensive bone loss of the distal femur was observed and APC was fixed to the host bone with a Dall-Miles cable. **c** The right knee was similar operative finding to that of the left knee and APC was fixed to the host bone in the same way as the left knee

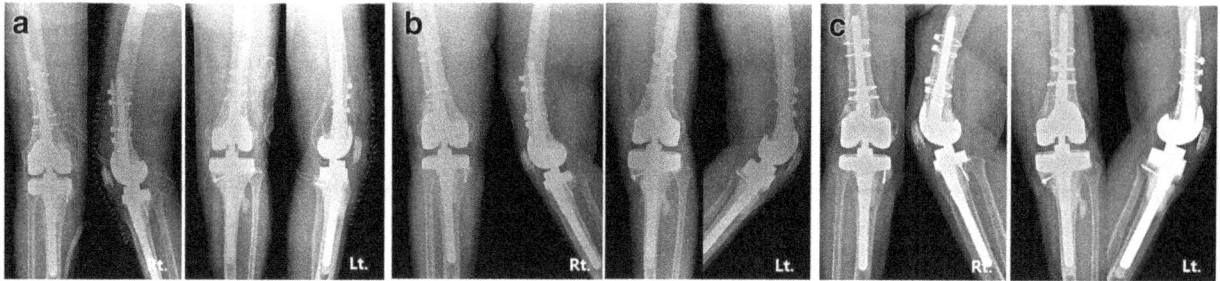

Fig. 5 A series of radiographs. **a** anteroposterior and lateral radiographys of both knees at post RTKA, **b** 5 years follow-up, **c** 10 years follow-up showing good allograft incorporation

reaction (from prosthesis wear particles); the resulting osteolysis, stress-shielding effect, and loosening of the prosthesis can result in bone loss and infection [3]. Few options are available to the surgeon for reconstruction of massive bone defects surrounding a failed TKA.

The application of allografts in RTKA is an attractive option. The use of femoral head allografts for the management of large bone defects in RTKA has been reported [4, 5]. There are few studies that simultaneously reconstruct large bone defects of distal femur and proximal tibia using allografts in RTKA [6]. Use of APC for distal femoral and massive proximal tibial allografts proved to be a successful mode of treatment with distinct advantages. In the case of relatively small size bone defects, filling a cement, impaction bone graft or metal augment can be used. In this case, this method could not be used because it was an uncontained type bone defect of entire femoral condyle. And compared to rotational hinge prosthesis and megaprosthesis, which are commonly thought of as large bone defects in general APC offers great healing capacity in terms of attaching to the host bone, which contributes to avoid massive rotational stress between them. Also, in our case, the anterior cortex of the distal femur was too slender and a rotating hinge prosthesis was not appropriate. In the megaprosthesis has the disadvantage of additional bone resection, reconstruction of the patella tendon may be difficult when using the proximal tibial component, and it is relatively difficult to preserve the original joint line. In addition, since the host bone is designed according to the prosthesis, bone loss may be greater than APC, which designs the prosthesis according to the host bone. Therefore, we used APC and there was no problem after 10 years of follow-up. However, disadvantages are not commonly available, the early recovery of range of motion and slower full weight-bearing compared to other methods. So, this case was non weight-bearing for 6 weeks after surgery, followed by 6 weeks of partial weight-bearing, then full weight-bearing with a walker starting at 12 weeks postoperatively.

Griffin et al. [7] reported that the second-generation design had a wear-related failure rate of 1.1%, compared with 8.3% in the first-generation design. Moreover, 10-year survival was was 97% with the second-generation design, compared with 87.7% for the first-generation. Peter et al. [8] also reported that wear of polyethylene could cause osteolytic lesions around the prosthesis, and this could cause eventual failure of TKA. We also observed severe polyethylene wear, despite proper soft tissue balance, femur-tibia angle, and cement use in our case. The polyethylene used in this study is a first-generation product, and osteolysis in our study seems to be one of the causes of polyethylene wear.

The thickness of polyethylene is a key factor determining the distribution of contact stress, which is inversely proportional to the degree of early wear [9]. We thought that the patient's relatively young age (59 years old) and active lyfestyles, as well as use of 8 mm-thick polyethylene, could have caused polyethylene the wear in our case. One study reported that contact stress in polyethylene implants increases rapidly as the thickness of the implant decreases [10]. For thin polyethylene inserts, a slight further reduction in thickness increases the contact stress significantly. The study concluded that a polyethylene thickness of more than 8 mm should be used in TKA. Polyethylene inserts less than 10 mm in thickness were associated with early fatigue failure. Therefore, a thickness of at least 8 mm, but preferably 10 mm, is recommended for TKA. We used 17 mm polyethylene in RTKA. Polyethylene wear and osteolysis were not observed 10 years after surgery.

Analyses of periprosthetic tissue retrieved during revision of failed total joint replacements showed that ultra-high-molecular-weight polyethylene (UHMWPE) wear debris is the most frequent type of debris around failed hip, knee and shoulder total joint replacements, whether or not the implants were cemented [11]. Macrophages activated by wear particle debris release an array of cytokines and proinflammatory mediators in joint fluid. This leads to recruitment, proliferation, differentiation and maturation of osteoclast precursors, and subsequent

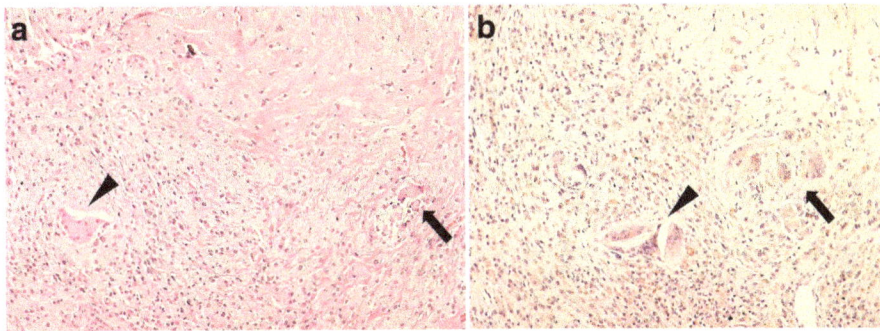

Fig. 6 Histology of synovial tissue with macrophages, giant cells (black arrows), and giant cell- polyethylene particles (black arrowheads). **a** Hematoxylin-eosin staining (× 10), **b** Immunohistochemical staining for CD-68 (× 10)

bone resorption eventually leads to implant loosening [12]. In our study, macrophages, giant cells, and foreign material, thought to be polyethylene particles, were found in inflamed synovial tissue (Fig. 6).

The use of APC enabled a stable and durable reconstruction in this uncommon presentation with large femoral bone deficiencies encountered during a RTKA. At-ten-year follow-up, we found no infection, graft failure or loosening of implants, in spite of using massive structural allografts in bilateral RTKA. Further follow-up with a larger number of patients is necessary to determine the long-term outcomes of these allografts.

Abbreviations
APC: Allograft–prosthesis composites; RTKA: Revision total knee arthroplasty; TKA: Total knee arthroplasty; VVC: Varus-valgus constrained

Acknowledgements
Not applicable.

Funding
No funding was received.

Authors' contributions
SL, SN: Conception and design, Acquisition, analysis and interpretation of data, preparation of the manuscript. KC: Acquisition, analysis and interpretation of data, critical revision of the manuscript. JH: Conception and design, preparation and revision of radiographs and intraoperative photographs. CC: Conception and design, analysis of data, revising the manuscript, supervision. Revising the manuscript and given final approval of the version to be published. All authors read and approved the final manuscript.

Competing interests
The authors declare that they have no competing interests.

Author details
[1]Department of Orthopedic Surgery, School of Medicine, Wonkwang University Hospital, Muwang-ro 895, Iksan, Jeollabuk-do, South Korea. [2]College of Sports Science, Chung-Ang University, Anseong, South Korea.

References
1. Mow CS, Wiedel JD. Structural allografting in revision total knee arthroplasty. J Arthroplast. 1996;11:235–41.
2. Engh GA, Parks NL. The management of bone defects in revision total knee arthroplasty. Instr Course Lect. 1997;46:227–36.
3. Insall JN. Revision of total knee replacement. Instr Course Lect. 1986; 35:290–6.
4. Bae DK, Kwon CH, Shin DJ, Shin NC. Use of structural allograft in revision total knee arthroplasty. Knee Surg Relat Res. 2000;12:19–24.
5. Kim KH, Kho DH, Shin JY, Lee JH, Kim DH. Revision total knee arthroplasty using femoral head allograft. Knee Surg Relat Res. 2007;19:51–6.
6. Chun CH, Kim JW, Kim SH, Kim BG, Chun KC, Kim KM. Clinical and radiological results of femoral head structural allograft for severe bone defects in revision TKA-a minimum 8-year follow-up. Knee. 2014;21:420–3.
7. Griffin WL, Fehring TK, Pomeroy DL, Gruen TA, Murphy JA. Sterilization and wear-related failure in first- and second-generation press-fit condylar total knee arthroplasty. Clin Orthop Relat Res. 2007;464:16–20.
8. Peter PC, Engh GA, Dwyer KA, Vinh TN. Osteolysis after total knee arthroplasty without cement. J Bone Joint Surg. 1992;74:864–76.
9. Feng EL, Stulberg DS, Wixon RS. Progressive subluxation and polyethylene wear in total knee replacement with flat articular surfaces. Clin Orthop. 1993;299:60–71.
10. Bartel DL, Bicknell VL, Wright TM. The effect of conformity, thickness and material on stresses in ultra-high molecular weight components for total joint replacement. J Bone Joint Surg. 1986;68:1041–51.
11. Mirra JM, Marder RA, Amstutz HC. The pathology of failed total joint arthroplasty. Clin Orthop Relat Res. 1982;170:175–83.
12. Nich C, Takakubo Y, Pajarinen J, Ainola M, Salem A, Sillat T, Rao AJ, Raska M, Tamaki Y, Takagi M, Konttinen YT, Goodman SB, Gallo J. Macrophages–key cells in the response to wear debris from joint replacements. J Biomed Mater Res A. 2013;101:3033–45.

Periprosthetic tibial fractures in total knee arthroplasty – an outcome analysis of a challenging and underreported surgical issue

Anna Janine Schreiner[1], Florian Schmidutz[1,2], Atesch Ateschrang[1], Christoph Ihle[1], Ulrich Stöckle[1], Björn Gunnar Ochs[3*] and Christoph Gonser[1]

Abstract

Background: Periprosthetic fractures after total knee arthroplasty (TKA) are an increasing problem and challenging to treat. The tibial side is commonly less affected than the femoral side wherefore few studies and case reports are available. The aim of this study was to analyze the outcome of periprosthetic tibial fractures and compare our data with current literature.

Methods: All periprosthetic tibial TKA fractures that were treated at our Level 1 Trauma Center between 2011 and 2015 were included and analyzed consecutively. The Felix classification was used to assess the fracture type and evaluation included the radiological and clinical outcome (Knee Society Score/KSS, Oxford Knee Score/OKS).

Results: From a total of 50 periprosthetic TKA fractures, 9 cases (7 female, 2 male; 2 cruciate retaining, 7 constrained TKAs) involving the tibial side were identified. The mean age in this group was 77 (65–85) years with a follow-up rate of 67% after a mean of 22 (0–36) months. The Felix classification showed type IB ($n = 1$), type IIB ($n = 2$), type IIIA ($n = 4$) and type IIIB ($n = 2$) and surgical intervention included ORIF ($n = 6$), revision arthroplasty ($n = 1$), arthrodesis ($n = 1$) and amputation ($n = 1$). The rate of adverse events and revision was 55.6% including impaired wound healing, infection and re-fracture respectively peri-implant fracture. Main revision surgery included soft tissue surgery, arthrodesis, amputation and re-osteosynthesis. The clinical outcome showed a mean OKS of 29 (19–39) points and a functional/knee KSS of 53 (40–70)/41 (17–72) points. Radiological analyses showed 4 cases of malalignment after reduction and plate fixation.

Conclusions: Periprosthetic tibial fractures predominantly affect elderly patients with a reduced bone quality and reveal a high complication rate. Careful operative planning with individual solutions respecting the individual patient condition is crucial. If ORIF with a plate is considered, restoration of the correct alignment and careful soft tissue management including minimal invasive procedures seem important factors for the postoperative outcome.

Keywords: Periprosthetic fractures, Total knee arthroplasty, Felix, Malalignment

* Correspondence: ochsgunnar@gmx.de
[3]Department of Orthopedics and Trauma Surgery, Medical Center, Faculty of Medicine, Albert-Ludwigs-University of Freiburg, Hugstetter Str. 55, 79106 Freiburg, Germany
Full list of author information is available at the end of the article

Background

Periprosthetic fractures constitute an upcoming challenge in revision arthroplasty. Reasons include increasing numbers of total knee arthroplasty (TKA), longer life expectancy and implant survival as well as patient related risk factors such as osteoporosis and sarcopenia [1].

The overall incidence of periprosthetic fractures after TKA is estimated to range between 0.3 to 2.5% [2–4]. The vast majority involves the distal femur (2%) whereas the proximal tibia is less frequently affected (0.3–0.5%) and thus has received little attention in the past [5]. The intraoperatively rate of periprosthetic TKA fractures is given with about 4% [6], but is likely to be underreported. Nevertheless, the majority of periprosthetic TKA fractures usually occur 2–4 years postoperatively after TKA and increases after revision TKA up to 38% [4].

Risk factors for periprosthetic TKA fractures include patient related factors like osteoporosis, age, female sex, revision and osteolysis. Specific surgical risk factors are the use of long tibial stems, cementless press-fit fixation, malalignment or malrotation of the tibial component, previous osteotomy e.g. of the tibial tuberosity and osseous defects in revision arthroplasty [5, 7, 8]. Besides, periprosthetic tibial fractures seem to be closely related to the implant design.

Periprosthetic fractures are a life-threatening condition for many of the predominantly elderly patients with a previous study reporting a one-year mortality rate between 11 to 44.8% [9, 10]. Therefore, the main object is to achieve early mobilization with a good functionality to reduce mortality [11]. Further aims include restoration of leg axis, bone-implant union and a stable joint which is influenced by patients' general condition as well as the type of TKA.

In contrast to periprosthetic TKA fractures of the femur, only few studies with limited numbers of patients have analysed periprosthetic fractures of the tibia. Therefore, the aim of this study was to analyse functional and radiological outcomes after periprosthetic TKA fractures and compare our data with those reported in the current literature providing present information to better anticipate prospective developments in revision arthroplasty in especially geriatric patients in the long-term.

Methods

This consecutive analysis included all patients who were initially treated or revised for a tibial periprosthetic TKA fracture in the Department of Arthroplasty at our Level 1 Trauma Centre between 2011 and 2015. Classification of the periprosthetic tibial fractures was done according to the widespread Felix classification which is also known as the Mayo classification [12]. The classification was introduced by Felix et al based on an analysis of 102 periprosthetic tibial fractures [13] and includes 4 types

related to the major anatomic pattern (I = tibial plateau, II = adjacent to the stem, III = distal to the prosthesis, IV = tibial tubercle) as well as 3 subcategories regarding fixation and time of fracture (A = prosthesis well fixed, B = loose prosthesis, C = intraoperative) [13]. While a loose prosthesis (Felix type B) usually indicates revision arthroplasty, Felix A and C fractures may be addressed by operative or non-operative fracture management [12].

All fractures were analysed radiologically and if the patients were available also examined clinically within the study. The standardized clinical examination was performed by one examiner comprising range of motion, pain, stability of the affected knee and palpation of the TKA site as well as outcome rating with the established Knee Society Score [14] and Oxford Knee Score [15, 16].

Radiological examinations consisted of standardized radiographs of the knee and/or the lower leg in two planes (anteroposterior and lateral views) and were analysed for tibial malalignment, union rate and implant failure. A deviation on fracture reduction and/or fixation of ≥5° in both planes as well as a deviation ≥5° of the 90° tibial slope angle were rated pathological. Malalignment regarding the tibial slope was expressed as exceeding tilt angle of the tibial plateau. Measurements were performed with the commercially available evaluation tool mediCAD® (HECTEC GmbH, Landshut, Germany) which is imbedded in the clinical image data base IMPAX® (Agfa HealthCare GmbH, Bonn, Germany).

Apart from radiological and outcome measurements, additional patient information such as previous history and surgery or any other adverse events before and after surgery were captured from the digital patient charts of our hospital. The last preceding medical procedure before the periprosthetic fracture was rated as index surgery which could either be primary or revision arthroplasty.

In case of loss of follow-up because of decease of the patient or drop-out the latest patient file data and radiographs available were analysed retrospectively. Insufficient data was graded as exclusion criteria. Patients suffering from dementia, with insufficient knowledge of the study language or incapability of participation in the study due to severe health conditions e.g. were excluded as well. The study protocol was approved by the local ethics committee (622/2015B02) and patients gave their written consent to participate in the study. Statistical analysis including patient demographics and data displayed as mean, standard deviation and range was performed with Microsoft Excel 2016 (Microsoft Corporation, Redmond, USA).

Results

Overall, 50 periprosthetic fractures associated to TKA were identified, from which 9 cases (18%) showed a periprosthetic tibial TKA fracture. Figure 1 displays the distribution according to the Felix classification. No case had to be excluded according to our exclusion criteria. The cohort (7 female, 2 male) showed a mean age of 77.1 ± 6.0 (65–85) years and a BMI of 28.5 ± 3.7 (25–36) kg/m^2 at the time of surgery due to their periprosthetic fracture. The total mean follow-up was 22.3 ± 10.5 (0–36) months with a follow-up rate of 67% (2 drop-outs and 1 death due to internal medical reasons). All patients suffered from comorbidities with a mean of 2.3 ± 1.6 (0–5) orthopaedic and 4.6 ± 2.5 (1–10) internal side diagnoses. Mean time between index surgery and periprosthetic tibial fracture was 59.7 ± 64.1 (0.25–209) months. Retrospectively, there were 2 intraoperative fractures which were diagnosed with a delay of 6 days and 4 months, respectively. Time period between occurrence of the periprosthetic tibial fracture and revision surgery was 1.1 ± 1.6 (0–5) months. The primary TKA was performed between 1997 and 2015.

Surgical history of the patients was uneventful in 3 cases with 6 cases having a low grade periprosthetic joint infection (PJI), aseptic loosening, mechanical failure, wound healing disorder, unicompartimental knee arthroplasty (UKA) and patellectomy with partly several revisions before index surgery. In summary, 67% of all patients had 1.3 times preceding surgery. The cohort comprised 2 cruciate retaining prostheses and 7 semi- or fully constrained total knee arthroplasties.

There were 7 cases of low energy trauma and 2 cases related to osteolysis causing the periprosthetic tibial fracture. Mean duration of hospital stay was 22.8 ± 13.0 (8–51) days and mean duration of surgery was 109.9 ± 41.4 (63–169) minutes with a transfusion rate of 43%. Surgery due to the periprosthetic tibial fracture comprised $n = 6$ open reduction and internal fixation (ORIF), $n = 1$ revision arthroplasty, $n = 1$ arthrodesis and $n = 1$ amputation (Fig. 2).

One case (Felix type IIIB) had been treated with ORIF at another hospital first and was revised at our hospital due to PJI with loosening of the TKA. The type IB fracture was successfully revised with revision arthroplasty. This patient also survived an intraoperative lung arteries embolism. One of the type IIB fractures resulted in an amputation due to an extensive PJI with a wound healing disorder in the course. The other type IIB fracture was treated with ORIF and finally lead to arthrodesis due to wound healing disorders, loosening and infection. One of the IIIA fractures was successfully treated with ORIF with a wound healing disorder that could be handled conservatively. The other type IIIA fracture was followed by 5 revisions including re-ORIF with additional autologous bone grafting following re-fracture, non-union, wound healing disorders and a peri-implant fracture. The other 2 type IIIA fractures showed no adverse events after osteosynthesis. One of the type IIIB fractures was treated with ORIF followed by 6 revision surgeries due to implant failure, infection and wound healing disorder and finally resulting in amputation. The other type IIIB fracture was successfully treated with arthrodesis. In total, the rate of adverse events as well as revision was 55.6% ($n = 5$ each). Osteosynthesis was applied by the majority (66.7%, $n = 6$). Amputation as well as arthrodesis were treatment options in the first place due to an infectious constellation in one case and extensive bone loss in the other case always also regarding patients' age and demands.

Main complications were wound healing disorders (41.7%), infection (16.7%) and re-fracture or peri-implant

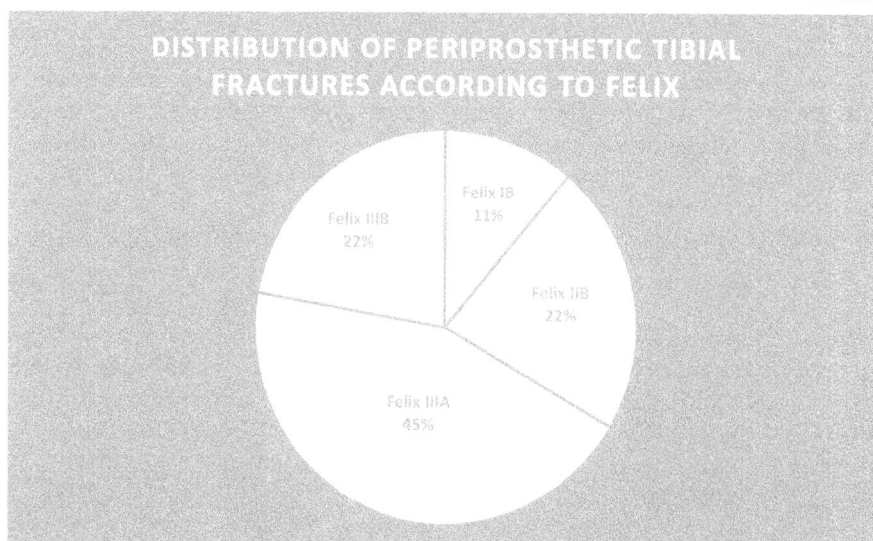

Fig. 1 Distribution of periprosthetic fractures according to Felix (Felix IB $n = 1$, IIB $n = 2$, IIIA $n = 4$, IIIB $n = 2$)

Periprosthetic tibial fractures in total knee arthroplasty – an outcome analysis of a challenging...

177

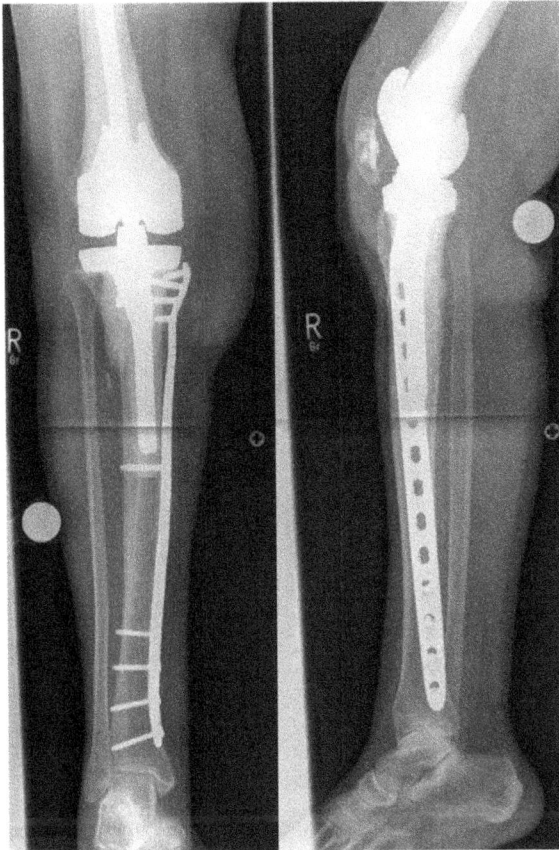

Fig. 2 ORIF with a long medial plate in a periprosthetic tibial fracture around a hinged TKA

fracture (16.7%) with 0.5 adverse events per patient. Loosening, implant failure and non-union occurred in 8.3% each. Main revision surgery included soft tissue surgery (28.6%), arthrodesis (28.6%), amputation (14.2%) and re-osteosynthesis (28.6%) with 1.5 revisions per patient. Table 1 gives an overview of the treatment of the periprosthetic fractures of the tibia in our cohort.

Mean Oxford Knee Score was 28.8 ± 6.6 (19–39) points. The functional Knee Society Score and the knee Knee Society Score showed a mean of 53.3 ± 13.7 (40–70) points and 41.3 ± 17 (17–72) points, respectively. Clinical examination comprising pain, stability of the affected knee and palpation of the site showed no relevant results. Mean range of motion at the time of follow-up was 0-0-100°.

Radiological evaluation revealed 2 cases of malalignment after ORIF with a plate in the coronal plane (6° and 7° varus malalignment) as well as 2 cases of malalignment in both planes (both 5° malalignment in the frontal plane as well as 8° and 5° in the sagittal plane). Figure 3 shows a case with combined malalignment in both planes. No case showed an isolated malaligned tibial slope in comparison to isolated malalignments in the frontal plane after plate fixation as described above. The other cases were $n = 4$ amputations/arthrodesis and $n = 1$ correct alignment. There was no implant failure and the healing rate was 100% (for $n = 5$ ORIF) at the time of follow-up.

Discussion

Periprosthetic tibial fractures represent a rare but potentially fatal complication after TKA. In this study, we present a consecutive series of tibial TKA fractures, confirming the challenging treatment associated with a high complication rate. To the best of our knowledge, this is the only current study on PubMed evaluating the treatment and outcome of tibial Felix type fractures after TKA. Only Kim et al. reported a series with minimally invasive plate osteosynthesis (MIPO) [17]. Like previous reports, our data are limited by the small case number which does not allow present statistical statements so far.

In the original report of Felix et al., type I fractures represent the main fracture type ($n = 61/102$), while Felix type III fractures (n = 6/9) were the most frequent ones observed in ours [13]. Furthermore, we recorded no type

Table 1 Overview of periprosthetic tibial fractures regarding treatment, adverse events and revision surgery

Felix	n	Treatment	Adverse Events	Revision Surgery
IB	1	Revision Arthroplasty	–	–
IIB	2	ORIF	Wound healing disorder, infection, loosening	Arthrodesis
		Amputation	Wound healing disorder	Soft tissue revision
IIIA	4	ORIF	Wound healing disorder	–
		ORIF	Re-fracture, non-union, wound healing disorder, peri-implant fracture	Several Re-ORIF, autologous bone grafting
		ORIF	–	–
		ORIF	–	–
IIIB	2	ORIF	Implant failure, infection, wound healing disorder	Several Re-ORIF, amputation with soft tissue revision
		Arthrodesis	–	–

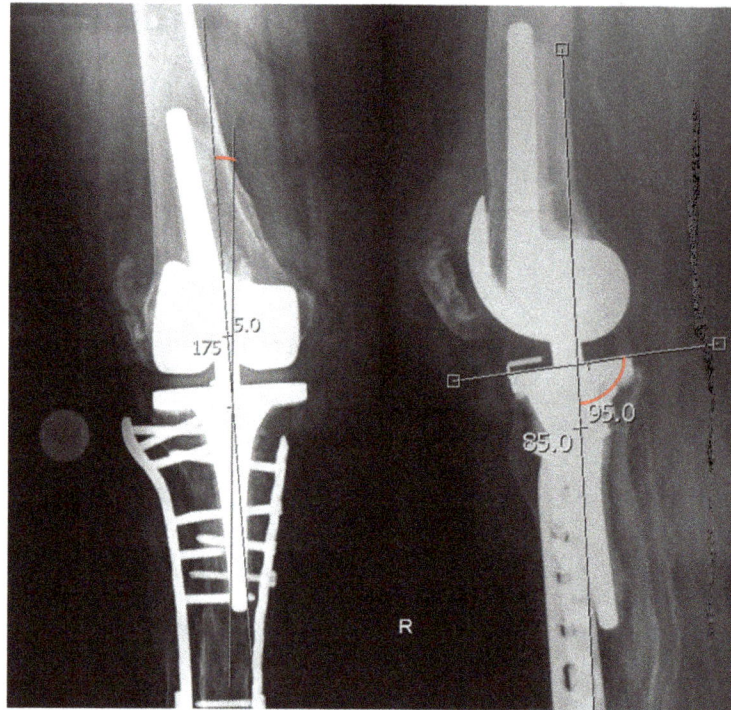

Fig. 3 Malalignment after double plate fixation of a periprosthetic tibial fracture (Frontal plane: 5° varus malalignment; sagittal plane: 5° anterior tibial slope)

4 fracture which complies with the low incidence ($n = 2/102$) as reported before [13]. Accordingly, most tibial TKA fractures occurred in our cohort postoperatively ($n = 7/9$). Felix et al. further described a predominate pattern of type IB and IIB fractures that were usually treated by revision surgery [13]. In our series, these Felix types (IB $n = 1$; IIB $n = 2$) were treated with revision surgery, osteosynthesis and amputation respectively. It is important to notice that even though individual cases of Felix type B fractures can be handled with ORIF, usually revision surgery is required. Intraoperative fractures were observed in 18.6% ($n = 19/102$) by Felix et al. [13] which confirms our findings of 22.2% (n = 2/9). Both intraoperative fractures were diagnosed with a delay, supporting the assumption of a high rate of underreported cases.

Postoperative fractures are predominantly observed in females and usually associated with a low-energy trauma [13]. Felix et al. figured out that the fracture type and the related proportion of a loose implant is predictive for the treatment success; while Felix type I fractures had the lowest survival rates, Felix type III fractures revealed the highest. Similarly, we observed a complication rate of 67% in type III fractures ($n = 6$), but no adverse event with our Felix type I fracture.

In this content it must be noted, that Felix et al. developed their algorithm for a heterogenous collective retrospectively. The subgroups were also classified regarding

their related treatment which makes it difficult to compare the outcome of the fracture types. Patients who underwent immediate revision in the Felix cohort type Ib required later revision in 22.2% ($n = 6/27$), type IIIa were usually treated conservatively and type IIIb delayed for revision for health reasons [13].

Aside from Felix et al., there are only 3 original articles currently reported on the outcome of periprosthetic tibial TKA fractures, all with a limited number of 7–16 patients (Table 2) [13, 17–20]. Another study biomechanically evaluated the treatment options of periprosthetic tibial plateau fractures during UKA [20]. The authors found a significantly higher fracture stability for angle-locking plates compared to cannulated screws [20] which seems to be transferable to tibial TKA fractures.

Kim et al. could treat 16 tibial TKA fractures (Felix type II $n = 6$, Felix type III $n = 10$) with a locking plate in MIPO technique and achieved satisfactory results [17]. The authors emphasized the importance of a rigid proximal fixation, as fewer than 8 cortices giving purchase to screws showed higher failure rates [17]. Considering the high rate of postoperative wound healing disorders in this fracture entity, the use of MIPO techniques seems favourable.

The aspect of plating can also be extended to the question of single vs double plating respectively mono vs polyaxial locking plates in periprosthetic fractures as mono axial plates often used in combination with double

Table 2 Original articles analysing periprosthetic tibial fractures

Author	Year	Title	n	Central message
Our study	2018	Periprosthetic tibial fractures in total knee arthroplasty –an outcome analysis of a challenging and underreported surgical issue	9	Soft tissue management, correct alignment and minimal invasive procedures are important for the outcome of old and osteoporotic patients associated with a high complication rate
Kim et al	2016	Successful outcome with minimally invasive plate osteosynthesis for periprosthetic tibial fracture after total knee arthroplasty.	16	Minimally invasive plate osteosynthesis with locking plates can achieve satisfactory results regarding union, alignment, range of motion and functional outcome
Seeger et al	2013	Treatment of periprosthetic tibial plateau fractures in unicompartimental knee arthroplasty: plates versus cannulated screws.	12	Biomechanical analysis of matched fresh frozen tibiae demonstrating that angle stable plates show significantly higher fracture loads than fixation with cannulated screws and should be preferred
Tabutin et al	2007	Tibial diaphysis fractures below a total knee prosthesis	6	Successful results with intramedullary nailing in osteoporotic bone stock regarding bone healing and knee function
Thompson et al	2001	Periprosthetic tibial fractures after cementless low contact stress total knee arthroplasty.	7	Correct alignment and possible cement fixation regarding tibial component insertion is important in primary TKA as malalignment and osteopenia are risk factors for periprosthetic fractures

plating was preferred in some cases so far. Hanschen et al. could demonstrate that single plating with polyaxial locking plates in complex distal femur fractures leads to good functional and clinical results [21]. Regarding the soft tissue management as well as the outcome in the treatment of Felix fractures so far, the transfer of this aspect to the tibial side should be well considered.

Similarly, Tabutin et al. treated 6 tibial diaphysis fractures after TKA (all Felix type IIIB) successfully with less invasive intramedullary nailing [18]. Although not applicable on all cases, this offers a less invasive technique when the lateral radiograph shows enough space for the nail between the prosthesis keel and the anterior tibial tuberosity [18].

Thompson et al. described 7 tibial fractures (Felix type I) after changing from a cemented to a cementless TKA, which were successfully treated conservatively ($n = 3$) or with a long cemented stem ($n = 4$) [19]. Risk factors for the occurrence were a preoperative neutral or valgus knee axis and osteopenia whereas age, gender and diagnosis were not [19]. The authors underline the importance of tibial cement fixation and a correct alignment [19]. The importance of correct tibial alignment is confirmed by Felix et al. and our results. Furthermore, several studies on periprosthetic TKA fractures clearly identified a varus malalignment as a risk factor for periprosthetic fractures [22–24].

We further identified 4 case reports in the literature reporting on periprosthetic tibial TKA fractures. Fonseca et al. present the case of periprosthetic tibial fracture (Mayo Clinic type I) associated with a tibial stem fracture [25]. Their finite-element CAD analysis revealed that the implant breakage occurred due to tibial

overloading at the plate/stem transition zone [25]. The patient was successfully revised with a longer stem and the authors emphasize the importance of respecting local bone quality. Beharrie et al. combined a long tibial stem in a periprosthetic tibial fracture with additional impaction bone grafting similar as known from acetabular or femoral reconstruction [26, 27].

Similarly, Kumar et al. reported a periprosthetic tibial fracture after lateral UKA following a trivial fall resulting in a loose component and a large tibial bone defect [28]. Revision required long stems as well as proximal structural tibial allograft and the authors emphasized the importance of meticulous analysis and preoperative planning [28]. Furthermore, it has to be noted that UKA goes along with an incidence of 0.2% up to 5% of tibial fractures related to the tibial saw cuts [12, 20, 29].

Surgical treatment of periprosthetic fractures is associated with high rates of adverse events and further revisions, wherefore alternative options should always be considered. Doorgakant et al. treated a Type IIa fracture conservatively with pulsed electromagnetic stimulation [30]. Bone union was achieved after 7 months with asymptomatic fully weight-bearing after 14 months. Although this appears to be a viable therapy, the long immobilization as well as other factors such as the fracture pattern, bone loss, patient biology and general condition have to be respected [30].

Complication rates for periprosthetic fractures in TKA is high and differs depending on type of fracture, degree of osteoporosis and applied implant. Fractures at the tibia are connected with a clearly higher rate of adverse events than those at the femur including non-union, malalignment, re-fractures, PJI, arthrofibrosis and implant failure [31, 32]. The outcome is further related to the fracture location, with fractures distal to the implant (Felix type III) revealing a 5-year-survival rate of 87%, while the rate decreases to 51% and 2.5% for Felix type I and II. The high rates of implant failure after type I and II fractures underline the difficulty of treating these periprosthetic fractures [13]. Our data can also confirm the results of Felix et al. reporting a high rate of adverse events and further revisions.

Unfortunately, the low incidences and the poor representation in the literature currently makes it impossible to present statistical valid data for this serious medical problem. Burnett et al. assume that the increasing numbers of TKA together with the longer implant and patient survival will clearly increase the number of periprosthetic fractures. This will be further aggravated by the demographic changes with patients presenting a more complex medical background including multiple revisions or PJI amongst other medical side diagnoses which will additionally increase the preexisting high risk for complications. The conversion rate to arthrodesis and amputation shows the huge impact of those fractures and sometimes can also be a treatment option in the first place for old and multimorbid patients, especially considering the high number of wound healing disorders and infection in this and other studies.

The impact of tibial TKA fractures is further reflected by the low functional outcome according to our outcome scores. In this context, careful soft tissue management and if applicable minimal invasive procedures seem advantageous. However, we could also demonstrate that malalignment after osteosynthesis in periprosthetic fractures is a risk factor for further complications and thus should be avoided. Altogether, the impact and complication rate of periprosthetic tibial TKA fractures suggest that this entity should be treated in a centre with expertise in both revision and arthroplasty and traumatology. Further studies are needed to give more evidence regarding the treatment strategy and outcome of the single fracture entities.

Conclusions

Periprosthetic tibial fractures are less common and only insufficiently reported in the current literature compared to periprosthetic fractures of the distal femur. These fractures are predominantly recorded in old patients with reduced bone stock and show a high complication rate. In our study we can confirm the classification and treatment options according to Felix et al. Nevertheless, individual solutions must be considered facing epidemiological developments and complex settings in revision arthroplasty. In case of plate fixation, correct alignment and soft tissue management are considerable factors for the postoperative outcome and should favour minimal

invasive procedures if possible. Further studies are required to properly evaluate and address periprosthetic tibial fractures.

Abbreviations
MIPO: Minimally invasive plate osteosynthesis; ORIF: Open reduction and internal fixation; PJI: Periprosthetic joint infection; TKA: Total knee arthroplasty; UKA: Unicompartimental knee arthroplasty

Funding
No funding was obtained for this study.

Authors' contributions
AJS and BGO raised, analysed and interpreted the clinical and radiological patient data. AJS, FS, and BGO were major contributors in writing the manuscript. CG, CI, AA and US evaluated the data and wrote the manuscript. All authors read and approved the final manuscript.

Consent for publication
Not applicable.

Competing interests
The authors declare that they have no competing interests.

Author details
[1]BG Trauma Center Tübingen, Eberhard Karls University Tübingen, Schnarrenbergstrasse 95, 72076 Tübingen, Germany. [2]Department of Orthopaedic Surgery, Physical Medicine and Rehabilitation, University of Munich (LMU), Marchioninistraße 15, 81377 Munich, Germany. [3]Department of Orthopedics and Trauma Surgery, Medical Center, Faculty of Medicine, Albert-Ludwigs-University of Freiburg, Hugstetter Str. 55, 79106 Freiburg, Germany.

References
1. Della Rocca GJ, Leung KS, Pape HC. Periprosthetic fractures: epidemiology and future projections. J Orthop Trauma. 2011;25(Suppl 2):S66–70.
2. Frosch K-H, Madert J. Kniegelenksnahe Frakturen bei Knie-TEP. OP-J. 2015;31:62.
3. Su ET, DeWal H, Di Cesare PE. Periprosthetic femoral fractures above total knee replacements. J Am Acad Orthop Surg. 2004;12:12–20.
4. Ritter MA, Thong AE, Keating EM, et al. The effect of femoral notching during total knee arthroplasty on the prevalence of postoperative femoral fractures and on clinical outcome. J Bone Joint Surg Am. 2005;87:2411–4.
5. Burnett RS, Bourne RB. Periprosthetic fractures of the tibia and patella in total knee arthroplasty. Instr Course Lect. 2004;53:217–35.
6. Alden KJ, Duncan WH, Trousdale RT, Pagnano MW, Haidukewych GJ. Intraoperative fracture during primary total knee arthroplasty. Clin Orthop Relat Res. 2010;468:90–5.
7. Diehl P, Burgkart R, Gollwitzer H. Periprothetische Frakturen nach Knietotalendoprothetik. Orthopäde. 2006;35:961–74.
8. Erhardt JB, Kuster M-S. Periprothetische Frakturen am Kniegelenk. Orthopäde. 2010;39:97–108.
9. Drew JM, Griffin WL, Odum SM, et al. Survivorship after Periprosthetic femur fracture: factors affecting outcome. J Arthroplast. 2016;31:1283–8.

10. Jennison T, Yarlagadda R. Mortality in patients sustaining a periprosthetic fracture following a previous extracapsular hip fracture fixation. Injury. 2018; 49:702–4. https://doi.org/10.1016/j.injury.2018.01.001.

11. Fakler JKM, Ponick C, Edel M, et al. A new classification of TKA periprosthetic femur fractures considering the implant type. BMC Musculoskelet Disord. 2017;18:490.

12. Hanssen AD, Stuart MJ. Treatment of periprosthetic tibial fractures. Clin Orthop Relat Res. 2000;(318):91–8.

13. Felix NA, Stuart MJ, Hanssen AD. Periprosthetic fractures of the tibia associated with total knee arthroplasty. Clin Orthop Relat Res. 1997;(345):113–24.

14. Insall JN, Dorr LD, Scott RD, Scott WN. Rationale of the knee society clinical rating system. Clin Orthop Relat Res. 1989;(248):13–4.

15. Dawson J, Fitzpatrick R, Murray D, Carr A. Questionnaire on the perceptions of patients about total knee replacement. J Bone Joint Surg Br Vol. 1998;80:63–9.

16. Murray DW, Fitzpatrick R, Rogers K, et al. The use of the Oxford hip and knee scores. J Bone Joint Surg Br Vol. 2007;89:1010–4.

17. Kim HJ, Park KC, Kim JW, Oh CW, Kyung HS, Oh JK, et al. Successful outcome with minimally invasive plate osteosynthesis for periprosthetic tibial fracture after total knee arthroplasty. Orthop Traumatol Surg Res. 2016; 103:263–8. https://doi.org/10.1016/j.otsr.2016.10.007.

18. Tabutin J, Cambas PM, Vogt F. Tibial diaphysis fractures below a total knee prosthesis. Rev Chir Orthop Reparatrice Appar Mot. 2007;93:389–94.

19. Thompson NW, McAlinden MG, Breslin E, et al. Periprosthetic tibial fractures after cementless low contact stress total knee arthroplasty. J Arthroplast. 2001;16:984–90.

20. Seeger JB, Jaeger S, Rohner E, et al. Treatment of periprosthetic tibial plateau fractures in unicompartmental knee arthroplasty: plates versus cannulated screws. Archives of orthopaedic and traumatic surgery. Arch Orthop Unfallchir. 2013;133:253–7.

21. Hanschen M, Aschenbrenner IM, Fehske K, et al. Mono- versus polyaxial locking plates in distal femur fractures: a prospective randomized multicentre clinical trial. Int Orthop. 2014;38:857–63.

22. Rand JA, Coventry MB. Stress fractures after total knee arthroplasty. J Bone Joint Surg Am Vol. 1980;62:226–33.

23. Lotke PA, Ecker ML. Influence of positioning of prosthesis in total knee replacement. J Bone J Surg Am Vol. 1977;59:77–9.

24. Wilson FC, Venters GC. Results of knee replacement with the Walldius prosthesis: an interim report. Clin Orthop Relat Res. 1976;(120):39–46.

25. Fonseca F, Rebelo E, Completo A. Tibial periprosthetic fracture combined with tibial stem stress fracture from total knee arthroplasty. Rev Bras Ortop. 2011;46:745–50.

26. Beharrie AW, Nelson CL. Impaction bone-grafting in the treatment of a periprosthetic fracture of the tibia: a case report. J Bone Joint Surg Am. 2003;85-a:703–7.

27. Slooff TJ, Buma P, Schreurs BW, Schimmel JW, Huiskes R, Gardeniers J. Acetabular and femoral reconstruction with impacted graft and cement. Clin Orthop Relat Res. 1996;(324):108–15.

28. Kumar A, Chambers I, Wong P. Periprosthetic fracture of the proximal tibia after lateral unicompartmental knee arthroplasty. J Arthroplast. 2008;23:615–8.

29. Berger RA, Meneghini RM, Jacobs JJ, et al. Results of unicompartmental knee arthroplasty at a minimum of ten years of follow-up. J Bone Joint Surg Am. 2005;87:999–1006.

30. Doorgakant A, Bhutta MA, Marynissen H. Management of a tibial periprosthetic fracture following revision knee arthroplasty using a pulsed electromagnetic field stimulation device: a case report. Cases J. 2009;2:8706.

31. Mittelmeier T, Stöckle U, Schaser K. Periprothetische Frakturen nach Knietotalendoprothetik. Unfallchirurg. 2005;108:481–95.

32. Schaser K. Voraussetzungen für eine erfolgreiche Osteosynthese. AE Bulletin 2011: Periprothetische Frakturen des Hüft- und Kniegelenkes. 2011;2:11–8.

23

Combined use of topical intraarticular tranexamic acid and rivaroxaban in total knee arthroplasty safely reduces blood loss, transfusion rates, and wound complications without increasing the risk of thrombosis

Yong Tae Kim[1], Min Wook Kang[1], Joon Kyu Lee[2], Young Min Lee[1] and Joong Il Kim[1]*

Abstract

Background: Blood loss and deep vein thrombosis (DVT) are important complications after total knee arthroplasty (TKA). Topical tranexamic acid (TXA) effectively reduces wound bleeding but may elevate the risk of DVT. In contrast, rivaroxaban potently prevents DVT but has been associated with bleeding complications. The simultaneous use of topical TXA and rivaroxaban in TKA has not been much investigated.

Methods: A retrospective cohort study was conducted with two consecutive groups of patients who underwent TKA. Intraoperatively, one group (RVTX group) received topical, intraarticular TXA, while the other (RV group) did not. Both groups were administered rivaroxaban postoperatively for 14 days and underwent Doppler ultrasound for DVT screening. After propensity score matching, both groups consisted of 52 patients (104 patients in total) and were compared regarding total drain output, nadir haemoglobin (Hb), maximum Hb decrease, calculated total blood loss, transfusion rate, and incidence of DVT and wound complications.

Results: Both groups showed no significant differences in the propensity-matched variables of age, sex, body mass index, American Society of Anesthesiologists physical status score, and preoperative Hb. The RVTX group showed a significantly higher nadir Hb ($p < 0.001$), lower drain output ($p < 0.001$), Hb decrease ($p = 0.015$), total blood loss ($p < 0.001$), and rate of transfusion ($p < 0.001$) and fewer wound complications ($p = 0.027$). However, the incidence of DVT ($p = 1.000$) did not differ significantly between the two groups, and all cases were asymptomatic.

Conclusions: The combined use of intraarticular topical TXA with rivaroxaban in patients undergoing TKA is a safe and effective method to reduce blood loss, the need for transfusion, and wound complications without elevating the risk of DVT.

Keywords: Total knee replacement, Tranexamic acid, Rivaroxaban, Blood loss, Transfusion, Wound complication, Deep vein thrombosis

* Correspondence: jungil@hanmail.net
[1]Department of Orthopaedic Surgery, Hallym University Kangnam Sacred Heart Hospital, 1, Singil-ro, Yeongdeungpo-gu, Seoul 150-950, South Korea
Full list of author information is available at the end of the article

Background

Total knee arthroplasty (TKA) involves a significant amount of blood loss due to extensive bone cuts and soft tissue dissection. Persistent bleeding may increase the risk of infection, worsen the postoperative wound condition, cause transfusion-related complications such as immunologic rejection and disease transmission, and increase costs [1–4]. Among the various options in addition to standard tourniquet use, the antifibrinolytic agent tranexamic acid (TXA) has shown promising results due to its ease of use, relatively low cost, and high haemostatic potency [5–7]. However, concerns exist regarding its possible systemic effect on elevating thrombotic risk, especially when no or a weak concurrent thromboprophylaxis regimen is used [8]. Thus, topical application of TXA has been investigated and found to be comparable to intravenous injection for decreasing transfusion rates [9].

Deep vein thrombosis (DVT) is of a major concern in TKA because it is the main cause of postoperative pulmonary embolism, a potentially life-threatening complication. The natural incidence of DVT after TKA without prophylaxis is reported to be as high as 45–56% [10, 11]. Therefore, thromboprophylaxis, traditionally using low molecular weight heparin (LMWH), warfarin, and aspirin, has long been a standard postoperative protocol. However, oral agents such as rivaroxaban, apixaban, and dabigatran have recently been introduced due to their advantages of easier administration, no need for monitoring, and increased or equivalent potency compared to classic anticoagulants. Among these oral drugs, rivaroxaban demonstrated the most effective protection against DVT [12]. However, studies have shown higher incidences of wound bleeding and deep surgical site infection [13, 14] in patient groups who were given rivaroxaban after TKA.

Though TXA and rivaroxaban are each highly effective for their approved purposes, the benefits may be overshadowed by higher risks of DVT and wound complications, respectively [8, 13, 14]. However, it is plausible that when TXA and rivaroxaban are used together, the actions of one drug may compensate for the adverse effects of the counterpart drug. Nevertheless, many studies regarding the use of TXA in TKA involved a thromboprophylaxis regimen other than rivaroxaban [15–19]; only a few analysed the concurrent use of TXA with rivaroxaban in TKA [20–22]. In most of these studies, TXA was administered intravenously, although topical TXA has been shown to be noninferior to intravenous injections in reducing blood loss, with a minimal resultant systemic concentration [19, 23]. Thus far, the concurrent use of topical TXA and rivaroxaban has not yet been investigated extensively.

The objective of this study is to evaluate the efficacy and safety of the combined regimen of topical TXA with rivaroxaban in TKA by comparing groups with or without topical TXA use, both with thromboprophylaxis via rivaroxaban. The main hypothesis was that the intraarticular injection of TXA after capsule closure, combined with rivaroxaban use for thromboprophylaxis, would result in a smaller postoperative haemoglobin (Hb) decrease, fewer transfusions and wound complications, and no increase in DVT risk.

Methods

Inclusion and exclusion criteria

After the approval by the Institutional Review Board of the authors' institute (HUKSHH IRB 2017–10-010) and in accordance with the Declaration of Helsinki, a single-centre retrospective cohort study was performed on patients who (1) received primary unilateral TKA for degenerative arthritis, (2) received postoperative rivaroxaban for thromboprophylaxis, and (3) either received or did not receive topical TXA for haemostasis.

In February 2015, rivaroxaban was selected as the primary pharmacologic DVT prophylactic agent after TKA in the authors' institute. Previously, LMWH was the first line treatment, and for patients who refused subcutaneous injection, aspirin was offered. Starting in March 2017, due to growing reports of postoperative bleeding, intraarticular injection of TXA after capsule closure was added to the routine surgical procedure. There was no bias in case selection when using TXA, as consecutive patients underwent the default perioperative protocol solely depending on the operation date.

The published contraindications [24, 25] for each drug were strictly obeyed; patients who could not receive rivaroxaban or topical TXA were not included in the study. Patients who could not meet the preoperative Hb requirements (> 10 g/dL) and required preoperative transfusion were excluded. Patients who received implants other than those specified in the latter section due to a previous contralateral implant of another design were excluded. Cases in which patellar resurfacing was impossible due to an overly thin or small patella were also excluded. Such exclusions were made to minimize the confounding factors and set the use of topical TXA as the only independent variable.

The total number of patients included was 106 for the rivaroxaban-only (RV) group, and 52 for the rivaroxaban plus topical TXA (RVTX) group.

Surgical intervention

All operations were performed through a standard medial parapatellar approach under spinal anaesthesia. A pneumatic tourniquet was inflated to 300 mmHg immediately before incision. All patients received the same cemented posterior stabilized implant (Persona®, Zimmer, Warsaw, IN), and the patella was resurfaced.

After final implant fixation and removal of excess cement, gauze packing was performed, and the tourniquet was deflated. Manual compression around the surgical field was applied until the cement had completely hardened, and bleeding foci evident after gauze removal were identified and cauterized. A clamped closed suction drain (Barovac®, Sewoon Medical, Cheonan, Korea) was placed inside the joint, and a watertight closure of the capsule was performed. At this point, the RVTX group received an intraarticular injection of 1 g of TXA (Tranexamsan®, Shinpoong Pharmaceutical, Seoul, Korea) mixed in 50 mL normal saline (Fig. 1). The solution was left in the joint with the drain clamped. After the injection, the knee was moved throughout the range of motion to confirm the watertight closure of the capsule. In both groups, the drain was unclamped after two hours and was removed 48 h after the surgery. No preoperative autologous blood transfusions or intraoperative blood salvage were performed.

Postoperative management
Both groups shared the same postoperative protocol. Immediately after surgery, an intermittent pneumatic compression pump (Flowtron®, ArjoHuntleigh, Addison, IL) was applied, and gentle compressive dressing of the operated leg was maintained until drain removal at 48 h postoperatively. Then, the compressive dressing was changed to a light adhesive dressing, and continuous passive motion was initiated. Tolerable weight bearing and early mobilization were encouraged.

Postoperative fluid replacement included standardized daily administration of 500 mL of hydroxyethyl starch volume expander (Volulyte®, Fresenius Kabi, Bad Homburg, Germany) on postoperative days (POD) 1 and 2. Transfusion of allogeneic blood was indicated only

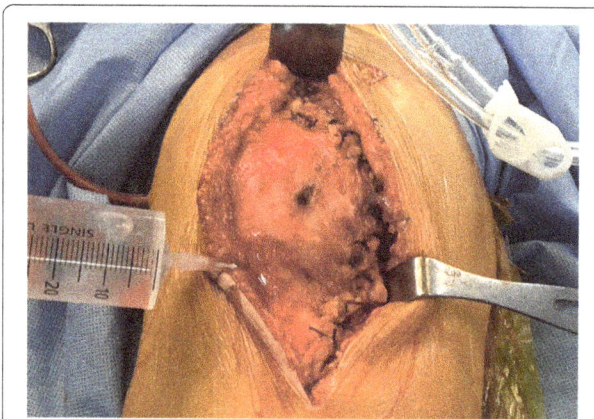

Fig. 1 Intraarticular injection of tranexamic acid after capsule closure. After watertight capsule closure, a solution of 1 g tranexamic acid in 50 mL normal saline was injected intraarticularly into the knee joint. Leakage of the solution was further monitored through the range of motion. Note the clamped drainage tube

when the Hb concentration decreased below 8 g/dL. Laboratory tests including Hb were performed on the day before surgery and on POD 1, 2, 4, and 6.

From POD 2 to 14, patients received a daily dose of 10 mg rivaroxaban (Xarelto®, Bayer HealthCare AG, Wuppertal, Germany). On POD 6, all patients, regardless of the presence of clinical symptoms of DVT, underwent a bilateral diagnostic Doppler ultrasound examination. If the findings were negative, patients were discharged on POD 7. Wound complications including wound dehiscence, hematoma, and surgical site infection were monitored during the hospital stay and after discharge until four weeks postoperatively at the outpatient clinic.

Data collection
The following data were retrieved retrospectively from medical records: demographic data including age, sex, and body mass index (BMI); physical status-related parameters including preoperative Hb (in g/dL) and American Society of Anesthesiologists physical status classification (ASA-PS); outcome measures related to blood loss including total drain output (in mL), nadir Hb during the hospital stay, maximum decrease in Hb (calculated by the nadir Hb subtracted from the preoperative Hb), total blood loss (in mL, calculated by the formulas published by Nadler et al. [26] and Good et al. [7]), and postoperative records of transfusion; routine Doppler ultrasound results; and wound complications.

Statistical analysis
To minimize possible confounding factors, both groups underwent propensity score matching prior to analysis. The variables matched included demographic data including age and sex and preoperative physical status data including BMI, ASA-PS, and preoperative Hb. The match tolerance, the maximum difference between propensity scores of any matched pair, was set to 0.1. As the number of patients in the RV group ($n = 106$) was approximately twice that in the RVTX group ($n = 52$), every patient in the RVTX group was matched to a patient in the RV group (the RV group hereafter refers to the group of 52 patients who were each matched with a patient of the RVTX group).

Further analysis was performed with an identical number ($n = 52$) of patients in both groups. For continuous data, independent t-tests were applied to express results as means and 95% confidence intervals (CI). Pearson chi-square and Fisher's exact tests were used to compare percentages for binary data.

A p-value less than 0.05 was considered statistically significant. IBM SPSS Statistics for Windows, Version 24 (IBM Corp., Armonk, NY) was used for propensity score matching and subsequent statistical analyses.

Results

The propensity matched variables of age, sex, BMI, preoperative Hb, and ASA-PS were not significantly different between the two groups (Table 1).

However, the RVTX group demonstrated a significantly higher nadir Hb during the hospital stay ($p < 0.001$) and a lower total drain output ($p < 0.001$), maximum decrease in Hb ($p = 0.015$), and total blood loss ($p < 0.001$) (Table 2). The RVTX group also demonstrated a significantly lower rate of postoperative transfusion ($p < 0.001$) (Table 3).

The incidence of DVT was not significantly different between the two groups (Table 3). A total of five patients, two from the RV group and three from the RVTX group, were diagnosed with isolated distal DVT by routine ultrasound examinations. However, none of the patients complained of any clinical symptoms, and further studies also excluded pulmonary thromboembolism. All patients were treated uneventfully with an extended daily dose of 20 mg of rivaroxaban for three months. During follow-up, no wound complications occurred in these patients.

However, a significant difference was observed in the occurrence of wound complications (Table 3). Although no cases of wound dehiscence or surgical site infection occurred, six patients, all from the RV group, developed a subcutaneous hematoma. Three patients required wound revision including hematoma removal, while in the other three patients, the hematomas resolved spontaneously with ice application and gentle compression.

Discussion

The present study showed that the combined regimen of topical TXA and rivaroxaban significantly reduces postoperative blood loss, the transfusion rate, and wound complications, without increasing the risk of DVT.

Several studies so far have investigated the combined use of TXA and rivaroxaban in TKA. With intravenous TXA, Wang et al. [17] reported less blood loss and a lower rate of transfusion and wound complications in the rivaroxaban-IV TXA group, with no significant difference in DVT occurrence. Wood et al. [20] also reported a

significantly reduced need for transfusion in the same patient group. Similar results with intraarticular TXA were produced by Wang et al. [22] with a dose of 0.5 g in a 10 mL solution, and Yen et al. [27] with a dose of 3 g in a 100 mL solution.

The classic arsenal of chemical thromboprophylaxis has limitations such as the need for daily injections (LMWH, enoxaparin, fondaparinux), a narrow therapeutic window (warfarin), or insufficient protection (aspirin) [28, 29]. Therefore, surgeons are now focusing on novel agents with potency matching or exceeding the traditional options, ease of oral administration, and no need for constant monitoring [30]. These options include the direct factor Xa inhibitors rivaroxaban and apixaban, and the direct thrombin inhibitor dabigatran [25, 31, 32]. Gómez-Outes et al. [12] compared these three oral anticoagulants with enoxaparin and showed rivaroxaban to be the most effective agent.

However, rivaroxaban has been associated with complications related to bleeding due to its potent anticoagulant properties. Wang et al. [21] demonstrated that in patients given rivaroxaban alone after TKA, compared to patients with additional intravenous TXA, significantly higher incidences of ecchymoses and wound hematoma were recorded. Ricket et al. [14] compared patients who received either rivaroxaban or enoxaparin and described a higher rate of clinically relevant non-major bleeding, including surgical site bleeding and hematoma. In a study by Brimmo et al. [13], compared to patients who received thromboprophylaxis other than rivaroxaban, those who received rivaroxaban after lower extremity arthroplasty demonstrated a significantly higher rate of early deep surgical site infection. Although the present study did not report any case of infection, a significantly higher incidence of wound hematoma was observed in the RV group, confirming the previous findings in the literature. In the period during which rivaroxaban was used without TXA, the authors became aware of the increasing number of cases of wound bleeding and sought additional TXA administration.

Simultaneously achieving postoperative haemostasis and thromboprophylaxis is complex, as the respective

Table 1 Propensity score matched data

	Rivaroxaban only (n = 52)	Rivaroxaban + IA TXA (n = 52)	p-value
Age (years)[a]	70.4 (68.0–72.9)	72.0 (70.0–74.0)	0.320
Male:Female[b]	6: 46	8: 44	0.775
BMI (kg/m²)[a]	25.1 (24.2–26.1)	25.0 (24.4–25.7)	0.816
ASA-PS classification[a]	2.1 (1.9–2.2)	2.1 (2.0–2.3)	0.704
Preoperative Hb (g/dL)[a]	12.5 (12.1–12.9)	12.6 (12.2–13.0)	0.630

IA TXA Intraarticular tranexamic acid, *BMI* Body mass index, *ASA-PS* American Society of Anesthesiologists Physical Status, *Hb* Haemoglobin
[a]Values presented as means (95% confidence interval) and compared by independent t-tests
[b]Values presented as proportions and compared using Pearson's chi-square test

Table 2 Continuous outcome measures

	Rivaroxaban only (n = 52)	Rivaroxaban + IA TXA (n = 52)	p-value
Total drain output (mL)	1021.4 (893.9–1148.9)	419.1 (349.9–488.3)	< 0.001
Nadir Hb during hospital stay (mL)	8.2 (7.9–8.6)	9.0 (8.8–9.3)	< 0.001
Maximum decrease in Hb (g/dL)	4.2 (3.9–4.6)	3.6 (3.1–4.0)	0.015
Total blood loss (mL)	1260.1 (1168.7–1351.6)	1008.2 (910.3–1106.2)	< 0.001

All values presented as means (95% confidence interval) and compared using independent t-tests

drugs are expected to exert opposite effects of coagulation and anticoagulation. While chemical thromboprophylaxis has long been regarded as a part of the standard treatment, pharmacologic treatments of postoperative haemostasis are not as popular, mostly due to concerns that such treatments may contribute to thrombogenesis [33–35]. However, TXA is an antifibrinolytic agent and does not trigger a coagulation cascade, but instead exerts its haemostatic effect by inhibiting the degradation of fibrin already formed at the bleeding foci [36]. Therefore, the safety of using TXA in TKA, which resulted in no significant elevation in DVT risk, has been reported in the literature [15, 16, 37]. However, all these studies had some form of concurrent thromboprophylaxis, which may have masked the possible elevation of DVT risk due to TXA. Thus, Nishihara et al. [8] conducted a study of intravenous TXA use with only mechanical, but no chemical, thromboprophylaxis. The results showed that compared to the group not administered TXA, the intravenous TXA group showed a significantly higher incidence of isolated distal DVT.

Therefore, topical TXA was administered in the present study to reduce the effects of rivaroxaban at the surgical site while minimizing the possible systemic effects of TXA in elevating DVT risk. This decision was supported by Wong et al. [23], who showed that topical TXA, compared to intravenous injection, demonstrated a lower serum concentration while maintaining a maximum level at the surgical site. Regarding the efficacy of TXA, in a meta-analysis [9] of six studies comparing topical and intravenous TXA, topical TXA was similarly effective in decreasing blood loss after TKA. The present study also strengthened these findings, as patients treated with intraarticular injections of TXA showed

significantly less blood loss and lower rates of transfusion, without a significant elevation in DVT risk.

Currently, the optimal protocol for topical TXA administration has not been established in the literature. Intraarticular injection with or without drain clamping, impregnation for a given time and removal of the residual solution within the open joint, or irrigation with the solution have been investigated as viable methods, and all showed significantly less blood loss than with no TXA use [9, 19, 38]. However, in the present study, routine intraarticular injection with the drain clamped offered a method of confirming watertight capsule closure, which may have been helpful in preventing subcutaneous hematomas and retrograde infections. Moreover, unlike impregnation, which requires a certain amount of time before removal of the solution, intraarticular injection required no delays but still provided a long contact time, maximizing the local concentration. Although all methods were significantly effective, the dosages also varied within studies, from 1 to 3 g of TXA in 10 to 100 mL of normal saline [9]. The minimum required concentration is also reported in the literature to be 10 to 20 mg/mL [39, 40]. Such information was the basis for the protocol of intraarticular injection of 1 g TXA per 50 mL normal saline in the present study [9, 39, 40].

The limitations of the present study must be noted. The present study is a retrospective study, which may be subject to selection bias. However, the treatment decision of whether to include intraarticular TXA in the surgical protocol was based on the date of the surgery, not on other parameters. In addition, propensity score matching was employed to match the patients not only with demographic details but also using the physiological status reflected by preoperative Hb and ASA-PS.

Table 3 Binary outcome measures

	Rivaroxaban only (n = 52)	Rivaroxaban + IA TXA (n = 52)	p-value
Transfusions[a]	26 (50.0%)	8 (15.4%)	< 0.001
Ultrasound-diagnosed DVT[b]	2 (3.8%)	3 (5.8%)	1.000
Wound complications[b]	6 (11.5%)	0 (0%)	0.027

All values presented as the number of patients (percentage)
[a]Compared using Pearson's chi-square test
[b]Compared using Fisher's exact test

Haemodynamic outcome parameters and the need for transfusion, which is strictly triggered by the postoperative nadir Hb, can be greatly influenced by the preoperative status. Hence, the propensity score matching of preoperative Hb and ASA-PS was believed to have strengthened the results of the present study, which showed dramatic contrasts between the two groups. Another limitation of this study is the lack of an experimental group treated with TXA without rivaroxaban and a control group not treated with either TXA or rivaroxaban. However, as postoperative chemical thromboprophylaxis after TKA is now a standard of care, such a study design may have raised ethical issues.

Despite these limitations, this study is among the first to successfully prove the effectiveness and safety of the combined use of topical, intraarticular TXA with rivaroxaban. Previous publications have reported the high potency of the individual regimens and the limitations when not used in conjunction [13, 14, 21]. Therefore, the present study can be of value in choosing the optimal perioperative management for TKA patients, effectively lowering blood loss, and reducing transfusions and wound complications while offering the best protection available against DVT.

Conclusions

The combined use of topical, intraarticular TXA with rivaroxaban in patients undergoing TKA is a safe and effective approach to reduce blood loss, the need for transfusions and wound complications without elevating the risk of DVT.

Abbreviations

ASA-PS: American Society of Anesthesiologists physical status; BMI: Body mass index; CI: Confidence interval; DVT: Deep vein thrombosis; Hb: Haemoglobin; LMWH: Low molecular weight heparin; POD: Postoperative day; RV: Rivaroxaban-only; RVTX: Rivaroxaban plus topical TXA; TKA: Total knee arthroplasty; TXA: Tranexamic acid

Acknowledgements

The authors thank the Medical Research Collaborating Centre of Hallym University for the support in statistical analysis.

Funding

This research was supported by the Hallym University Research Fund 2017 (HURF-2017-47).

Authors' contributions

YTK collected the data, performed the measurement and analysis, participated in the study design and drafted the manuscript. JKL and YML participated in the study design, supervised the analysis and helped to draft the manuscript. MWK collected the data, performed the measurement. JIK designed the study, supervised the whole study process and helped to draft and review the manuscript. All authors read and approved the final manuscript.

Consent for publication

Not applicable.

Competing interests

The authors declare that they have no competing interests.

Author details

[1]Department of Orthopaedic Surgery, Hallym University Kangnam Sacred Heart Hospital, 1, Singil-ro, Yeongdeungpo-gu, Seoul 150-950, South Korea. [2]Department of Orthopaedic Surgery, Hallym University Sacred Heart Hospital, 22, Gwanpyeong-ro 170beon-gil, Dongan-gu, Anyang 431-796, South Korea.

References

1. Fiebig E. Safety of the blood supply. Clin Orthop Relat Res. 1998;357:6–18.
2. Gascón P. Immunologic abnormalities in patients receiving multiple blood transfusions. Ann Intern Med. 1984;100:173.
3. Heddle NM, Klama LN, Griffith L, Roberts R, Shukla G, Kelton JG. A prospective study to identify the risk factors associated with acute reactions to platelet and red cell transfusions. Transfusion. 1993;33:794–7.
4. Schreiber GB, Busch MP, Kleinman SH, Korelitz JJ. The risk of transfusion-transmitted viral infections. N Engl J Med. 1996;334:1685–90.
5. Seo J-GG, Moon Y-WW, Park S-HH, Kim S-MM, Ko K-RR. The comparative efficacies of intra-articular and IV tranexamic acid for reducing blood loss during total knee arthroplasty. Knee Surg Sport Traumatol Arthrosc. 2013;21:1869–74.
6. Zufferey P, Merquiol F, Laporte S, Decousus H, Mismetti P, Auboyer C, et al. Do Antifibrinolytics reduce allogeneic blood transfusion in orthopedic surgery? Anesthesiology. 2006;105:1034–46.
7. Good L. Tranexamic acid decreases external blood loss but not hidden blood loss in total knee replacement. Br J Anaesth. 2003;90:596–9.
8. Nishihara S, Hamada M. Does tranexamic acid alter the risk of thromboembolism after total hip arthroplasty in the absence of routine chemical thromboprophylaxis? Bone Jt. J. 2015;97-B(4):458–62.
9. Wang H, Shen B, Zeng Y. Comparison of topical versus intravenous tranexamic acid in primary total knee arthroplasty: a meta-analysis of randomized controlled and prospective cohort trials. Knee. 2014;21:987–93.
10. Kim Y-H, Kim J-SS. Incidence and natural history of deep-vein thrombosis after total knee arthroplasty. A prospective, randomised study. J. Bone Joint Surg. Br. 2002;84:566–70.
11. Stringer MD, Steadman CA, Hedges AR, Thomas EM, Morley TR, Kakkar VV. Deep vein thrombosis after elective knee surgery. An incidence study in 312 patients. J. Bone Joint Surg. Br. 1989;71:492–7.
12. Gómez-Outes A, Terleira-Fernández AI, Suárez-Gea ML, Vargas-Castrillón E. Dabigatran, rivaroxaban, or apixaban versus enoxaparin for thromboprophylaxis after total hip or knee replacement: systematic review, meta-analysis, and indirect treatment comparisons. BMJ. 2012;344:e3675.
13. Brimmo O, Glenn M, Klika AK, Murray TG, Molloy RM, Higuera CA. Rivaroxaban use for thrombosis prophylaxis is associated with early Periprosthetic joint infection. J Arthroplast. 2016;31:1295–8.
14. Ricket AL, Stewart DW, Wood RC, Cornett L, Odle B, Cluck D, et al. Comparison of postoperative bleeding in Total hip and knee arthroplasty patients receiving rivaroxaban or enoxaparin. Ann Pharmacother. 2016;50:270–5.
15. Alshryda S, Sarda P, Sukeik M, Nargol A, Blenkinsopp J, Mason JM. Tranexamic acid in total knee replacement: a systematic review and meta-analysis. Bone Joint J. 2011;93-B:1577–85.
16. Chen W-P. Effectiveness and safety of tranexamic acid in reducing blood loss in Total knee arthroplasty: a meta-analysis. J Bone Joint Surg Am. 2012;94:1153.

17. Panteli M, Papakostidis C, Dahabreh Z, Giannoudis PV. Topical tranexamic acid in total knee replacement: a systematic review and meta-analysis. Knee. 2013;20:300–9.

18. Gandhi R, Evans HMK, Mahomed SR, Mahomed NN. Tranexamic acid and the reduction of blood loss in total knee and hip arthroplasty: a meta-analysis. BMC Res. Notes. 2013;6:184.

19. Alshryda S, Sukeik M, Sarda P, Blenkinsopp J, Haddad FS, Mason JM. A systematic review and meta-analysis of the topical administration of tranexamic acid in total hip and knee replacement. Bone Joint J. 2014; 96–B:1005–15.

20. Wood AM, Smith R, Keenan A, Brenkel I, Walmsley P. Using a combination of tranexamic acid and rivaroxaban in total knee replacements reduces transfusion requirements: a prospective cohort study. J Arthrosc Jt Surg. 2014;1:76–81.

21. Wang J-W, Chen B, Lin P-C, Yen S-H, Huang C-C, Kuo F-C. The efficacy of combined use of rivaroxaban and tranexamic acid on blood conservation in minimally invasive Total knee arthroplasty a double-blind randomized, controlled trial. J Arthroplast. 2017;32:801–6.

22. Wang CG, Sun ZH, Liu J, Cao JG, Li ZJ. Safety and efficacy of intra-articular tranexamic acid injection without drainage on blood loss in total knee arthroplasty: a randomized clinical trial. Int J Surg Elsevier Ltd. 2015;20:1–7.

23. Wong J, Abrishami A, El Beheiry H, Mahomed NN, Roderick Davey J, Gandhi R, et al. Topical application of tranexamic acid reduces postoperative blood loss in Total knee arthroplasty. J Bone Joint Surg Am. 2010;92:2503–13.

24. Gómez-barrena E, Ortega-andreu M, Padilla-eguiluz NG, Hanna P. Topical intra-articular compared with intravenous tranexamic acid to reduce blood loss in primary Total knee replacement. J Bone Joint Surg Am. 2014;96:1937–44.

25. Turpie AGG, Fisher WD, Bauer KA, Kwong LM, Irwin MW, Kälebo P, et al. BAY 59-7939: an oral, direct factor Xa inhibitor for the prevention of venous thromboembolism in patients after total knee replacement. A phase II dose-ranging study. J Thromb Haemost. 2005;3:2479–86.

26. Nadler SB, Hidalgo JH, Bloch T. Prediction of blood volume in normal human adults. Surgery. 1962;51(2):224–32. [cited 2018 Jan 3]

27. Yen S-H, Lin P-C, Chen B, Huang C-C, Wang J-W. Topical tranexamic acid reduces blood loss in minimally invasive Total knee arthroplasty receiving rivaroxaban. Biomed Res Int. 2017;2017:1–8.

28. Warwick D. New concepts in orthopaedic thromboprophylaxis. J Bone Joint Surg Br. 2004;86:788–92.

29. Nicolaides AN, Breddin HK, Fareed J, Goldhaber S, Haas S, Hull R, et al. Prevention of venous thromboembolism. International consensus statement. Guidelines compiled in accordance with the scientific evidence. Int Angiol. 2001;20:1–37.

30. Kinov P, Tanchev PP, Ellis M, Volpin G. Antithrombotic prophylaxis in major orthopaedic surgery: an historical overview and update of current recommendations. Int Orthop. 2014;38:169–75.

31. Eriksson BI, Dahl OE, Rosencher N, Kurth AA, van Dijk CN, Frostick SP, et al. Oral dabigatran etexilate vs. subcutaneous enoxaparin for the prevention of venous thromboembolism after total knee replacement: the RE-MODEL randomized trial. J Thromb Haemost. 2007;5:2178–85.

32. Lassen MR, Davidson BL, Gallus A, Pineo G, Ansell J, Deitchman D. The efficacy and safety of apixaban, an oral, direct factor Xa inhibitor, as thromboprophylaxis in patients following total knee replacement. J Thromb Haemost. 2007;5:2368–75.

33. Yhim HY, Lee J, Lee JY, Lee JO, Bang SM. Pharmacological thromboprophylaxis and its impact on venous thromboembolism following total knee and hip arthroplasty in Korea: a nationwide population-based study. PLoS One. 2017;12:1–15.

34. Bala A, Huddleston JI, Goodman SB, Maloney WJ, Amanatullah DF. Venous thromboembolism prophylaxis after TKA: aspirin, warfarin, enoxaparin, or factor Xa inhibitors? Clin Orthop Relat Res. 2017;475:2205–13.

35. Lee G-C, Hawes T, Cushner FD, Scott WN. Current trends in blood conservation in Total knee arthroplasty. Clin Orthop Relat Res. 2005;440:170–4.

36. Dunn CJ. Tranexamic acid a review of its use in surgery and other indications. Drugs. 1999;57:1005–10032.

37. Tan J, Chen H, Liu Q, Chen C, Huang W. A meta-analysis of the effectiveness and safety of using tranexamic acid in primary unilateral total knee arthroplasty. J Surg Res. 2013;184:880–7.

38. Sarzaeem MM, Razi M, Kazemian G, Moghaddam ME, Rasi AM, Karimi M. Comparing efficacy of three methods of tranexamic acid administration in reducing hemoglobin drop following total knee arthroplasty. J Arthroplast. 2014;29:1521–4.

39. Yue C, Pei F, Yang P, Xie J, Kang P. Effect of topical tranexamic acid in reducing bleeding and transfusions in TKA. Orthopedics. 2015;38:315–24.

40. Zhao-yu C, Yan G, Wei C, Yuejv L, Ying-ze Z. Reduced blood loss after intra-articular tranexamic acid injection during total knee arthroplasty: a meta-analysis of the literature. Knee Surg. Sport. Traumatol. Arthrosc. 2014;22: 3181–90.

24

Perioperative multiple low-dose Dexamethasones improves postoperative clinical outcomes after Total knee arthroplasty

Yuangang Wu[1†], Xiaoxi Lu[2,3†], Yimei Ma[2,3], Yi Zeng[1], Xianchao Bao[1], Huazhang Xiong[1] and Bin Shen[1*]

Abstract

Background: The purpose of this study was to investigate the efficacy and safety of multiple low-dose dexamethasones in primary total knee arthroplasty (TKA).

Methods: One hundred fifty patients were equally randomized into 3 groups: Group A ($n = 50$) received 2 doses of normal saline only; Group B ($n = 50$) received with 1 dose of intravenous dexamethasone and 1 dose of normal saline; Group C ($n = 50$) received with 2 doses of intravenous dexamethasone. The clinical outcomes and complications were assessed.

Results: The CRP and IL-6 were significantly lower in Group C and B than Group A at 24, 48, and 72 h postoperatively ($P < 0.001$ for all). The intensity of postoperative nausea and vomiting (PONV) in Group C was lower than Group A at 24 ($P < 0.001$, $P = 0.002$), 48 ($P = 0.005$, $P = 0.041$) and 72 h ($P = 0.017$, $P = 0.031$) postoperatively and Group B at 24 h ($P = 0.027$, $P = 0.019$) postoperatively. Pain were significantly less in Group C than Group A at 24 ($P < 0.001$), 48 h ($P = 0.037$) postoperatively and Group B 24 h ($P = 0.030$) postoperatively. Patients in Group C had better range of motion (ROM) and satisfaction than Group A ($P < 0.001$, $P = 0.002$) and B ($P = 0.001$, $P = 0.043$). No differences were found in complications.

Conclusions: The administration of 10 mg dexamethasone 1 h before the surgery, and repeated at 6 h postoperatively can significantly reduce the level of postoperative CRP and IL-6 and the incidence of PONV, relieve pain, achieve an additional analgesic effect, and improve the early ROM compared with the other two groups in TKA.

Level of Evidence: Therapeutic Level I.

Keywords: Total knee arthroplasty, Dexamethasones, Clinical outcomes, Randomized controlled study

Background

Total knee arthroplasty (TKA) has become a successful surgical method for the treatment of severe knee diseases [1–3]. TKA, however, involves extensive osteotomy, soft tissue release and surgical trauma, which often lead to severe postoperative inflammatory reactions [4–6]. Consequently, patients can experience severe pain in the early postoperative period [7, 8], accompanied by postoperative nausea and vomiting (PONV) [9–11], and a prolonged length of stay (LOS) [12]. Pain and PONV may hinder the early recovery of TKA, resulting in patients dissatisfaction [13–16]. Therefore, it is better to improve the fast-track recovery of patients in reducing postoperative inflammation, relieving pain and preventing PONV.

Glucocorticoids, which have powerful anti-inflammatory and antiemetic effects, are widely used in perioperative management, such as abdominal [17, 18], gynaecologic [19], and TKA surgery [20–22], for reducing the postoperative inflammatory response, alleviating postoperative pain and preventing PONV. However, the most suitable protocol

---

* Correspondence: shenbin_1971@163.com
†Yuangang Wu and Xiaoxi Lu contributed equally to this work.
[1]Department of Orthopaedic Surgery, West China Hospital, West China Medical School, Sichuan University, Chengdu 610041, Sichuan Province, China
Full list of author information is available at the end of the article

for administration and dosage remains controversial. As previously reported, glucocorticoids were given at a single and low dose, with fewer samples in most previous studies [23–25]. In addition, concerns regarding the adverse effects of glucocorticoid therapy, including infection and gastro-intestinal bleeding, have potentially limited its widespread use in TKA [26]. Last, although the administration of the drug provides better pain and vomiting relief than traditional methods, many patients still suffer from it at the initial stage after surgery [19, 22, 27].

The current study was therefore designed to compare the effectiveness and safety of multiple low doses of dexamethasone in patients following primary TKA by evaluating: (1) whether multiple low doses of dexamethasone reduce postoperative inflammatory markers and the incidence of PONV; (2) whether multiple low doses of dexamethasone relieve pain and provide an additional analgesic effect, improving the range of motion (ROM) and patient satisfaction; and (3) whether multiple low doses of dexamethasone are safe in primary TKA.

Methods
Study design and patients
This randomized controlled trial was approved by the institutional ethics committee and written informed consent was obtained from each patient. The study was registered in the Chinese Clinical Trial Registry on 09/07/2018 (ChiCTR1800017036). All consecutive patients with a diagnosis of end-stage osteoarthritis following primary unilateral TKA were enrolled for inclusion in the study. The exclusion criteria were as follows: rheumatoid arthritis, revision surgery, allergy to the dexamethasone and tranexamic acid, administration of the glucocorticoid 3 months before surgery, alcohol dependence, a history with thrombosis, the severe liver and kidney deficiency and body mass index (BMI) > 35 kg/m^2. Patients were randomly assigned to three groups containing 50 patients with a list generated by a computer, and randomization was blind and performed with the use of sealed envelopes at a ratio of 1:1:1 to be opened just prior to surgery.

Patients in the Group A was given intravenously 2 mL of normal saline solution 1 h before the surgery and repeated 6 h after surgery. Patients in the Group B was given intravenously 10 mg dexamethasone (2 ml, Tianjin Kingyork group Co., Ltd., China) 1 h before the surgery and repeated intravenously 2 mL of normal saline solution 6 h after surgery. Patients in the Group C was given intravenously 10 mg dexamethasone solution 1 h before the surgery and repeated 6 h after surgery. To support the double-blind study, patients in group A were treated with 2 doses of a normal saline solution and patients in group B were treated also normal saline solution 6 h after surgery. All drugs were administered by a nurse

who was not involved in the study. The patients, investigators, and statisticians were all blind during the study.

Surgical technique
All patients were performed general anesthesia, which was administered by the same anesthetists. All TKAs were performed by 1 senior orthopedic surgeon through a midline skin incision, medial parapatellar approach. All patients have used the PFC Sigma PS (DePuy Orthopedics Inc., Warsaw, IN, USA) prosthesis. All of the wound closed at about 45°of knee bends. The arthrotomy closure was performed using an interrupted figure-of-eight #1 EthibondTM (Ethicon, Somerville, NJ, USA), a subdermal closure using interrupted buried simple 2–0 Monocryl TM (Ethicon) and staples for skin closure. All patients were given intraoperatively 20 mg/kg tranexamic acid (Chongqing Lummy Pharmaceutical Co., Ltd. China) 10 min before the skin incision, and repeated 3 h after surgery. No patients used the tourniquet, drainage tube, femoral nerve block and/or intravenous patient-controlled analgesia.

Postoperative care
All patients received cefuroxime 1.5 g 2 h before the operation to prevent infection. After the operation, the patient was transferred to the anesthesia recovery unit for 2 h and then sent to the inpatient ward. A cold pack was applied to the surgical site 2 days. Daily gait rehabilitation program and weight training were conducted by a physiotherapist on the first day after surgery.

All patients received the same management for pain and PONV. Multimodal oral analgesic drugs (200 mg q12 h celecoxib, 75 mg q8 h pregabalin) were administered for pre-emptive analgesia 1 day before the surgery. After the surgery, the pain levels of all patients were measured using a visual analogue scale (VAS, 0 - no pain, 10 - worst imaginable pain). The routine analgesia regimen remains the same as before surgery when the VAS level of the patient was lower than 4. Oral oxycodone (10 mg q8 h) was used when the VAS level of the patient was between 4 and 6, and intramuscular injection of pethidine hydrochloride (100 mg) was used when a patient reported pain greater than 6. The severity of nausea of all patients was measured using VAS (VAS, 0-on nausea, 10- worst imaginable nausea). Metoclopramide (10 mg) was injected intravenously as the first-line antiemetic rescue treatment when PONV occurred two or more times or the VAS level was greater than 4. An intramuscular injection of ondansetron (5 mg) can be used as the second-line antiemetic rescue option when severe nausea persists after two doses of metoclopramide for a 30-min interval.

All patients were given subcutaneously low molecular-weight heparin (LMWH, 0.2 mL, 2000 IU) at 6 h postoperatively, and repeated with a full dose at 24-h intervals

(0.4 mL, 4000 IU) until discharge. After discharge, 10 mg rivaroxaban (Xarelto, Bayer, Germany) was administered orally for 15 days to prevent thrombosis [28]. Intermittent pneumatic compression device was routinely applied on the calves of patients until walking. Doppler ultrasound examination was used assessing deep vein thrombosis (DVT) at the time of discharge and at 1, 3-month follow-up assessments, or at any time clinically suspected DVT. Pulmonary embolism (PE) was diagnosed on the basis of clinical symptoms and chest computed tomography (CT) scans.

Outcome measurements
The outcomes were evaluated including the inflammation reaction of CRP and IL-6, pain level (VAS score) and the number of patients requiring analgesic rescue drugs (Oxycodone and Pethidine hydrochloride), the severity of nausea (VAS score), the incidence of PONV and the number of patients requiring antiemetic rescue (Metoclopramide and Ondansetron). CRP, IL-6, pain level, the severity of nausea, and PONV were routinely tested preoperatively and at 24, 48, and 72 h postoperatively. Nausea was defined as a subjective feeling of unpleasant related to awareness of the urge to vomit. Vomiting is the forcible discharge of stomach contents from the mouth. ROM and a six-point satisfaction questionnaire [5] was assessed at the time of discharge. The LOS and wound-related complications were recorded carefully.

Statistical analysis
The sample size of the current study was calculated, as previously described by Lunn [24], using VAS score as the primary outcome; it was determined that, for 90% power and a significance level of 0.05, requiring 24 patients in each group. With the consideration of exclusion, we decided to include 50 patients in each group. One-way ANOVA and Tukey's post-hoc were used to compare the quantitative data, such as CRP, IL-6, pain level, the severity of nausea, and ROM. The Pearson chi-square test or Fisher exact test was used for comparing qualitative data, such as the incidence of PONV, patient satisfaction, and complications. All analyses were performed using SPSS version 22.0, significance was set at $P < 0.05$.

Results
Baseline characteristics
During the recruitment period from January 2017 to October 2017, 165 patients with osteoarthritis requiring unilateral primary TKA were scheduled. Among these patients, 15 of these patients were excluded for the following reasons: 6 patients with glucocorticoid 3 months before surgery, 3 had alcohol dependence, 5 declined to participate, 1 had an infection. Thus, 150 patients were eventually included in the analysis, 50 patients were randomized to each group (Fig.1).

No patients were lost during the follow-up. Table 1 summarizes the baseline characteristics of the 3 groups. There were no statistically significant differences in age, gender, BMI, American Society of Anesthesiologists, preoperative Hb, Hct, CRP, IL-6, ROM and VAS among the 3 groups of patients.

Inflammation marks
The mean CRP and IL-6 increased postoperatively in all patients after the surgery. The mean level of CRP peaked 48 h postoperatively among the 3 groups. It was significantly lower in Group C and Group B than Group A at 24 ($P < 0.001$, $P < 0.001$), 48 ($P < 0.001$, $P < 0.001$), and 72 h ($P < 0.001$, $P < 0.001$) postoperatively. The mean level of CRP in Group C was lower than Group B at 24 h ($P < 0.001$) postoperatively, however, it was no statistical significance at 48 ($P = 0.081$) and 72 h ($P = 0.057$) postoperatively (Fig.2).

The mean level of IL-6 peaked in Group C and B at 48 h postoperatively compared with Group A at 24 h postoperatively. It was significantly lower in Group C and Group B than Group A at 24 ($P < 0.001$, $P < 0.001$), 48 ($P < 0.001$, $P < 0.001$), and 72 h ($P < 0.001$, $P < 0.001$) postoperatively. Although, the mean level of IL-6 in Group B was slightly greater than Group C at 24 ($P = 0.133$), 48 ($P = 0.073$), and 72 h ($P = 0.075$) postoperatively, it was no statistical significance (Fig.3).

Pain level and rescue analgesic
The postoperative mean VAS pain score was significantly lower in Group C than in Group A at 24 h ($P < 0.001$), 48 h ($P = 0.037$) postoperatively and compared with B 24 h ($P = 0.030$) postoperatively. The differences were also statistically significant between Groups B and A at 24 h ($P = 0.012$) postoperatively (Fig. 4).

Similar to the pain level, the number of patients requiring oxycodone and pethidine hydrochloride was lower in Group C compared with Group A at 24 h ($P < 0.001$, $P < 0.001$) and 48 h ($P = 0.003$, $P < 0.001$) postoperatively, and it was also lower in Group B than Group A at 24 h postoperatively ($P = 0.027$, $P = 0.034$). The level of pethidine hydrochloride was less in Group C than B at 24 h postoperatively ($P = 0.003$) (Table 2).

Intensity of nausea, PONV, and rescue antiemetic
The intensity of nausea in Group C was lower than Group A at 24 ($P < 0.001$), 48 ($P = 0.005$) and 72 h ($P = 0.017$) postoperatively and compared with Group B at 24 h ($P = 0.027$) postoperatively, and it was also lower in Group B than Group A at 24 h postoperatively ($P = 0.041$) (Table 3).

Similar to the intensity of nausea, the incidence of PONV was lower in Group C than Group A at 24 ($P = 0.002$), 48 ($P = 0.041$) and 72 h ($P = 0.031$) postoperatively, and there

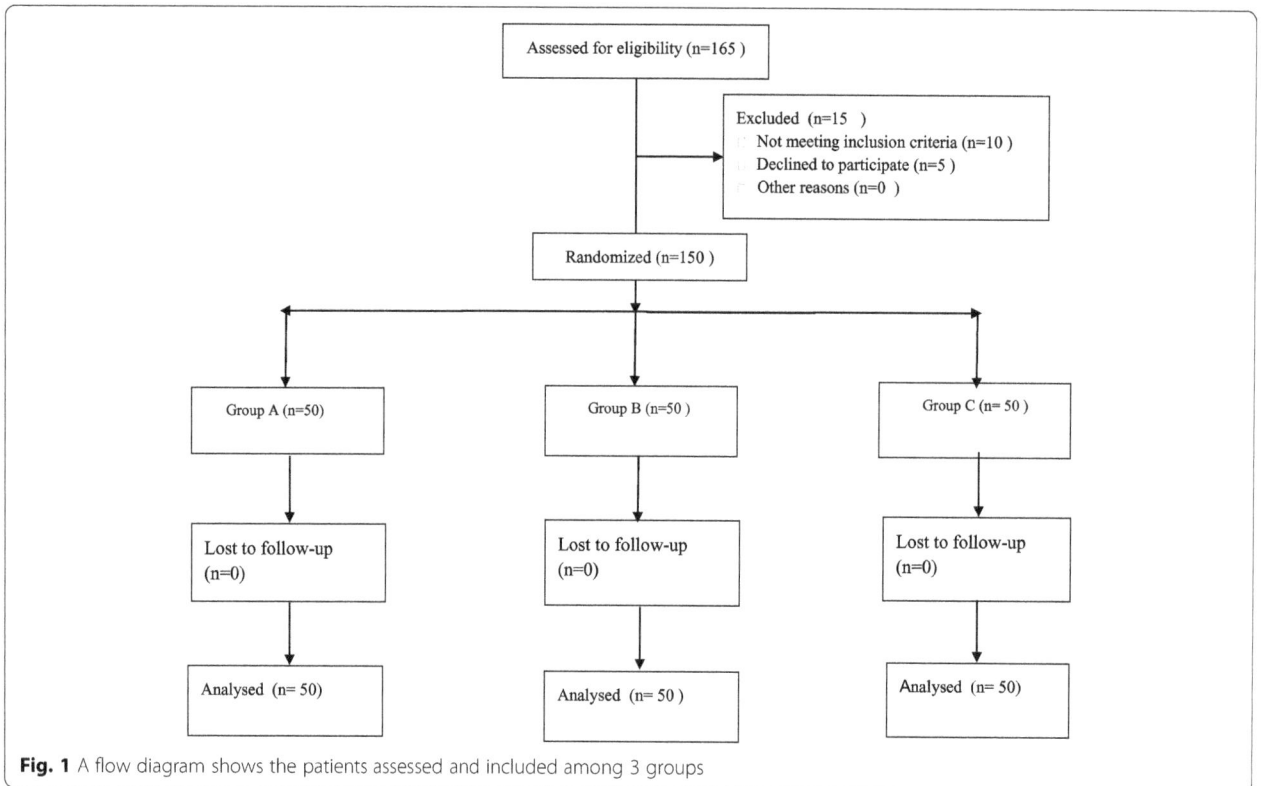

Fig. 1 A flow diagram shows the patients assessed and included among 3 groups

was also a significant difference between Groups B and A at 24 h ($P = 0.019$) postoperatively (Table 3).

The number of patients requiring metoclopramide was lower in Group C compared with Group A at 24 ($P < 0.001$), 48 ($P = 0.025$) and 72 h ($P = 0.035$) postoperatively, and it

was also lower in Group B than Group A at 24 h ($P = 0.017$) postoperatively (Table 2).

No three-group differences in the number of patients requiring ondansetron were found at 24 ($P = 0.064$), 48 ($P = 0.132$) and 72 h ($P = 1$) postoperatively (Table 2).

Table 1 Preoperative demographics

Variables	Group A ($n = 50$)	Group B ($n = 50$)	Group C ($n = 50$)	P Value
Age (y)*	67.40 ± 3.34	66.90 ± 4.62	66.38 ± 3.38	0.414
Gender‡ (M/F)	32/18	33/17	30/20	0.818
Weight (kg)*	65.52 ± 4.99	65.22 ± 4.81	66.38 ± 3.84	0.423
Hight (cm)*	159.38 ± 6.76	158.06 ± 5.81	157.92 ± 6.86	0.465
BMI (kg/m²)*	25.85 ± 2.08	26.14 ± 1.98	26.70 ± 2.08	0.109
ASA*	1.98 ± 0.65	1.94 ± 0.65	2.02 ± 0.62	0.824
Preop.Hb (g/L)*	13.42 ± 0.55	13.45 ± 0.53	13.39 ± 0.56	0.858
Preop.Hct (L/L)*	39.84 ± 1.26	39.87 ± 1.17	39.74 ± 1.25	0.867
Preop.CRP (mg/L)*	3.23 ± 0.96	3.29 ± 0.76	3.25 ± 0.93	0.950
Preop.IL-6 (pg/mL)*	4.05 ± 1.10	4.15 ± 1.15	4.11 ± 0.47	0.859
Preop. ROM*	94.54 ± 3.40	93.90 ± 3.42	93.89 ± 4.15	0.594
Preop. VAS*	5.16 ± 0.68	5.32 ± 0.82	5.22 ± 0.68	0.542
Duration of surgery (min)*	66.84 ± 3.30	67.92 ± 3.30	68.02 ± 2.83	0.120

Abbreviations: *y* years, *M* male, *F* female, *R* right, *L* left, *BMI* body mass index, *ASA* American Society of Anesthesiologists, *Preop* preoperative, *Hb* hemoglobin, *Hct* hematocrit, *CRP* C-reactive protein, *IL-6* interleukin 6, *ROM* range of motion, *VAS* visual analogue scale
P value indicates a significant difference among the groups
*was analyzed by the one-way ANOVA;
‡ was analyzed by the Pearson chi-square test or the Fisher exact test

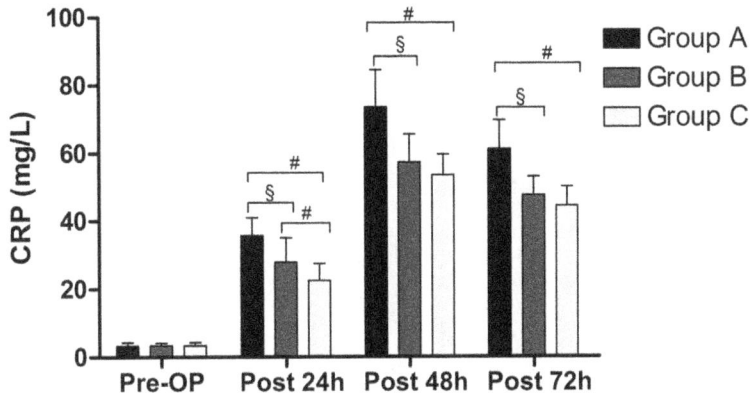

Fig. 2 The level of CRP in all groups. Pre-OP = preoperative, post = postoperative. A significant difference among the 3 groups as calculated with one-way ANOVA. ‡ Significantly different from the Group B. # Significantly different from the Group C

ROM, LOS, patient satisfaction, and complications

At the time of discharge, the ROM in Group C was better than in Group A ($P < 0.001$) and B ($P = 0.001$), but it was no differenced in the other subgroup in another subgroup. The average LOS in Group A, B, C were 5.02 ± 0.62, 4.94 ± 0.84, and 4.82 ± 0.72 days respectively, no differences were found ($P = 0.393$). Patients in Group C had significantly higher satisfaction ratings than Groups A ($P = 0.002$) and B ($P = 0.043$) (Table III), no benefits in Group B relative to Group A was found ($P = 0.298$) (Table 3).

No DVT and PE was found in any of the patients, however, 9 patients (group A, 3 cases, group B, 3 cases, group C, 5 cases) developed intramuscular venous thrombosis. 2 patients from Group C and 1 patients from Group B had superficial infection during the 3-month follow-up period, which was controlled by dressing change and oral antibiotics. No gastrointestinal hemorrhage occurred (Table 3).

Discussion

The most important finding of this study is that patients in Group C who were intravenously administered 10 mg dexamethasone 1 h preoperatively and repeated 10 mg at 6 postoperatively can significantly reduce the postoperative level of CRP and IL-6, decrease the incidence of PONV and receive additional analgesic and antiemetic effects, and achieve a better ROM and patient satisfaction, without increasing the risk of wound-related complications when compared with patients in Group A and B.

TKA is one of the most effective methods to treat knee diseases [1, 2]. However, surgical trauma following TKA often results in severe postoperative inflammation, which is associated with postoperative pain and PONV [8, 9]. As a result, the fast-track treatment of the patients was hampered postoperatively. Glucocorticoids are known for their analgesic, anti-inflammatory, and anti-emetic effects, although the mechanisms are unclear. In using corticosteroids, therefore, its pharmaceutical ingredients enter the surrounding tissue and reduce the inflammatory response at the site of surgical trauma, thus providing effective pain relief. Dexamethasone is a kind of synthetic glucocorticoid with high bioavailability and long acting time. In the current study, significant increases in CRP and IL-6 levels

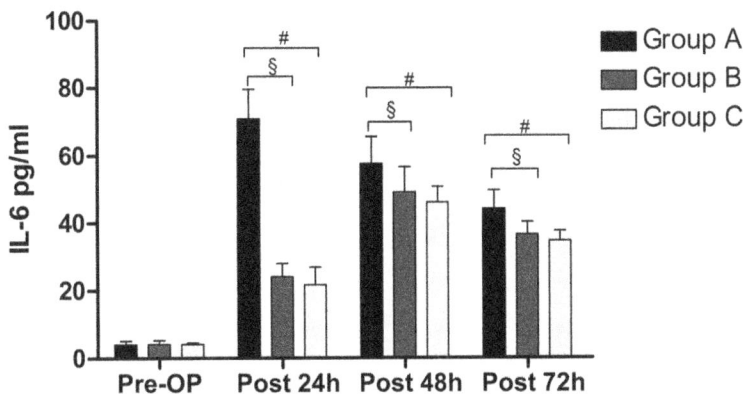

Fig. 3 The level of IL-6 in all groups. Pre-OP = preoperative, post = postoperative. A significant difference among the 3 groups as calculated with one-way ANOVA. ‡ Significantly different from the Group B. # Significantly different from the Group C

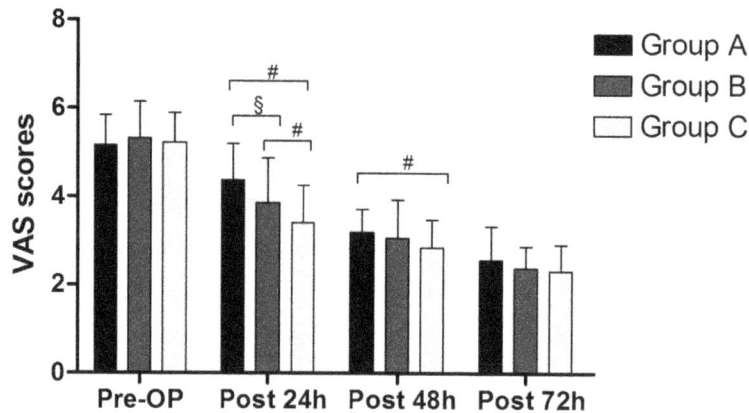

Fig. 4 The level of pain in all groups. Pre-OP = preoperative, post = postoperative. A significant difference among the 3 groups as calculated with one-way ANOVA. ‡ Significantly different from the Group B. # Significantly different from the Group C

were found in the three treatment groups, however, CRP and IL-6 levels increased significantly less in Groups C and B compared with Group A at 24, 48, and 72 h. It was also observed to be lower in Group C than in Group B. Thus, our findings suggest that intravenous dexamethasone administered 1 h preoperatively and repeated at 6 h postoperatively reduced the postoperative inflammatory response compared to Groups A and B.

Compared with the level of pain preoperatively, pain declined after TKA among the three groups. As previously reported, the analgesic effect of glucocorticoid is achieved by inhibiting phospholipase, thus blocking the pathway of cyclooxygenase and lipoxygenase in the inflammatory chain reaction [29]. At the same time, it can also inhibit the level of bradykinin [30] in tissues and the release of neuropeptides from nerve endings [31], both of which

may enhance the sense of injury in inflammatory tissues and surgical wounds. An Randomized Controlled Trial (RCT) performed by Koh et al. [22] prospectively evaluated 269 TKAs randomized to receive dexamethasone (10 mg) combined with ramosetron or ramosetron alone. These results suggest that patients with dexamethasone experienced lower pain and consumed fewer opioids during the 6 to 24 h postoperative. Similarly, another RCT study by Xu et al. [32] involving 108 TKA patients divided into 2 groups of 54 patients. The two treatment groups were either given two doses of 10 mg IV dexamethasone or placebo, the study found that the pain at rest and walking was lower at 24 h postoperatively in the dexamethasone group. The results in current study echo those findings. We showed a statistically significant reduction of the VAS score of pain in Group C than Group A at 24 and

Table 2 The the number of patients of requiring rescue analgesic and antiemetic

Variables	Group A (n = 50)	Group B (n = 50)	Group C (n = 50)	P Value
Oxycodone-post 24 h (n)‡	28§#	17 #	8	0.001
Oxycodone-post 48 h (n)‡	19 #	11	6	0.009
Oxycodone-post 72 h (n)‡	8	5	3	0.265
Pethidine hydrochloride-post 24 h (n)‡	22§#	12	6	0.001
Pethidine hydrochloride-post 48 h (n)‡	14 #	7	2	0.004
Pethidine hydrochloride-post 72 h (n)‡	3	1	0	0.166
Metoclopramide-post 24 h (n)‡	21§#	10	7	0.003
Metoclopramide-post 48 h (n)‡	12 #	7	3	0.039
Metoclopramide-post 72 h (n)‡	6 #	2	0	0.025
Ondansetron-post 24 h (n)‡	7	3	1	0.064
Ondansetron-post 48 h (n)‡	2	0	0	0.132
Ondansetron-post 72 h (n)‡	0	0	0	1

Abbreviations: *post* postoperative, *h* hours, *n* number
‡ was analyzed by the Pearson chi-square test or the Fisher exact test
P value indicates a significant difference among the groups
§Significantly different from the Group B. # Significantly different from the Group C

Table 3 The clinical outcomes and complications among the 3 groups

Variables	Group A (n = 50)	Group B (n = 50)	Group C (n = 50)	P Value
Intensity of Nausea-post 24h*	2.96 ± 1.24§#	2.38 ± 1.07#	1.76 ± 1.24	0.001
Intensity of Nausea-post 48h*	1.66 ± 0.82#	1.38 ± 0.90	1.12 ± 0.82	0.008
Intensity of Nausea-post 72h*	1.18 ± 0.77#	0.94 ± 0.73	0.74 ± 0.85	0.023
PONV-post 24 h‡	22§#	11	8	0.004
PONV- post 48 h‡	14 #	8	5	0.058
PONV- post 72 h‡	10 #	4	2	0.026
Satisfaction level (n)‡				0.007
Very satisfied	18 #	23 #	35	
Somewhat satisfied	14	17	11	
Neither satisfied nor dissatisfied	11	6	4	
Somewhat dissatisfied	7	4	0	
Very dissatisfied	0	0	0	
ROM*	99.66 ± 2.60 #	100.70 ± 2.37 #	102.48 ± 1.99	0.001
LOS (days)*	5.02 ± 0.62	4.94 ± 0.84	4.82 ± 0.72	0.393
DVT (n)‡	0	0	0	1
PE (n)‡	0	0	0	1
Intramuscular thrombosis (n)‡	3	3	5	0.675
Superficial infection (n)‡	0	1	2	0.360
Gastrointestinal hemorrhage (n)‡	0	0	0	1

Abbreviations: *Post* postoperative, *h* hours, *n* number, *PONV* postoperative nausea and vomiting, *ROM* range of motion, *LOS* length of stay, *DVT* deep vein thrombosis, *PE* Pulmonary embolism

*was analyzed by the one-way ANOVA;

‡ was analyzed by the Pearson chi-square test or the Fisher exact test

P value indicates a significant difference among the groups

§Significantly different from the Group B. # Significantly different from the Group C

48 h postoperatively and Group B at 24 h postoperatively. Furthermore, the requirements of oxycodone and pethidine hydrochloride were significantly lower in Group C.

The antiemetic effects of dexamethasone were well documented [17, 19, 22, 32] and supported in our study. However, the mechanism by which glucocorticoids relieve PONV is not fully understood. Its effect may be mediated by the inhibition of prostaglandin synthesis or the inhibition of endogenous opioid release [33]. The current study showed that two doses of dexamethasone were more effective in preventing the PONV and reducing the intensity of nausea than the single dose or without dexamethasone groups. The results are consistent with previous studies [10, 22, 32] suggesting that dexamethasone has a better antiemetic effect. In a recent meta-analysis of 3 randomized controlled trials [34], dexamethasone not only reduces postoperative pain level and opioid consumption within 48 h but also reduces postoperative PONV. Although few previous studies have investigated the antiemetic efficacy of two doses of low-dose dexamethasone after TKA. The current results as well as previous studies [10, 32] suggest that the use of multiple low doses of dexamethasone has a stronger antiemetic effect on the early stage of PONV than a

single dose of dexamethasone. The results therefore suggest that the repeated administration of dexamethasone 6 h postoperatively can effectively reduce the incidence of PONV. Additionally, functional outcome assessments in our study demonstrated a better ROM in Group C. The outcomes might explain the significantly higher satisfaction ratings of patients in Group C at the time of discharge.

However, the optimal routes and doses of dexamethasone remain controversial. A range of doses from 4 to 10 mg in primary TKA has been established in most studies [22, 35]. Barnes et al. [36] suggested that glucocorticoids bind to intracellular glucocorticoid receptors, which are mainly mediated by the synthesis of transcriptional proteins. Therefore, the starting time of biological action is generally 1–2 h [29], and it was reasonable to give dexamethasone 1 h before the surgery so that it reached its plasma concentration at the beginning of resuscitation in this study. In addition, since early media-activated metabolic reaction occurs immediately after surgical incision [37], it is also reasonable to give dexamethasone 1 h before the surgery to obtain a potential therapeutic effect postoperatively. As previously reported [22, 27], patients still have to deal with pain and PONV with single-dose dexamethasone. Thus, we added an additional 10-mg dose of dexamethasone at 6 h post-operatively, assuming that it would have a meaningful clinical benefit.

Although TKA is associated with thrombosis [3, 38], and glucocorticoids are associated with wound healing and postoperative infection, previous studies using low or high doses of glucocorticoids have not shown that glucocorticoids are associated with these complications during the perioperative period [22, 32, 34]. In our study, we also found that the additional low dose of dexamethasone was given at 6 postoperatively, and no patients had an obvious adverse effect and/or complication during postoperative follow-up. It is known that synthetic glucocorticoids,such as dexamethasone, prescribed in daily care can induce hypertension. However, the exact mechanism by which glucocorticoids may induce hypertension is unclear [39]. Some evidence supports the fact that glucocorticoids may actually have nothing to do with elevated blood pressure in the first few weeks. Gabriel et al. [40] reported that 15.3% of 124 patients with rheumatoid polymyalgia prescribed glucocorticoid treatment for hypertension, and 26.3% of 57 patients who received non-steroidal anti-inflammatory drugs had hypertension. Furthermore, Fardet et al. [41] also sugessted that the increase of blood pressure during the first months of exposure to synthetic glucocorticoids seems clinically nonsignificant. At the same time, there was also no evidence that perioperative dexamethasone administration is associated with increased postoperative glucose levels (> 200 mg/dl) or higher maximum glucose levels in total joint arthroplasty [42]. Therefore, we believe that there is evidence to support that two doses of low-dose preoperative treatment with dexamethasone are safe in TKA procedures.

This study had some limitations. The follow-up period for assessing functional outcome was 24 h, 48 h and 72 h postoperatively; therefore, this study does not show the long-term effects of dexamethasone. Second, although this study showed a lower incidence of wound-related complications, a larger sample size is required to adequately assess the significant differences in adverse events. Third, two doses of low-dose dexamethasone showed better clinical results, but the best method and dose of dexamethasone and whether a further use is needed to produce additional results remain unclear.

Conclusions

The administration of 10 mg dexamethasone 1 h before the surgery, and repeated at 6 h postoperatively can significantly reduce the level of postoperative CRP and IL-6 and the incidence of PONV, relieve pain, achieve an additional analgesic effect, and improve the early ROM compared with the other two groups in TKA.

Abbreviations
BMI: Body mass index; CRP: C-reactive protein; DVT: Deep vein thrombosis; IL-6: Interleukin 6; LOS: Length of stay; PBV: Patient's blood volume; PE: Pulmonary embolism; PONV: Postoperative nausea and vomiting; ROM: Range of motion; TKA: Total knee arthroplasty; VAS: Visual analogue scale

Acknowledgements
The authors would like to thank Dr. Li Chen (chenli930@scu.edu.cn) from Analytical & Testing Center Sichuan University for her help with image processing and data analysis, and I would also like to thank Dr. Shuting Li (447623681@qq.com) from Department of Ultrasonography, West China Hospital, Sichuan University, for providing diagnosis of venous thrombosis.

Funding
This study was funded by the National Natural Science Foundation of China Program (No. 81601936, No. 81672219), for providing support of design and drafted the manuscript; and it was funded by the Science and Technology Department of Sichuan Province (No. 2017FZ0056 and No. 2018HH0141), for providing support of data acquisition and language modification; and it was also funded by the Health Department of Sichuan Province (N0.18ZD016), for providing support of interpreted the data and revised the manuscript.

Authors' contributions
BS, YZ and YGW conceived, designed and coordinated the experiments and drafted the manuscript. BS, YGW, YZ, XCB and HZX contributed to data acquisition.YZ, YGW, HZX, XXL and YMM analysed and interpreted the data. XCB, HZX, XXL and YMM revised the manuscript. XXL and YMM corrected language. All authors read and approved the final manuscript.

Consent for publication
Not applicable.

Competing interests
The authors declare that they have no competing interests.

Author details
[1]Department of Orthopaedic Surgery, West China Hospital, West China Medical School, Sichuan University, Chengdu 610041, Sichuan Province, China. [2]Department of Pediatrics, West China University Second Hospital, Sichuan University, Chengdu 610041, Sichuan Province, China. [3]Key Laboratory of Birth Defects and Related Diseases of Women and Children (Sichuan University), Ministry of Education, Chengdu, China.

References
1. Wu Y, Zeng Y, Bao X, Xiong H, Hu Q, Li M, Shen B. Comparison of mini-subvastus approach versus medial parapatellar approach in primary total knee arthroplasty. Int J Surg. 2018;57:15–21.
2. Kurtz S, Ong K, Lau E, Mowat F, Halpern M. Projections of primary and revision hip and knee arthroplasty in the United States from 2005 to 2030. J Bone Joint Surg Am. 2007;89:780–5.
3. Wu Y, Zeng Y, Li C, Zhong J, Hu Q, Pei F, Shen B. The effect of postoperative limb positioning on blood loss and early outcomes after primary total knee arthroplasty: a randomized controlled trial. Int Orthop. Epub 2018 Oct 23.
4. Filos KS, Lehmann KA. Current concepts and practice in postoperative pain management: need for a change? Eur Surg Res. 1999;31:97–107.

5. Huang Z, Xie X, Li L, Huang Q, Ma J, Shen B, Kraus VB, Pei F. Intravenous and Topical tranexamic acid alone are superior to tourniquet use for primary Total knee arthroplasty: a prospective, Randomized Controlled Trial. J Bone Joint Surg Am. 2017;99:2053–61.

6. Shen H, Zhang N, Zhang X. Ji W. C-reactive protein levels after 4 types of arthroplasty. Acta Orthop. 2009;80:330–3.

7. Cui Z, Liu X, Teng Y, et al. The efficacy of steroid injection in total knee or hip arthroplasty. Knee Surg Sports Traumatol Arthrosc. 2015;23:2306–14.

8. Kehlet H, Jensen TS, Woolf CJ. Persistent postsurgical pain: risk factors and prevention. Lancet. 2006;367:1618–25.

9. Chen JJ, Frame DG, White TJ. Efficacy of ondansetron and prochlorperazine for the prevention of postoperative nausea and vomiting after total hip replacement or total knee replacement procedures: a randomized, double-blind, comparative trial. Arch Intern Med. 1998;158:2124–8.

10. Backes JR, Bentley JC, Politi JR, Chambers BT. Dexamethasone reduces length of hospitalization and improves postoperative pain and nausea after total joint arthroplasty: aprospective randomized controlled trial. J Arthroplast. 2013;28(8 Suppl):11–7.

11. Gan TJ, et al. Consensus guidelines for managing postoperative nausea and vomiting. Anesth Analg. 2003;97:62.

12. Aasvang EK, Luna IE, Kehlet H. Challenges in postdischarge function and recovery: the case of fast-track hip and knee arthroplasty. Br J Anaesth. 2015;115:861–6.

13. Polkowski GG 2nd, Ruh EL, Barrack TN, Nunley RM, Barrack RL. Is pain and dissatisfaction after TKA related to early-grade preoperative osteoarthritis? Clin Orthop Relat Res. 2013;471:162–8.

14. Gunaratne R, Pratt DN, Banda J, Fick DP, Khan RJK, Robertson BW. Patient dissatisfaction following Total knee arthroplasty: a systematic review of the literature. J Arthroplast. 2017;32:3854–60.

15. Dorr LD, Chao L. The emotional state of the patient after total hip and knee arthroplasty. Clin Orthop Relat Res. 2007;463:7–12.

16. Myles PS, Williams DL, Hendrata M, Anderson H, Weeks AM. Patient satisfaction after anaesthesia and surgery: results of a prospective survey of 10,811 patients. Br J Anaesth. 2000;84:6–10.

17. Zaghiyan K, Melmed GY, Berel D, Ovsepyan G, Murrell Z, Fleshner P. A prospective, randomized, noninferiority trial of steroid dosing after major colorectal surgery. Ann Surg. 2014;259:32–7.

18. Srinivasa S, Kahokehr AA, Yu TC, Hill AG. Preoperative glucocorticoid use in major abdominal surgery: systematic review and meta-analysis of randomized trials. Ann Surg. 2011;254:183–91.

19. Yang XY, Xiao J, Chen YH, Wang ZT, Wang HL, He DH, Zhang J. Dexamethasone alone vs in combination with transcutaneous electrical acupoint stimulation or tropisetron for prevention of postoperative nausea and vomiting in gynaecological patients undergoing laparoscopic surgery. Br J Anaesth. 2015;115:883–9.

20. Luna IE, Kehlet H, Jensen CM, Christiansen TG, Lind T, Stephensen SL, Aasvang EK. The effect of preoperative intra-articular methylprednisolone on pain after TKA: a randomized double-blinded placebo controlled trial in patients with high-pain knee osteoarthritis and sensitization. J Pain. 2017;18:1476–87.

21. Hartman J, Khanna V, Habib A, Farrokhyar F, Memon M, Adili A. Perioperative systemic glucocorticoids in total hip and knee arthroplasty: a systematic review of outcomes. J Orthop. 2017;14:294–301.

22. Koh IJ, Chang CB, Lee JH, Jeon YT, Kim TK. Preemptive low-dose dexamethasone reduces postoperative emesis and pain after TKA: a randomized controlled study. Clin Orthop Relat Res. 2013;471:3010–20.

23. Jules-Elysee KM, Lipnitsky JY, Patel N, et al. Use of low dose steroids in decreasing cytokine release during bilateral total knee replacement. Reg Anesth Pain Med. 2011;36:36–40.

24. Lunn TH, Kristensen BB, Andersen LO, et al. Effect of high-dose preoperative methylprednisolone on pain and recovery after total knee arthroplasty: a randomized, placebo-controlled trial. Br J Anaesth. 2011;106:230–8.

25. Miyagawa Y, Ejiri M, Kuzuya T, Osada T, Ishiguro N, Yamada K. Methylprednisolone reduces postoperative nausea in total knee and hip arthroplasty. J Clin Pharm Ther. 2010;35:679–84.

26. Horne G, Devane P, Davidson A, Adams K, Purdie G. The influence of steroid injections on the incidence of infection following total knee arthroplasty. N Z Med J. 2008;121:U2896.

27. Koh IJ, Chang CB, Jeon YT, Ryu JH, Kim TK. Does ramosetron reduce postoperative emesis and pain after TKA? Clin Orthop Relat Res. 2012;470:1718–27.

28. Wu Y, Zeng Y, Hu Q, Li M, Bao X, Zhong J, Shen B. Blood loss and cost-effectiveness of oral vs intravenous tranexamic acid in primary total hip arthroplasty: a randomized clinical trial. Thromb Res. 2018 Oct 6;171:143–8.

29. Sapolsky RM, Romero LM, Munck AU. How do glucocorticoids influence stress responses? Integrating permissive, suppressive, stimulatory and preparative actions. Endocr Rev. 2000;21:55–89.

30. Hargreaves KM, Costello A. Glucocorticoids suppress levels of immunoreactive bradykinin in inflamed tissue as evaluated by microdialysis probes. Clin Pharmacol Ther. 1990;48:168–78.

31. Hong D, Byers MR, Oswald RJ. Dexamethasone treatment reduces sensory neuropeptides and nerve sprouting reactions in injured teeth. Pain. 1993;55:171–81.

32. Xu B, Ma J, Huang Q, Huang ZY, Zhang SY, Pei FX. Two doses of low-dose perioperative dexamethasone improve the clinical outcome after total knee arthroplasty: a randomized controlled study. Knee Surg Sports Traumatol Arthrosc. 2018;26:1549–56.

33. Henzi I, Walder B, Tramer MR. Dexamethasone for the prevention of postoperative nausea and vomiting: a quantitative systematic review. Anesth Analg. 2000;90:186–94.

34. Fan ZR, Ma J, Ma XL, Wang Y, Sun L, Wang Y, Dong BC. The efficacy of dexamethasone on pain and recovery after total hip arthroplasty: a systematicreview and meta-analysis of randomized controlled trials. Medicine (Baltimore). 2018;97:e0100.

35. Fujii Y, Nakayama M. Effects of dexamethasone in preventing postoperative emetic symptoms after total knee replacement surgery: a prospective, randomized, double-blind, vehicle-controlled trial in adult Japanese patients. Clin Ther. 2005;27:740–5.

36. Barnes PJ. Anti-inflammatory actions of glucocorticoids: molecular mechanisms. Clin Sci (Lond). 1998;94:557–72.

37. Wang JJ, Ho ST, Tzeng JI, Tang CS. The effect of timing of dexamethasone administration on its efficacy as a prophylactic antiemetic for postoperative nausea and vomiting. Anesth Analg. 2000;91:136–9.

38. Wu Y, Yang T, Zeng Y, Si H, Cao F, Shen B. Tranexamic acid reduces blood loss and transfusion requirements in primary simultaneous bilateral total knee arthroplasty: a meta-analysis of randomized controlled trials. Blood Coagul Fibrinolysis. 2017 Oct;28(7):501–8.

39. PeppaM, KraniaM, Raptis SA. Hypertension and other morbidities with Cushing's syndrome associated with corticosteroids: a review. Integr Blood Press Control 2011;4:7–16.

40. Gabriel SE, Sunku J, Salvarani C, O'Fallon WM, Hunder GG. Adverse outcomes of antiinflammatory therapy among patients with polymyalgia rheumatica. Arthritis Rheum. 1997;40:1873–8.

41. Fardet L, Nazareth I, Petersen I. Synthetic glucocorticoids and early variations of blood pressure: a population-based cohort study. J Clin Endocrinol Metab. 2015;100(7):2777–83.

42. Nurok M, Cheng J, Romeo GR, Vecino SM, Fields KG, YaDeau JT. Dexamethasone and perioperative blood glucose in patients undergoing total joint arthroplasty: a retrospective study. J Clin Anesth. 2017;37:116–22.

25

Range of motion after total knee arthroplasty in hemophilic arthropathy

Radovan Kubeš[1*], Peter Salaj[2], Rastislav Hromádka[3] ⓘ, Josef Včelák[1], Aleš Antonín Kuběna[4], Monika Frydrychová[1], Štěpán Magerský[1], Michal Burian[1], Martin Ošťádal[1] and Jan Vaculik[1]

Abstract

Background: Outcomes of total knee replacement in cases of hemophilic patients are worse than in patients who undergo operations due to osteoarthritis. Previous publications have reported varying rates of complications in hemophilic patients, such as infection and an unsatisfactory range of motion, which have influenced the survival of prostheses. Our retrospective study evaluated the data of hemophilic patients regarding changes in the development of the range of motion.

Methods: The data and clinical outcomes of 72 total knee replacements in 45 patients with hemophilia types A and B were reviewed retrospectively. Patients were operated between 1998 and 2013. All of the patients were systematically followed up to record the range of motion and other parameters before and after surgery.

Results: The mean preoperative flexion contracture was $17° \pm 11°$ (range, 0°-40°), and it was $7° \pm 12°$ (range, 0°-60°) postoperatively. The mean flexion of the knee was $73° \pm 30°$ (range, 5°-135°) before the operation and $80° \pm 19°$ (range, 30°-110°) at the last follow-up. The mean range of motion was $56° \pm 34°$ (range, 0°-130°) before the operation and $73° \pm 24°$ (range, 10°-110°) at the last follow-up.

Conclusions: Statistical analysis suggested that the range of motion could be improved until the 9th postoperative week. The patient should be operated on until the flexion contracture reaches 22° to obtain a contracture < 15° postoperatively or until the contracture reaches 12° to obtain less than 5°. The operation generally does not change the flexion of the knee in cases of hemophilic patients, but it reduces the flexion contracture and therefore improves the range.

Keywords: Hemophilic arthropathy, Total knee replacement, Range of motion, Flexion contracture, Hemophilia, Orthopaedics

Background

The knee is the most commonly impaired joint in cases of patients with hereditary bleeding disorders [1]. Hemophilic patients have a reduced quality of life due to cartilage and bone damage, which causes loss of mobility. The pathological processes inside the joints remain subjects of different theories and remain unclear. Several papers have described good functional results and reduction of these problems after total knee arthroplasty (TKA). Previous reports have reported varying rate of complications, such as infection and flexion contracture, and survival [2–12] of TKA, which are much more frequent than in patient with osteoarthritis [1, 13, 14].

One of the most important parameters of the outcomes of surgery with a close correlation with quality of life (QOL) is the range of motion (ROM). In particular, extension of the knee, i.e., the level of postoperative flexion contracture, is important for the mobility of the patient [13]. Flexion contracture affects the function of the operated joint, but it also impairs the gait and the day living activities (Fig. 1).

This retrospective study evaluated the data from hemophilic patients regarding the range of motion. The aim of this study was to provide information about preoperative and postoperative parameters that can delineate the functional outcomes of TKA. Parameters, such as flexion contracture, flexion and range of motion, were

---

* Correspondence: rastho@gmail.com
[1]Department of Orthopaedics, 1st Faculty of Medicine, Charles University and Na Bulovce Hospital, Budínova 2, 180 81 Prague 8, Czech Republic
Full list of author information is available at the end of the article

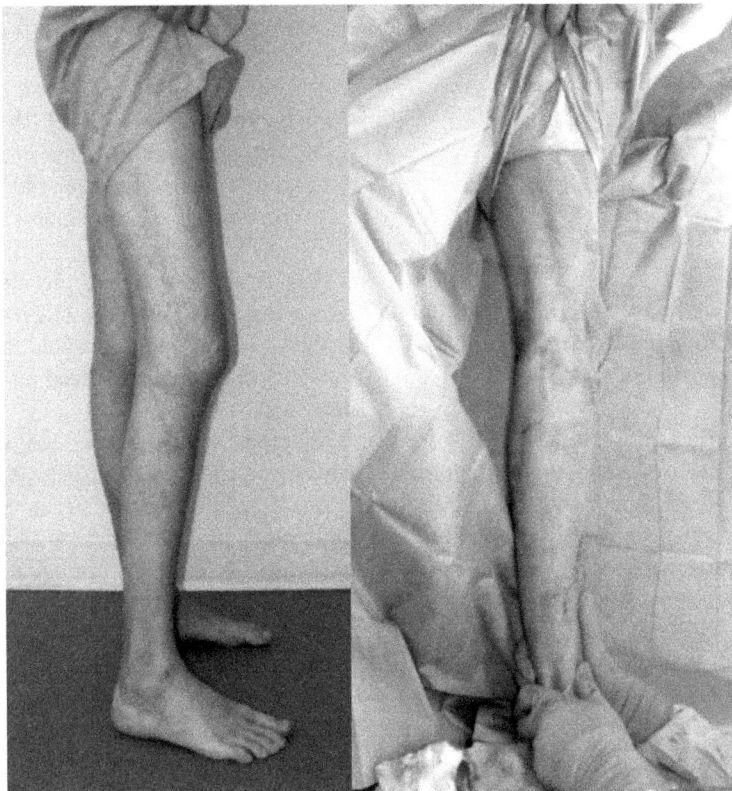

Fig. 1 Clinical view of the same knee - preoperative extension deficiency and its correction after implantation of the TKR

followed before and after implantation to provide detailed information about their development.

Methods

The data and clinical outcomes of 72 TKAs in 45 patients with hemophilia A and B were reviewed retrospectively. The patients were operated on over a period of 15 years between 1998 and 2013 by one surgeon (RK). The main objective criteria for surgery were recurrent bleeding conditions, pain and difficult mobility in normal daily activities or a rapid progression of flexion contracture and the subjective will of the patient to improve the QOL. However, all of the patients were strongly warned that TKR has a limited survival rate, and all of the patients had to sign an informed consent form.

Preoperatively, hematological and biochemical analyses were performed. The hematological status, grade of failure, and type of coagulation disorder were known from the hematologic history. Everything was checked prior to the operation to find any changes, especially regarding the level of coagulation activity and the detection and level of inhibitors. The traditional classification of hemophilia severity was used to distribute the patients into three groups: severe (less than 1% activity of the factor), moderate (1 to 5%) and mild (5 to 40%) [1, 15]. Distribution of our patients is shown in Table 1. The

status of HIV and hepatitis activity was determined in every case.

Management before the surgery involved assessing the nature and frequency of bleeding and the patient history taken by the surgeon. The following parameters were evaluated on follow-ups: recurrence of bleeding episodes into the joint and physical examination of range of motion (ROM), i.e. extension (flexion contracture) and flexion. X-rays of the joint were routinely obtained (Fig. 2). All of the patients included in the study were severely affected with recurrent hemarthroses of the knee joint. The Knee Society score [16] was used for evaluation of patients before and after the operations at every follow up.

The hematologic part of the operation was fully under the control of our cooperating hematologic department (Institute of Clinical and Experimental Hematology, UHKT); in the most difficult cases, a hematologist was also a member of our operation group and cooperated with the anesthesiologist.

Currently, we prefer the model of a short preoperative rehabilitation program under full coverage of prophylactic therapy to prevent any bleeding close to surgery and improve muscle function and prepare patients for postoperative activity. We know that the first postoperative days are usually very painful, and we cannot expect

Table 1 Number of patients according severity of haemophilia

		Hemophilia A	Hemophilia B
No. of Patients		42	3
Severity	Severe	24	1
	Moderate	16	2
	Mild	2	–
No. of TKA		67	5

much muscle activity. This physical therapy (PT) is done in our cooperating hematologic department (UHKT) and helps to predict the postoperative behavior of our patients.

The preoperative examination standardly involved physical and X-ray evaluation of all of the large joints, i.e. the shoulder, elbow, hip, knee and ankle joints which facilitated the planning of multiple operations. In these cases, we always considered that postoperative PT programs and, especially, walking activity were very important to the status of the upper extremities for the possibility of walking with the help of crutches, especially in cases of bilateral procedures.

The standard implantation of TKA involved midline incision and a medial parapatellar approach. A tourniquet is usually used only in the phase of the procedure when all resections are done and gaps are balanced - i.e. just before implantation (cementing) when we clean and "dry" (ideally with the help of "pulsation" jet lavage) resected surfaces.

The limited time of tourniquet use strategy, according to our recommendation, has these reasons:

- Usually very complicated bone and soft tissue status prevents to finish operation during 60 min.
- Meticulous hemostasis is possible and fully advisable - esp. during release of soft tissue adhesions.
- In cases of release of soft tissue flexion contracture, when we manipulate full extension, we could cause traction tears of the popliteal vessels, which could be immediately diagnosed and solved.

This strategy also has the disadvantage of increased blood loss, both initially and overall, and worse initial visibility of the operation field, but gives less risk of immediate postoperative bleeding complications for your patients.

All types of cemented TKA implants were used, according to the type of impairment of the knee. Standard cruciate retaining or posterior stabilized implants were implanted, and in 7 cases, revision TKA or hinged knees implants for primary implantation were used (Fig. 3). The patients with all types of implants were used as a single group for the statistics. Separated groups of patients were statistically not significant when compare to each other. Second-generation cephalosporin was used as antibiotic prophylaxis, with one dose administered before and 2 doses after the operation.

Unilateral TKA or bilateral TKA was performed with a single admission in one or two procedures. Bilateral operations were performed in 18 patients (36 TKAs). The procedures were performed in parallel or sequentially on both knees at a single procedure in these cases. In 8 cases, hip replacement was performed sequential to knee replacement. In 9 patients, both knees were

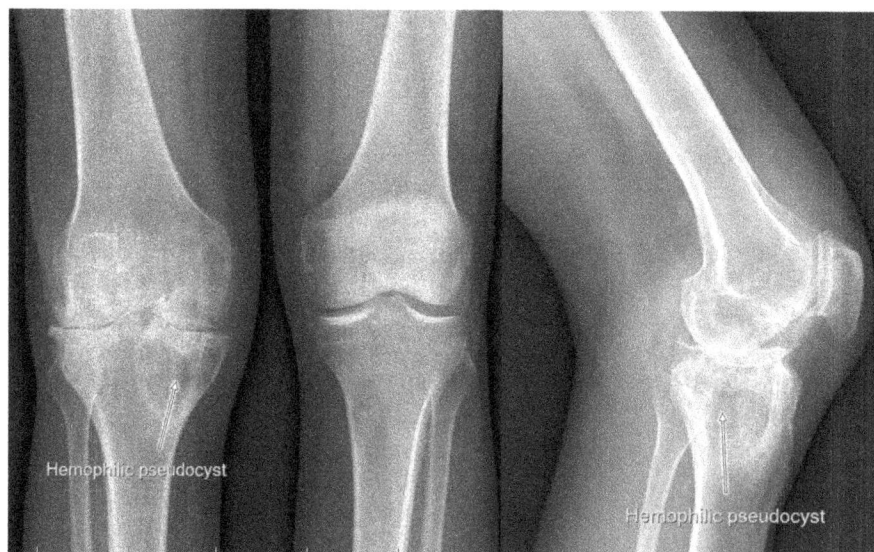

Fig. 2 Preoperative X-ray of the typical hemophiliac arthropathy of the right knee with hemophiliac pseudocyst of the proximal tibia

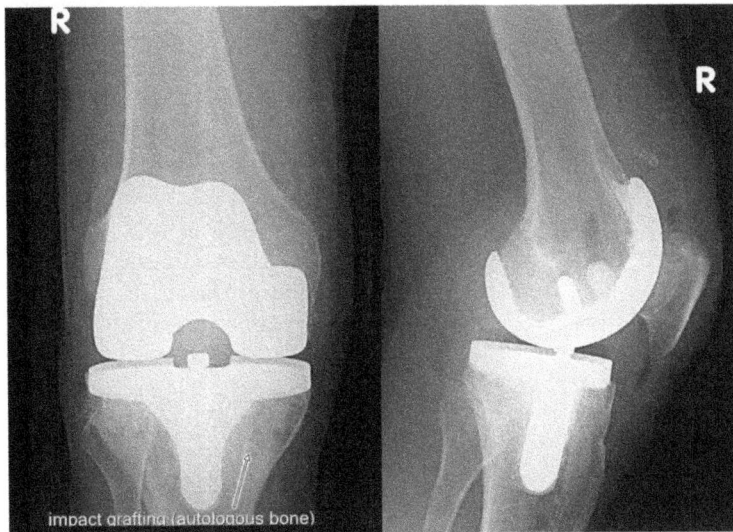

Fig. 3 Postoperative X-ray of the same knee with impact grafting of the haemophiliac pseudocyst (cemented standard CR implant)

operated on (18 TKAs), but the TKAs were implanted in two admissions. The patients were discharged from hospital when finish postoperative protocol of the physiotherapy and their haemophilia was stabilized.

Patients were assessed at follow-ups at 6 weeks, 3 months, 6 months, and 12 months and then every 12 months after discharge from the hospital. X-rays were obtained routinely at each follow-up, and the ROM of the operated knee joint (joints) was measured. The Knee Society score was evaluated at every follow-up.

Results

The median age of the patients at the time of the operation was 47.4 ± 13.3 years (range, 35–55). The patients were followed up for a median of 8.9 ± 4.3 years (range 6.3–13.1). The median time of hospitalization of a patient after the TKA surgery was 30 ± 12.5 days (range, 24–36 days).

The mean preoperative flexion contracture was $17° \pm 11°$ (median 15°, range 0°- 40°), and it was $7° \pm 12°$ (median 0°, range 0° to 60°) postoperatively (Fig. 4). The mean flexion of the knee was $73° \pm 30°$ (range 5°-135°) before the operation and $80° \pm 19°$ (range 30°-110°) at the last follow up - Fig. 5. The mean ROM was $56° \pm 34°$ (range 0° - 130°) before the operation and $73° \pm 24°$ (range 10°- 110°) at the last follow up.

The Knee Society Score [16] was used in all 72 cases to evaluate the outcomes of TKA before and after the operation. The mean clinical score before surgery was 28 (range, 13–36), and after TKA at the last follow up, it was 72 (range 62 to 80). The average functional score before the operation was 37 (range 15 to 50), and after the operation, it was 70 (range 50 to 80) in Table 2.

Complications were evaluated retrospectively according to the standardized list of the Knee Society [17].

Deep infection, superficial infection and loosening of the implants were recorded in 9 cases (12.5%). We did not register any case of nerve palsy, bleeding or vascular injury or other complications associated with TKA in this study. There was no occurrence of the development of clotting factor inhibitors in reviewing this group of patients.

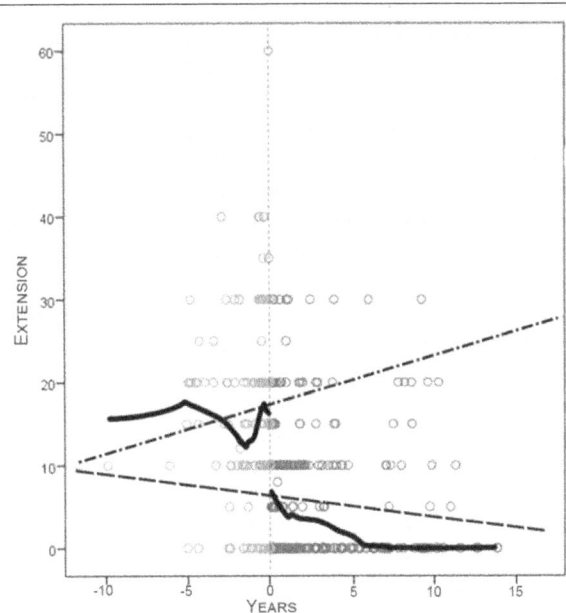

Fig. 4 The extension of the knee before and after the implantation of TKA. Lines represent increasing tendency (dash-dotted line) of the average value of preoperative flexion contracture and postoperative decrease in the parameter (dash line). Irregular solid curves show the medians of the parameters pre- and postoperatively. Small circles represent measured values

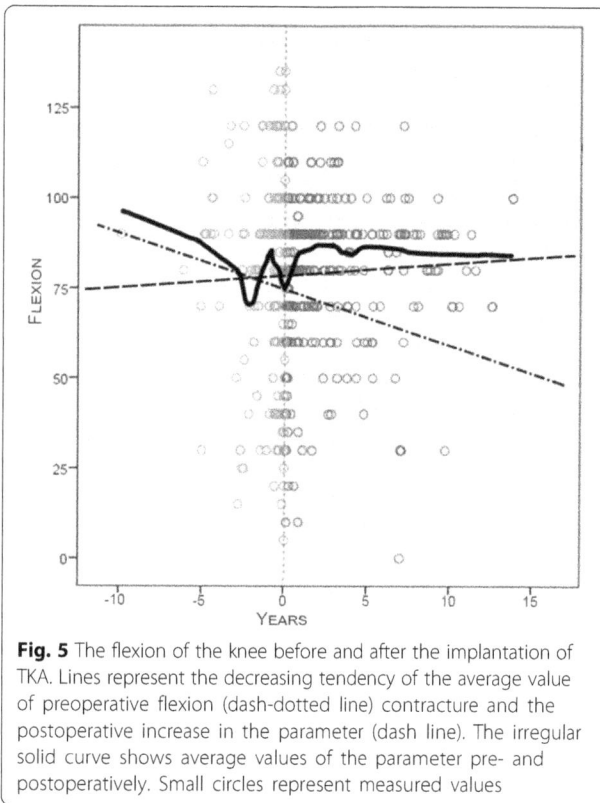

Fig. 5 The flexion of the knee before and after the implantation of TKA. Lines represent the decreasing tendency of the average value of preoperative flexion (dash-dotted line) contracture and the postoperative increase in the parameter (dash line). The irregular solid curve shows average values of the parameter pre- and postoperatively. Small circles represent measured values

In the study, 2 patients had proven HIV. The patients acquired the virus from infected clotting factors before the beginning of the study.

Discussion

The surgery for TKA in a patient with hemophilia is a complex procedure. The outcomes of the surgery depend of many factors. Typical for a patient with hemophilia is the progressive deterioration of the knee joint after bleeding episodes, which leads to a restriction of the joint's range of motion. Although the main goal of the TKA is to reduce pain, the range of motion is important for satisfactory outcomes.

Patients with hemophilia and severe knee arthritis frequently present with tree plane knee deformities [13]. The typical deformity is flexion on the sagittal plane, with contracture and external rotation. Destruction of joint surfaces on the lateral side leads to valgus deformity and dorsal subluxation of the tibia, which limit the of

range of motion and cause fibrosis of the surrounding soft tissue. These deformities, together with the presence of periarticular osteopenia and cysts, cause postoperative flexion contractures [13, 18] (Figs. 1, 2). The average range of motion of hemophilic patients after total knee replacement is less than that in cases of patients with osteoarthritis. Intra-capsular fibrotic changes and extra-capsular muscle contractures are typical problems that affect the operative outcomes after TKA [19]. The attention in preoperative planning should be focused on flexion contracture [13].

The flexion contracture of the knee joint, especially its rapid progression, is one of the important indication criteria for TKA surgery. The level of postoperative contracture is important for successful outcomes of surgery as well. Goddard [1] reported that the contracture improved from 18° (range, 0° to 50°) to 8° (range, 0° to 30°) at the time of the latest follow-up. Bae [18] published an average flexion contracture of 22.7° before implantation and 5.7° after surgery. Ernstbrunner et al. [11] published an average flexion contracture of 18° before implantation and 6° after operation. Atilla [13] argued that 27.5° preoperative flexion contracture led to extensive flexion contracture of 15° postoperatively, which significantly affected the gait. The operation in hemophiliacs should be not postponed when the contracture level reaches 15° [13].

In our study, the operation was usually performed due to the rapid progression of flexion contracture within the last year before implantation. We retrospectively and systematically evaluated the residual lack of extension. The flexion contracture develops in association with bleeding episodes. The graph (Fig. 4) shows the values of extension limitations. The average value of contracture generally tends to increase by 0.95° per year until surgery. The figure shows that the median contracture in cases of hemophilic patients slowly decreases over the years, but then it suddenly changes its course and increases. The operation should be planned with regard to changing the course of development of the contracture.

The contracture decreases rapidly in the first two months after TKA surgery and then significantly slows. Although the average lack of extension in our study was 7° at the last follow up, the median was 0° overall. The tendency of this parameter is to decrease after surgery, as shown in Fig. 1.

The flexion tended to decrease over time preoperatively in all cases over years (Fig. 5). Evaluation of the data showed a paradoxical increase in flexion, while the lack of the extension increased several months before surgery. After surgery, the flexion did not change significantly ($p = 0.435$). The profit was only 7° at the last follow up in the group of patients. A patient could not

Table 2 The Knee Society Score; outcomes of 72 TKA before and after the operation

	Age	Clinic Score		Functional Score	
		Before	After	Before	After
Score	41	28	72	37	70
(Range of Score)	30–62	13–36	68–80	15–50	50–80

expect better flexion of the joint, but the pain was decreased [20]. The patient could expect an improvement of ambulation because the surgery improved the ability to extend the joint [13]. Song [10] et al. reported average improvement of the flexion 4.9° after the operation.

The ROM of the knee was calculated as the subtraction of the extension from the flexion in our study. Goddard [1] published that the ROM was 68° (20° to 130°) preoperatively and 79° (20° to 120°) at the final follow-up. Bae [18] reported that the average preoperative range of motion was 73.4°, whereas the average postoperative range of motion increased to 92.3°. Atilla [13] reported an average range of motion of 37.6°, which improved to 57.1° postoperatively. All of these studies reported only a slight improvement in ROM. In our study, the pre- and postoperative ROMs were comparable to these results, and the average total flexion arc improved from 56° to 73°.

The postoperative range of motion compared to TKR in non-hemophilic patients is more limited. The implantation of TKA mostly affects and reduces the flexion contracture. The ROM of the knee improves, mostly due to the decrease in the flexion contracture. The operation significantly ($p < 0.001$) increased of the ROM, and the increase in this parameter was 17° in this group of patients.

The implantation affects the ROM, but often, the flexion contracture persists at some level. A contracture of the lower extremity joint affects the gait pattern [21]. Atilla et al. [13] reported that a flexion contracture of < 15° of the knee is satisfactory in cases of hemophilic patients. In this group of patients, we attempted to propose a threshold for the operation on the affected knee joint to reach a satisfactory level of contracture. The evaluation of the data showed that preoperative flexion contracture < 22° led to postoperative contracture < 15°, and preoperative contracture < 12° resulted in postoperative contracture < 5°. In our group, the rates were 72 and 50% of patients, respectively. We believe that TKA should be implanted until the flexion contracture is 22°.

The outcomes of the operations were evaluated by the Knee Society functional score (KSS) in our study Tab. 2. The clinical part of the KSS showed an average improvement of 44 points. The patients demonstrated satisfactory pain control because all of the patients rated the pain as better than moderate and improved. The suboptimal improvement in motion (see above) associated with satisfactory reduction of the knee pain was acceptable for most of the patients with hemophilia. The limited flexion was balanced by improvement of the flexion contracture. The average improvement in the functional score was 33 points. None of the patients referred to being housebound.

The outcomes were comparable with other studies. Bae [18] reported that the average preoperative knee score increased from 18.6 points (range, 3–29) to 82.8 points (range, 44–99). The average preoperative knee function score increased from 41.4 points (range, 20–60 points) to 75.8 points (range, 45–95 points). Goddard [1] used the HSS score in 49 patients (60 TKRs). The mean clinical score after surgery was 82 (70 to 95), and 95% of the TKAs had good or excellent results. Ernstbrunner [11] reported that the preoperative average clinical and the functional knee score increased from 36 and 62 points to 73 and 78 points after the operation, respectively.

Conclusion
Total knee replacement improves the mobility of hemophilic patients, especially the functional range of motion, and it provides satisfactory pain relief. The operation generally does not change the flexion of the knee, but it reduces the flexion contracture and therefore improves the range of motion. Statistical analysis suggested that the range of motion could be improved until the ninth postoperative week.

Abbreviations
PT: physical therapy; QOL: Quality of life; ROM: Range of motion; TKA: Total knee arthroplasty

Funding
The data processing and the study was funded by the authors' own resources.

Authors' contributions
RK designed the study, performed the research; main surgeon, PS haematologist of the study, RH analysed the data and wrote the paper; surgeon of the study, JV clinical examination of patients, data collecting, database cleaning, AAK designed the study, analysed the data (the main statistician), MF evaluated the data; surgeon of the study, SM clinical examination of patients, data collecting, database cleaning, MB clinical examination of patients, data collecting, database cleaning, MO clinical examination of patients, data collecting, database cleaning, JaV clinical examination of patients, data collecting, database cleaning. All authors read and approved the final manuscript.

Competing interests
The authors declare that they have no competing interests.

Author details
[1]Department of Orthopaedics, 1st Faculty of Medicine, Charles University and Na Bulovce Hospital, Budínova 2, 180 81 Prague 8, Czech Republic. [2]Institute of Clinical and Experimental Hematology, First Faculty of Medicine, Charles University and Institute of Hematology and Blood Transfusion, U Nemocnice 1, 12802 Prague 2, Czech Republic. [3]Department of Orthopaedics, 1st Faculty of Medicine, Charles University and Motol University Hospital, Úvalu 84, 15006 Prague 5, Czech Republic. [4]Department of Social and Clinical Pharmacy, Faculty of Pharmacy, Charles University, Akademika Heyrovského 1203, 500 05 Hradec Králové, Czech Republic.

References

1. Goddard NJ, Mann HA, Lee CA. Total knee replacement in patients with end-stage haemophilic arthropathy: 25-year results. J Bone Joint Surg Br. 2010;92:1085–9.

2. Norian JM, Ries MD, Karp S, Hambleton J. Total knee arthroplasty in hemophilic arthropathy. J Bone Joint Surg Am. 2002;84-A:1138–41.

3. Hicks JL, Ribbans WJ, Buzzard B, Kelley SS, Toft L, Torri G, et al. Infected joint replacements in HIV-positive patients with haemophilia. J Bone Joint Surg Br. 2001;83:1050–4.

4. Chiang CC, Chen PQ, Shen MC, Tsai W. Total knee arthroplasty for severe haemophilic arthropathy: long-term experience in Taiwan. Haemophilia. 2008;14:828–34.

5. Sikkema T, Boerboom AL, Meijer KA. Comparison between the complications and long-term outcome of hip and knee replacement therapy in patients with and without haemophilia; a controlled retrospective cohort study. Haemophilia. 2011;17:300–3.

6. Cohen I, Heim M, Martinowitz U, Chechick A. Orthopaedic outcome of total knee replacement in haemophilia a. Haemophilia. 2000;6(2):104–9.

7. Chevalier Y, Dargaud Y, Lienhart A, Chamouard V, Negrier C. Seventy-two total knee arthroplasties performed in patients with haemophilia using continuous infusion. Vox Sang. 2013;104(2):135–43.

8. Panotopoulos J, Ay C, Trieb K, Schuh R, Windhager R, Wanivenhaus HA. Outcome of total knee arthroplasty in hemophilic arthropathy. J Arthroplast. 2014;29(4):749–52.

9. Westberg M, Paus AC, Holme PA, Tjonnfjord GE. Haemophilic arthropathy: long-term outcomes in 107 primary total knee arthroplasties. Knee. 2014; 21(1):147–50.

10. Song SJ, Bae JK, Park CH, Yoo MC, Bae DK, Kim KI. Mid-term outcomes and complications of total knee arthroplasty in haemophilic arthropathy: a review of consecutive 131 knees between 2006 and 2015 in a single institute. Haemophilia. 2017;

11. Ernstbrunner L, Hingsammer A, Catanzaro S, Sutter R, Brand B, Wieser K, Fucentese SF. Long-term results of total knee arthroplasty in haemophilic patients: an 18-year follow-up. Knee Surg Sport Tr A. 2017; 25(11):3431–8.

12. Mortazavi SM, Haghpanah B, Ebrahiminasab MM, Baghdadi T, Toogeh G. Functional outcome of total knee arthroplasty in patients with haemophilia. Haemophilia. 2016;22(6):919–24.

13. Atilla B, Caglar O, Pekmezci M, Buyukasik Y, Tokgozoglu AM, Alpaslan M. Pre-operative flexion contracture determines the functional outcome of haemophilic arthropathy treated with total knee arthroplasty. Haemophilia. 2012;18:358–63.

14. Rodriguez-Merchan EC. Total knee replacement in haemophilic arthropathy. J Bone Joint Surg Br. 2007;89:186–8.

15. White GC, 2nd, Rosendaal F, Aledort LM, Lusher JM, Rothschild C, Ingerslev J, et al. Definitions in hemophilia. Recommendation of the scientific subcommittee on factor VIII and factor IX of the scientific and standardization committee of the international society on thrombosis and Haemostasis. Throm Haemostasis 2001; 85: 560.

16. Insall JN, Dorr LD, Scott RD, Scott WN. Rationale of the knee society clinical rating system. Clin Orthop Relat R 1989: 13–14.

17. Healy WL, Della Valle CJ, Iorio R, Berend KR, Cushner FD, Dalury DF, et al. Complications of total knee arthroplasty: standardized list and definitions of the knee society. Clin Orthop Relat R. 2013;471:215–20.

18. Bae DK, Yoon KH, Kim HS, Song SJ. Total knee arthroplasty in hemophilic arthropathy of the knee. J Arthroplast. 2005;20:664–8.

19. Goddard NJ, Rodriguez-Merchan EC, Wiedel JD. Total knee replacement in haemophilia. Haemophilia. 2002;8:382–6.

20. Silva M, Luck JV, Jr. Long-term results of primary total knee replacement in patients with hemophilia. J Bone Joint Surg Am 2005; 87: 85–91.

21. Kagaya H, Ito S, Iwami T, Obinata G, Shimada Y. A computer simulation of human walking in persons with joint contractures. Tohoku J Exp Med. 2003; 200:31–7.

Permissions

The contributors of this book come from diverse backgrounds, making this book a truly international effort. This book will bring forth new frontiers with its revolutionizing research information and detailed analysis of the nascent developments around the world.

We would like to thank all the contributing authors for lending their expertise to make the book truly unique. They have played a crucial role in the development of this book. Without their invaluable contributions this book wouldn't have been possible. They have made vital efforts to compile up to date information on the varied aspects of this subject to make this book a valuable addition to the collection of many professionals and students.

This book was conceptualized with the vision of imparting up-to-date information and advanced data in this field. To ensure the same, a matchless editorial board was set up. Every individual on the board went through rigorous rounds of assessment to prove their worth. After which they invested a large part of their time researching and compiling the most relevant data for our readers.

The editorial board has been involved in producing this book since its inception. They have spent rigorous hours researching and exploring the diverse topics which have resulted in the successful publishing of this book. They have passed on their knowledge of decades through this book. To expedite this challenging task, the publisher supported the team at every step. A small team of assistant editors was also appointed to further simplify the editing procedure and attain best results for the readers.

Apart from the editorial board, the designing team has also invested a significant amount of their time in understanding the subject and creating the most relevant covers. They scrutinized every image to scout for the most suitable representation of the subject and create an appropriate cover for the book.

The publishing team has been an ardent support to the editorial, designing and production team. Their endless efforts to recruit the best for this project, has resulted in the accomplishment of this book. They are a veteran in the field of academics and their pool of knowledge is as vast as their experience in printing. Their expertise and guidance has proved useful at every step. Their uncompromising quality standards have made this book an exceptional effort. Their encouragement from time to time has been an inspiration for everyone.

The publisher and the editorial board hope that this book will prove to be a valuable piece of knowledge for researchers, students, practitioners and scholars across the globe.

List of Contributors

Peter Feczko and Jacobus J. Arts
Department Orthopaedic Surgery, Research School Capri, Maastricht University Medical Centre, P. Debyelaan 25, 6229 HX Maastricht, The Netherlands

Lutz Engelmann
Heinrich-Braun-Krankenhaus Zwickau, Städtisches Klinikum, Zwickau, Germany

David Campbell
Repatriation General Hospital, Adelaide, Australia

Young Shil Park
Department of Pediatrics, Kyung Hee University Hospital at Gangdong, School of Medicine, Kyung Hee University, 892, Dongnam-ro, Gangdong-Gu, Seoul 05278, Korea

Won-Ju Shin
Department of Orthopedic Surgery, Kyung Hee University Medical Center, 23, Kyungheedae-ro, Dongdaemun-gu, Seoul 0244, Korea

Kang-Il Kim
Department of Orthopedic Surgery, Kyung Hee University Hospital at Gangdong, School of Medicine, Kyung Hee University, 892, Dongnam-ro, Gangdong-Gu, Seoul 05278, Korea

Maren Falch Lindberg and Anners Lerdal
Department of Surgery, Lovisenberg Diakonale Hospital, Pb 4970 Nydalen, 0440 Oslo, Norway
Department of Nursing Science, Institute of Health and Society, Faculty of Medicine, University of Oslo, Pb 1072 Blindern, 0316 Oslo, Norway

Tone Rustøen
Department of Nursing Science, Institute of Health and Society, Faculty of Medicine, University of Oslo, Pb 1072 Blindern, 0316 Oslo, Norway
Department of Research and Development, Division of Emergencies and Critical Care, Oslo University Hospital, Pb 4956 Nydalen, 0424 Oslo, Norway

Christine Miaskowski
School of Nursing, University of California, San Francisco, UCSF, San Francisco, CA 94143, USA

Leiv Arne Rosseland
Department of Research and Development, Division of Emergencies and Critical Care, Oslo University Hospital, Pb 4956 Nydalen, 0424 Oslo, Norway
Institute of Clinical Medicine, University of Oslo, Pb 1072 Blindern, 0316 Oslo, Norway

Joong Il Kim
Department of Orthopaedic Surgery, Hallym University Kangnam Sacred Heart Hospital, 1, Singil-ro, Yeongdeungpo-gu, Seoul 150-950, Korea

Jak Jang, Ki Woong Lee, Hyuk Soo Han, Sahnghoon Lee and Myung Chul Lee
Department of Orthopaedic Surgery, Seoul National University Hospital, 101 Daehak-ro, Jongno-gu, Seoul 110-744, Korea

P. Z. Feczko, L. M. Jutten, P. J. Emans and J. J. Arts
Department of Orthopaedic Surgery, CAPHRI Research School, Maastricht University Medical Centre, P. Debyelaan 25, 6229 HX Maastricht, the Netherlands

M. J. van Steyn
Reynaert Private Hospital, Maastricht, the Netherlands

P. Deckers
Department of Orthopaedic Surgery, Zuyderland Hospital, Heerlen, the Netherlands

Laurie J. Goldsmith
Faculty of Health Sciences, Simon Fraser University, Blusson Hall 10506, 8888 University Drive, Burnaby, BC V5A 1S6, Canada

Nitya Suryaprakash
Centre for Clinical Epidemiology and Evaluation, Vancouver Coastal Health Research Institute, 7th floor, 828 West 10th Avenue, Vancouver, BC V5Z 1M9, Canada

Ellen Randall and Stirling Bryan
Centre for Clinical Epidemiology and Evaluation, Vancouver Coastal Health Research Institute, 7th floor, 828 West 10th Avenue, Vancouver, BC V5Z 1M9, Canada
School of Population and Public Health, University of British Columbia, 2206 East Mall, Vancouver, BC V6T 1Z3, Canada

Jessica Shum
Centre for Clinical Epidemiology and Evaluation, Vancouver Coastal Health Research Institute, 7th floor, 828 West 10th Avenue, Vancouver, BC V5Z 1M9, Canada
Department of Experimental Medicine, Faculty of Medicine, University of British Columbia, 10th Floor, 2775 Laurel Street, Vancouver, BC V5Z 1M9, Canada

Valerie MacDonald
Burnaby Hospital & Surgical Network, Fraser Health, 3935 Kincaid Street, Burnaby, BC V5K 2X6, Canada

Richard Sawatzky
School of Nursing, Trinity Western University, 7600 Glover Road, Langley, BC V2Y 1Y1, Canada
Centre for Health Evaluation and Outcome Sciences, Providence Health Care Research Institute, St. Paul's Hospital, 588-1081 Burrard Street, Vancouver, BC V6Z 1Y6, Canada

Samar Hejazi
Department of Evaluation and Research Service, Fraser Health, Suite 400, Central City Tower, 13450 102 Avenue, Surrey, BC V3T 0H1, Canada

Jennifer C. Davis
Department of Physical Therapy, Faculty of Medicine, University of British Columbia, 212 Friedman Building, 2177 Wesbrook Mall, Vancouver, BC V6T 1Z3, Canada
Aging, Mobility and Cognitive Neurosciences Lab, University of British Columbia, Djavad Mowafaghian Centre for Brain Health, 2215 Wesbrook Mall, Vancouver, BC V6T 1Z3, Canada

Patrick McAllister
Rebalance MD, 104-3551 Blanshard Street, Victoria, BC V8Z 0B9, Canada

L. L. Jasper, C. A. Jones and L. A. Beaupre
Department of Physical Therapy, University of Alberta, Rm 2-50 Corbett Hall, Edmonton, AB T6G 2G4, Canada

J. Mollins
Alberta Health Services, Edmonton, Canada

S. L. Pohar
Canadian Agency for Drugs and Technologies in Health, Ottawa, Canada

Amelia R. Winter
Orthopaedic and Arthritis Center for Outcomes Research (OrACORe), Department of Orthopedic Surgery, Boston, MA, USA

Jamie E. Collins
Orthopaedic and Arthritis Center for Outcomes Research (OrACORe), Department of Orthopedic Surgery, Boston, MA, USA
Harvard Medical School, Boston, MA, USA

Jeffrey N. Katz
Orthopaedic and Arthritis Center for Outcomes Research (OrACORe), Department of Orthopedic Surgery, Boston, MA, USA
Division of Rheumatology, Immunology and Allergy, Brigham and Women's Hospital, 60 Fenwood St, Suite 5016, Boston, MA 02115, USA
Harvard Medical School, Boston, MA, USA
Departments of Epidemiology and Environmental Health, Harvard T. H. Chan School of Public Health, Boston, MA, USA

Stefan Rahm, Roland S. Camenzind, Andreas Hingsammer, Christopher Lenz, David E. Bauer, Mazda Farshad and Sandro F. Fucentese
Orthopaedic Department, Balgrist University Hospital, University of Zurich, Forchstrasse 340, 8008 Zurich, CH, Switzerland

Jung-Ro Yoon, In-Wook Seo and Young-Soo Shin
Department of Orthopedic Surgery, Veterans Health Service Medical Center, 61 Jinhwangdoro-gil, Gangdong-Gu, Seoul 134-791, Korea

Josefine E. Naili and Eva W. Broström
Department of Women's and Children's Health, Karolinska Institutet, MotorikLab, Q2:07, Karolinska University Hospital, 171 76 Stockholm, Sweden

Per Wretenberg
Department of Orthopedics, School of Medical Sciences, Örebro University and Örebro University Hospital, Örebro, Sweden

Viktor Lindgren
Department of Molecular Medicine and Surgery, Karolinska Institutet, L1:00, Karolinska University Hospital, 171 76 Stockholm, Sweden

Maura D. Iversen
Department of Women's and Children's Health, Karolinska Institutet, MotorikLab, Q2:07, Karolinska University Hospital, 171 76 Stockholm, Sweden
Department of Physical Therapy, Movement & Rehabilitation Sciences, Bouve College of Health Sciences, Northeastern University, 360 Huntington Avenue, Boston, MA 02115, USA
Division of Rheumatology, Immunology and Allergy, Brigham and Women's Hospital, Harvard Medical School, Boston, MA, USA

Margareta Hedström
Department of Clinical Science, Intervention and Technology, Karolinska Institutet, Karolinska University Hospital, K54, 141 86 Stockholm, Sweden

Ilana M. Usiskin, Heidi Y. Yang, Bhushan R. Deshpande, Jamie E. Collins, Griffin L. Michl, Savannah R. Smith, Kristina M. Klara, Faith Selzer, Jeffrey N. Katz and Elena Losina
Orthopaedic and Arthritis Center for Outcomes Research, Department of Orthopaedic Surgery, Brigham and Women's Hospital, 75 Francis Street, BC-4016, Boston, MA 02115, USA

Paul J. P. van der Ven, Sebastiaan van de Groes, Jorrit Zelle and Gerjon Hannink
611 Orthopaedic Research Laboratory, Department of Orthopaedics, Radboud University Medical Center, 6500HB Nijmegen, The Netherlands

Sander Koëter
Department of Orthopaedics, Canisius-Wilhelmina Hospital, Nijmegen, The Netherlands

Nico Verdonschot
611 Orthopaedic Research Laboratory, Department of Orthopaedics, Radboud University Medical Center, 6500HB Nijmegen, The Netherlands Laboratory for Biomechanical Engineering, University of Twente, Enschede, The Netherlands

Zhenyang Mao, Bing Yue, You Wang, Mengning Yan and Kerong Dai
Shanghai Key Laboratory of Orthopaedic Implants, Shanghai Ninth People's Hospital, Shanghai Jiaotong University School of Medicine, Shanghai, People's Republic of China
Department of Orthopaedic Surgery, Shanghai Ninth People's Hospital, Shanghai Jiaotong University School of Medicine, 639 Zhizaoju Road, Shanghai 200011, People's Republic of China

Flemming K. Nielsen, Niels Egund and Anne Grethe Jurik
Department of Radiology, Aarhus University Hospital, Noerrebrogade 44, 8000 Aarhus, Denmark

Anette Jørgensen
Department of Rheumatology, Aarhus University Hospital, Noerrebrogade 44, 8000 Aarhus, Denmark

M. T. Berninger
Joint Replacement Institute, Garmisch-Partenkirchen Medical Center, Auenstr. 6, 82467 Garmisch-Partenkirchen, Germany
Department of Trauma Surgery, BG Trauma Center Murnau, Prof.-Küntscher Str. 8, 82418 Murnau, Germany

J. Friederichs and V. Bühren
Department of Trauma Surgery, BG Trauma Center Murnau, Prof.-Küntscher Str. 8, 82418 Murnau, Germany

W. Leidinger
Department of Anesthesiology and Intensive Care, Garmisch-Partenkirchen Medical Center, Auenstr. 6, 82467 Garmisch-Partenkirchen, Germany

P. Augat
Institute of Biomechanics, BG Trauma Center Murnau, Prof.-Küntscher Str. 8, 82418 Murnau, Germany
Institute of Biomechanics, Paracelsus Medical University, Strubergasse 21, 5020 Salzburg, Austria

C. Fulghum and W. Reng
Joint Replacement Institute, Garmisch-Partenkirchen Medical Center, Auenstr. 6, 82467 Garmisch-Partenkirchen, Germany

Duan Wang, Wei-Kun Meng, Hao-Yang Wang, Ze-Yu Luo, Fu-Xing Pei, Qi Li and Zong-Ke Zhou
Department of Orthopedics, West China Hospital/West China School of Medicine, Sichuan University, 37# Wuhou Guoxue road, Chengdu 610041, People's Republic of China

Hui Zhu
Out-patient department, West China Second University Hospital, Sichuan University, Chengdu 610041, People's Republic of China
Key Laboratory of Birth Defects and Related Disease of Woman and Children (Ministry of Education), West China Second University Hospital, Sichuan University, Chengdu 610041, People's Republic of China

Jonathan R. B. Hutt, Avtar Sur, Hartej Sur and Aine Ringrose
Department of Trauma and Orthopaedics, St George's University Hospitals NHS Foundation Trust, London, UK

Mark S. Rickman
Department of Orthopaedics and Trauma, The University of Adelaide and Royal Adelaide Hospital, Adelaide, Australia

Sung-Hyun Lee, Sung-Hyun Noh, Keun-Churl Chun and Churl-Hong Chun
Department of Orthopedic Surgery, School of Medicine, Wonkwang University Hospital, Muwang-ro 895, Iksan, Jeollabuk-do, South Korea

Joung-Kyue Han
College of Sports Science, Chung-Ang University, Anseong, South Korea

Anna Janine Schreiner, Atesch Ateschrang, Christoph Ihle, Ulrich Stöckle and Christoph Gonser
BG Trauma Center Tübingen, Eberhard Karls University Tübingen, Schnarrenbergstrasse 95, 72076 Tübingen, Germany

Florian Schmidutz
BG Trauma Center Tübingen, Eberhard Karls University Tübingen, Schnarrenbergstrasse 95, 72076 Tübingen, Germany
Department of Orthopaedic Surgery, Physical Medicine and Rehabilitation, University of Munich (LMU), Marchioninistraße 15, 81377 Munich, Germany

Björn Gunnar Ochs
Department of Orthopedics and Trauma Surgery, Medical Center, Faculty of Medicine, Albert-Ludwigs-University of Freiburg, Hugstetter Str. 55, 79106 Freiburg, Germany

Yong Tae Kim, Min Wook Kang, Young Min Lee and Joong Il Kim
Department of Orthopaedic Surgery, Hallym University Kangnam Sacred Heart Hospital, 1, Singil-ro, Yeongdeungpo-gu, Seoul 150-950, South Korea

Joon Kyu Lee
Department of Orthopaedic Surgery, Hallym University Sacred Heart Hospital, 22, Gwanpyeong-ro 170beon-gil, Dongan-gu, Anyang 431-796, South Korea

Yuangang Wu, Yi Zeng, Xianchao Bao, Huazhang Xiong and Bin Shen
Department of Orthopaedic Surgery, West China Hospital, West China Medical School, Sichuan University, Chengdu 610041, Sichuan Province, China

Xiaoxi Lu and Yimei Ma
Department of Pediatrics, West China University Second Hospital, Sichuan University, Chengdu 610041, Sichuan Province, China
Key Laboratory of Birth Defects and Related Diseases of Women and Children
(Sichuan University), Ministry of Education, Chengdu, China
Radovan Kubeš, Josef Včelák, Monika Frydrychová, Štěpán Magerský, Michal Burian, Martin Ošťádal and Jan Vaculik
Department of Orthopaedics, 1st Faculty of Medicine, Charles University and Na Bulovce Hospital, Budínova 2, 180 81 Prague 8, Czech Republic

Peter Salaj
Institute of Clinical and Experimental Hematology, First Faculty of Medicine, Charles University and Institute of Hematology and Blood Transfusion, U Nemocnice 1, 12802 Prague 2, Czech Republic

Rastislav Hromádka
Department of Orthopaedics, 1st Faculty of Medicine, Charles University and Motol University Hospital, Úvalu 84, 15006 Prague 5, Czech Republic

Aleš Antonín Kuběna
Department of Social and Clinical Pharmacy, Faculty of Pharmacy, Charles University, Akademika Heyrovského 1203, 500 05 Hradec Králové, Czech Republic

Index